THE
SOUTH BEACH
DIET
WAKE-UP CALL

THE
SOUTH BEACH
DIET
WAKE-UP CALL

7 Real-Life Strategies for Living
Your Healthiest Life Ever

Arthur Agatston, MD

RODALE.

First published in hardcover by Rodale Inc. in 2011.

© 2011 by Dr. Arthur Agatston
The South Beach Diet® is a Registered Trademark of the SBD Holdings Group Corp.

Rodale books may be purchased for business or promotional use or for special sales.
For information, please write to:
Special Markets Department, Rodale Inc., 733 Third Avenue, New York, NY 10017.

Printed in the United States of America
Rodale Inc. makes every effort to use acid-free ♾, recycled paper ♾.

Book design by Christina Gaugler
Photos by Hilmar

Library of Congress Cataloging-in-Publication Data: 2011041469
ISBN 978–1–60961–893–3   paperback

Distributed to the trade by Macmillan
2   4   6   8   10   9   7   5   3   1   paperback

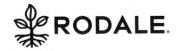

We inspire and enable people to improve their lives, and the world around them.
rodalebooks.com

To the Super Moms and Dads,
who are truly changing the way America eats and lives.
And, as always, to my Super Family—my wife, Sari,
and sons, Evan and Adam.

CONTENTS

Acknowledgments ix

PART 1: THE HEALTH OF OUR NATION: CONDITION CRITICAL!

CHAPTER 1. The Ticking Time Bomb 3
CHAPTER 2. Getting Old before Our Time 15
CHAPTER 3. The Perils of Progress 41
CHAPTER 4. What's Wrong (and Right) with "Diets" 56
CHAPTER 5. Eat to Live . . . Well 71
CHAPTER 6. New Concerns about Gluten 96
CHAPTER 7. The Power of the Dining Table 108
CHAPTER 8. The High Cost of Inactivity 123
CHAPTER 9. Wake Up and Get Some Sleep! 143

PART 2: THE SOUTH BEACH DIET WAKE-UP PROGRAM: 7 SIMPLE STRATEGIES FOR BETTER HEALTH

STRATEGY #1. Control the Clutter, Free Your Mind 169
STRATEGY #2. Make Every Meal Matter 177
STRATEGY #3. Shop Right! 191
STRATEGY #4. Cook As If Your Life Depends on It 211
STRATEGY #5. Eat In More, Dine Out Smart 216
STRATEGY #6. Get Moving, Get Fit 224
STRATEGY #7. Sleep Better, Live Longer 241

PART 3: MEGAFOODS AND MEGARECIPES FOR HEALTHY EATING

MegaFoods for Healthy Eating 254
MegaRecipes for Healthy Eating 259

Master Shopping List for a Healthy Diet 307
Online Resources 314
Select Bibliography 318
Index 328

ACKNOWLEDGMENTS

I have many to thank for encouraging and facilitating the evolution of my thinking, which has led to *The South Beach Diet Wake-Up Call*. To begin chronologically, I vividly recall a lecture in the mid-1990s by the late Dr. Fred Pashkow (who was then director of the Preventive Cardiology Program at the Cleveland Clinic). That lecture first sparked my interest in the concept that when it comes to our modern lifestyle, we should focus on how our DNA was designed as reflected in the way our hunter-gatherer ancestors lived. Reading the work of Dr. S. Boyd Eaton and Dr. Loren Cordain has also greatly advanced my education in this area.

My research colleagues, Drs. Keith Webster, Paul Kurlansky, and Robert Superko, were very helpful in expanding my knowledge of the pivotal roles that inflammation, stem cells, and genomics play in the modern degenerative diseases of the West.

Pediatricians David Ludwig of Children's Hospital Boston and Ricardo Restrepo of Miami Children's Hospital increased my understanding of the terrible toll poor nutrition is having on the health of our kids. And Dr. Andrea Vazzana of the NYU Child Study Center was invaluable in contributing her expertise to the parenting sections of this book.

I am very grateful for the tireless work of Danielle Hollar, PhD, Michelle Lombardo, and Sarah Messiah, PhD, and my nutrition director, Marie Almon, MS, RD, who were incredible forces behind our Healthier Options for Public Schoolchildren (HOPS) research program. Marie continues to be invaluable in keeping me up to date on the latest nutrition science.

Ira Harkavy, PhD, Frank Johnson, PhD, and program director Danny Gerber are the engines that have advanced the work of the Agatston Urban Nutrition Initiative at the University of Pennsylvania's Netter Center for University Community Partnerships.

The work of Jamie Oliver has been an inspiration. I first met and listened to Jamie several years ago, when he participated in our Childhood Obesity

Initiative symposium in Miami Beach, and I have been consistently impressed by his persistence and creativity over the years in improving nutrition, first in the UK and now in the United States.

My gluten adventure actually began with some basic education from my uncle, Dr. Robert Agatston, a retired geologist now in his late eighties, who learned he had celiac disease many years ago. He was the first to tell me that gluten was the cause of a much larger health problem than was appreciated by the medical community, and he was right. His tutelage increased my awareness of gluten sensitivities, which helped me recognize the reason for many of the health benefits of the gluten-free first phase of the South Beach Diet. I have since learned a great deal from the writings and research of Dr. Peter H. R. Green, director of the Celiac Disease Center at Columbia University, and from my colleague at the University of Miami, pediatrican Dr. Natalie Geary, who increased my understanding about the difference between celiac disease and gluten intolerance and the extent of wheat and gluten sensitivities in children.

Dr. Holly Atkinson, a fabulous internist, has done a wonderful job in keeping me and our research team current on all the medical areas discussed in this book, providing daily literature reviews and helpful discussions.

While I read more about the serious health effects of missing a good night's sleep, it was sleep specialist and longtime colleague Dr. Alejandro Chediak, the medical director of the Miami Sleep Disorders Center, who brought me up to speed in this area.

I learned a lot about how we grow and raise our food from personal conversations with Maria Rodale, publisher of this book, and from the writings of Michael Pollan. My friend Leonard Abess, an avid organic gardener and producer of organic maple syrup, also taught me a great deal about methods of organic farming.

My agents, Mel Berger and Eric Zohn, have provided me with excellent guidance and support along the way. Our publicist, Sandi Mendelson, has been an exceptional resource in advancing my message of prevention and health. Sandi, along with Cathy Gruhn of Hilsinger-Mendelson, has made my mission her mission.

At Rodale, I would like to thank executive vice president and general manager Karen Rinaldi for her unflagging support of our books, and Pam Krauss, vice president and publishing director, who has added her expert advice to this project. Diane Salvatore, editor in chief of *Prevention,* has also been a great supporter of my mission and enthusiastic about getting my message out. Thanks also to project editor Nancy N. Bailey and designer Christina Gaugler for their work on the book and to Amy King, executive director of art and design, who spent many hours creating a cover that would help convey the book's message. I also extend thanks to Kate Slate and Sandra Rose Gluck for their help in developing and testing the healthy recipes.

Finally, I have had constant and invaluable input from my live-in editor— my wife, Sari—and from our South Beach editorial director, Marya Dalrymple, who, in addition to editorial support, has worked tirelessly on keeping me focused on moving forward with the manuscript and in bringing the book to completion.

PART I

The Health
of Our Nation:

CONDITION CRITICAL!

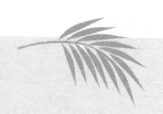

CHAPTER I

THE TICKING TIME BOMB

Americans are fatter and sicker than ever. We are eating horrendously, moving and exercising less, and not getting enough sleep. This has made us fatigued, depressed, irritable, achy, and generally miserable. And if feeling terrible isn't bad enough, these habits are also making us sick—with diseases like diabetes, heart disease, and cancer, to name just a few. We compensate by taking a lot of pills and supplements and resort to fad diets and other quick fixes that work temporarily or not at all. If we stay on this course, things are only going to get worse. If you don't believe me, keep reading. Even if you do believe me, but feel helpless to do anything about it, keep reading. My goal is to "wake" you up so that you can understand how we got to this sorry state and how you can turn things around for yourself, your family, your community, and, yes, for your country.

First let me introduce you to Marianne B. whose story illustrates the challenges we face.

Marianne, a 30-year-old nurse, is scared that the small Midwestern town where she and her husband are raising their two school-age children is literally dying before her eyes. What she's worried about is something that should be obvious, even to someone who's not a health-care professional. Nearly everyone in her town is either overweight or obese—including the kids. Diabetes is rampant. Heart disease is on the rise, especially among young adults. And at the hospital where she works, she is seeing more cases of severe allergies, chronic sinus and ear infections, asthma, and potentially life-threatening lung ailments than ever before.

It's no mystery to Marianne why so many people in her community are sick. "It's primarily the sedentary lifestyle and the poor diet, but people seem to be oblivious to the impact that their lifestyle is having on their health," she explains. What is perplexing to her is how many of them just don't get it.

Marianne's town isn't the only one that's in trouble—chances are your town is not much different from hers, and like the folks in her town, you too may have simply stopped noticing. That's hard to do, though, if you look at the maps on the Centers for Disease Control and Prevention Web site (www.cdc.gov/obesity/data/trends.html) that show obesity trends across the United States rising dramatically between 1985 and 2010. It really is astounding. In 1985, for all states for which there were data, the obesity rate was less than 15 percent, with many states having rates of less than 10 percent. Today, 36 states have obesity rates greater than 25 percent, with 12 of them at more than 30 percent! The state with the lowest obesity rate (21 percent) is Colorado. But if Colorado had the same obesity rate in 1985 that it has now, it would have been the fattest state in the Union instead of the thinnest. We've come a long way baby! Our country is headed for a medical and economic disaster.

A DOUBLE DEBT CRISIS

Every day we are witnessing the political battles over our national debt on TV, in the newspapers, and online. We have heard the debt crisis likened to a ticking time bomb, yet we continue to borrow money, seemingly without enough concern that we are just putting off the painful budget cuts that will have to be made later on. It appears that it will be our children and grandchildren who will have to pay for our lack of fiscal discipline today. That ticking time bomb will eventually blow up in our faces—or theirs.

We are unfortunately accumulating another national debt, and although it's not economic per se, the financial costs as well as the human costs could be insurmountable. It is also very much like a ticking time bomb that threatens us as individuals, as families, and as a nation. Our fast-food, sedentary lifestyle is wreaking havoc on our cells, tissues, and organs, and this will eventually lead to chronic diseases, some occurring sooner rather than later.

These changes begin in childhood (and some possibly in the womb; see "A Toxic Lifestyle Can Begin in the Womb," page 6). One example, and the one closest to my own experience and expertise, is coronary artery disease (atherosclerosis), which we know can begin in childhood. Atherosclerotic plaques arise in the walls of our arteries and progress silently. They usually cause no symptoms until the day one ruptures, potentially blocking a coronary artery and causing a heart attack. Most of us do not know how many of these ticking time bombs are growing in our vessels or when they will explode. As a society, what we also don't realize is that we are amassing other ticking time bombs that may well go off in the future and affect our health in different ways—some as strokes, others as cancers, Alzheimer's, macular degeneration, or myriad other diseases.

We are already experiencing the adverse health consequences of our poor lifestyle choices, and at the rate we're going, things will only get worse. The solution does not lie in health-care delivery once diseases become clinically apparent. Rather, it lies in the preventive lifestyle measures we can take long before. The hard truth is that whatever form health-care coverage ultimately takes—one-payer, multiple-payer, or a combination of coverages—it won't matter, because we won't be able to pay for it. If we do not make the positive lifestyle changes needed to halt and reverse the obesity epidemic now—today—our health-care system will be overwhelmed by a nation plagued by chronic disease. The system will be bankrupted by the sheer numbers of sick Americans.

THE SICKEST GENERATION

Journalist Tom Brokaw dubbed the men and women who lived through and fought in World War II the "greatest generation." If current trends continue, many adult readers of this book could have the dubious distinction of being remembered as the "sickest generation." If you are between the ages of 30 and 45, you should be very worried. You have the misfortune of being the first generation born into the fast-food, sedentary, screen-obsessed culture we have become. For the first time since I started practicing cardiology more than 30 years ago,

(continued on page 8)

A Toxic Lifestyle Can Begin in the Womb

Without immediate intervention, many children in the United States today are doomed to die prematurely. One out of six kids is currently so obese that he or she is vulnerable to a long list of diseases, like diabetes, heart disease, and nonalcoholic fatty liver disease, that open the door to a whole host of horrors, like limb amputation, kidney failure, and early death. If we continue along the same trajectory, one out of three babies born today will become diabetic at some point, and for the first time in modern history we will see a reduction in life span. We need to start protecting our children as early as possible, even before conception.

A woman who begins her pregnancy at a healthy weight and gains weight judiciously throughout its duration is doing herself and her baby a big favor. Unfortunately, half of all women who become pregnant are *already* overweight or obese. Obesity poses a health risk to pregnant women, predisposing them to preeclampsia (a potentially deadly type of high blood pressure), diabetes, premature delivery, and bigger babies (which increases the odds of having a C-section). It also makes it far more difficult to get down to a healthy weight after pregnancy, which, in turn, increases the risk of postpregnancy prediabetes, heart disease, and many different forms of cancer.

And now it appears that maternal obesity may be dangerous for the offspring later in life as well. Researchers in England assessed the cardiovascular risk of more than 5,000 9-year-old children and compared those results with their mothers' prepregnancy weight and subsequent weight gain during pregnancy. Their report, published in 2010 in the American Heart Association journal *Circulation,* shows a clear correlation between a high prepregnancy weight and/or excess weight gain during pregnancy and an increase in heart disease risk factors in the children of these mothers, as opposed to the children of mothers who gained only the recommended amount of weight. The children of mothers who were of excessive weight were themselves heavier and had larger waistlines, more body fat, higher systolic blood pressure, lower levels of good HDL cholesterol, and higher levels of inflammatory markers (chemicals in their blood that could predispose them to heart disease, cancer, arthritis, and a slew of other ailments when they get older). Now, the exact mechanism by which a mother's excess weight leads to heavier children isn't precisely understood at this time. It could be due to the mom's genetic or metabolic tendency to gain weight being passed on to her child; it could be the effect of excessive sweets and refined foods eaten during pregnancy on the developing fetus's metabolism; or it could be her lifestyle choices that influence her child during his or her early years—or a combination. Whatever the mechanism, it's not a great legacy to leave for your kids.

I'm not suggesting that a child's fate is necessarily sealed in the womb and that there's nothing that you can do later to make it right. Rather, I view this study and others like it as red flags reminding us of the important role that parents play in their children's health and well-being before, as well as after, they are born.

And here's a real surprise: It may not just be obese mothers who are passing the effects of their unhealthy condition on to their offspring. Paternal obesity may also be a factor in determining the health of children down the road—at least it is in rats. In a widely publicized study published in *Nature*, Australian researchers at the University of New South Wales in Sydney fed one group of male laboratory rats a high-fat diet to make them obese and induce prediabetes, and fed another group of male rats a normal diet. They mated both groups of male rats with normal-weight female rats, and they found that the female offspring of the obese male rats developed prediabetes by the time they were young adults, whereas the female offspring of the male rats who were fed the normal diet did not. (Whether similar effects emerge in male offspring remains to be seen.) Moreover, numerous studies confirm that obese parents are at much higher risk of having obese children, which probably has as much to do with the example they set for their children and the environment they create in their home as it does with any genetic factors.

heart attacks are on the rise for this age group, reversing decades of steady decline in deaths from heart disease in all age groups.

Recently, some very disturbing trends have been reported. In Olmsted County, Minnesota, home of the Mayo Clinic, autopsies have been performed since 1981 on young victims of unnatural deaths like accidents. For years, when doctors looked inside the coronary arteries of these young people, they saw a progressive *decrease* in the amount of atherosclerotic plaque that corresponded with a decrease in heart disease death rates. This decrease in both the amount of plaque and heart disease mortality continued until 1995, but then it began to slow down. The bad news is that since 2000, this slowdown has come to a halt: Plaque deposits in young people are no longer on the decline and are now *increasing*. These findings are consistent with the overall heart attack rates in Olmsted County and the rest of the country, where the decrease in heart attacks has plateaued and appears to be increasing among young Americans.

A 2007 study in the *New England Journal of Medicine* demonstrated that reduction in coronary artery disease deaths (mortality rates fell by more than 40 percent) from 1980 to 2000 would have been even more dramatic if not for the increase in deaths caused by obesity and resultant diabetes. It appears that since 2000 the skyrocketing increase in obesity and diabetes has halted the downward trend in heart attack deaths in young adults. Anecdotally, my colleagues and I, who screen for early vascular disease in our cardiology practices, are seeing more overweight young adults with the blood vessels typical of people decades older. I describe this phenomenon further in Chapter 2.

I call this generation of young adults the first fast-food, sedentary, computer-addicted, online-shopping, smart-phone-using, video-game-playing, social-networking generation. OK, let's just call them the "sickest generation," or "Generation S." The inescapable conclusion is that whatever we call them, *their fast-food, sedentary lifestyle is trumping the advances in medical science* that have been responsible for at least four decades of decreasing death rates from heart disease. And make no mistake: The same processes that are making our vessels prematurely old are also attacking the rest of our organs. And while their effects are becoming clinically apparent in the form of heart attacks and coronary artery disease in young adults, other manifestations are increasingly rearing their ugly heads in all age groups. In fact, our blood vessels and many of our organs are, in a sense, "rusting," and this process is beginning earlier and progressing faster than ever before.

MY JOURNEY

Soon after I first became interested in disease prevention in the 1980s, the early detection of atherosclerosis in the arteries of the heart became my focus. In the late 1980s and early 1990s, my colleagues and I pioneered the use of noninvasive computed tomography (CT) heart scanning to quickly and noninvasively image coronary atherosclerosis. Using this new technology, we began seeing atherosclerotic plaques in the arteries of young adults years before they were likely to cause heart attacks. I learned soon thereafter that the recently described metabolic syndrome (prediabetes) was a major cause of the progression of atherosclerosis to eventual heart attacks in my patients. I also learned that metabolic syndrome was a problem of lifestyle, not one that could be banished with medications. This piqued my interest in advances in nutrition science and led to the development of a healthy eating plan for my patients, which ultimately became the South Beach Diet.

Since then, I have come to appreciate that our nation's lifestyle problems are not just about heart and vascular disease. They encompass most of the chronic degenerative diseases of the Western world and now the Eastern world as well. Additionally, while I have always believed that exercise is very important to cardiovascular health, I have since learned that, like nutrition, it affects every aspect of our health and plays a role in many, if not most, maladies. I have also learned that optimal healthy exercise goes well beyond pounding the pavement. Our real understanding of the importance of core functional exercise and vigorous cardiovascular exercise—and why we should simply spend less time sitting—is relatively recent. I wrote a lot about this in my 2008 book, *The South Beach Diet Supercharged*. In the past several years, a large body of new research has introduced a third lifestyle area of great concern: sleep. While we have known of the link between sleep apnea and heart disease for some time, the importance of a good night's sleep in relation to many of our other health problems is just becoming apparent.

There has also been great progress in identifying the common threads that tie nutrition, exercise, sleep, and other lifestyle factors to our epidemic of chronic disease. The role of inflammation and its importance to our body's ability to repair tissues as we age is now coming into focus. Medical advances are showing us that our vessels and organs are rusting in a manner similar to a poorly maintained vehicle. Atherosclerosis in our vessels is just one indicator of this process. We now know that the amount of atherosclerosis we see on heart scans, along with other markers of inflammation like C-reactive protein, oxidative stress, and belly fat, are gauges of how fast our organs are aging. Consequently, they predict death not only from heart disease but from other chronic diseases like diabetes and cancer as well. We also know that good nutrition, proper exercise, and adequate sleep are all anti-inflammatory and anti-aging strategies that can halt and even reverse this so-called rusting process.

And there's more to understanding why our collective health has been deteriorating. Our DNA was designed to help us survive in the wild, not in our current high-tech environment. The physiologic mechanisms that helped our ancestors survive are killing us today. Understanding how this has happened is crucial if we are going to reverse our current downward spiral. When we veer from the way our forefathers ate, exercised, and slept, we do so at our own peril. This does not mean that we have to forfeit our modern technologies, but we do have to understand how they are affecting our health.

To better appreciate how our lifestyle is causing our chronic disease epidemics, we must look, at least briefly, at the technological and consequent economic changes that have led inextricably to our current unhealthy way of life. It is interesting and terribly disturbing to observe that as our fast-food, sedentary lifestyle has spread around the globe, the very same adverse health consequences have predictably followed.

Finally, I have learned, particularly from our work in elementary schools, that healthy changes must come from a holistic community approach. Obesity and diabetes, and their consequences, have too often been treated as clinical problems between patients and their doctors. Treatment at this stage occurs far too late and, as a result, is far too costly and not very effective. Our toxic lifestyle is a societal problem, and to be successful in addressing it, we have to treat it as such and very early in the game. For example, we need to alter school curriculums to teach healthy lifestyle education. This means incorporating nutrition and cooking classes and allowing sufficient time for physical education and recess. A later starting time and a nap time for preschoolers would also be very helpful, as kids would get more sleep. These changes will benefit children of all shapes and sizes and will only help, not hurt, academic performance. If kids eat healthy meals at school and learn about good nutrition and exercise, the weight will take care of itself. Skinny kids will gain weight and grow appropriately, and overweight kids will trim down.

MARIANNE'S WAKE-UP CALL

Despite the toxic time bomb in our midst, there is reason to be hopeful. It's possible for people and communities to change for the better. We can defuse the bomb if we put our minds to it. I know that it is possible to transform a harmful lifestyle into a healthy one because my colleagues and I have witnessed these changes in our clinical practices. I have also heard from people around the country who have done their homework and changed their lifestyles accordingly. Marianne B. is one of them.

In fact, Marianne B. is an excellent example of positive change. She began transforming her own life in 2006, when she turned to the South Beach Diet and lifestyle approach after she had gained a great deal of weight during pregnancy. Up until that time, she was living the same unhealthy lifestyle shared by many of her neighbors. She drank empty-calorie sodas throughout the day and typically reached for a convenient junk food snack when she was hungry. She drove everywhere and rarely walked, let alone exercised. Instead of cooking dinner for her family, she often picked up fast food at one of the dozens of franchises that lined the roads on her way home from work. Her wake-up call came when she found herself lugging around an extra 60 pounds after her second baby was born. This not only made her feel bad about herself but also, as she knew from her nursing experience, greatly increased her risk of diabetes and heart disease. It bothered her terribly that that she was not being a good role model for her children. Sick and tired of looking and feeling the way she did, and worried about her health, Marianne made a conscious decision to change for her own sake and the sake of her kids. She began cooking most of the family's meals at home, determined that her children would not be raised on a steady diet of cheeseburgers, french fries, and soft drinks. She made an effort to include more fresh fruits and vegetables, lean meats, chicken, and fish. She substituted baked sweet potatoes for the usual french fries and kept soda out of the house. Before long, her kids stopped asking for fast food. She also encouraged them to play outdoors, joining them whenever possible. And she put limits on how long they could play video games and watch TV.

Then she decided it was time to plant the seeds of her new healthy lifestyle throughout her community. She urged the women in her congregation to start bringing more wholesome dishes to church suppers, instead of the usual fried chicken and high-fat casseroles. She and other like-minded parents worked with the administration of their children's school to replace the typically starchy, fatty school lunches with healthier options. And she told anyone who'd listen that the conventional wisdom that kids won't eat vegetables, even if you serve them on a silver platter, is just plain wrong. The whole town heard Marianne say: "I have no trouble getting my kids to eat vegetables—they *love* their vegetables. They would be surprised if I served them a meal without vegetables."

FROM TOXIC TO HEALTHY

Marianne is one of the growing cadre of women I call Super Moms—women who are fighting back against the fast-food, sedentary way of life and its disastrous consequences, and who are transforming the culture within their homes, workplaces, schools, and communities. And this can also be said of the Super Dads, who are either the primary caregivers or who are partnering with their wives in clamoring for change.

While I do not want to sound sexist here, it has been my experience in my cardiology practice and the experience of my colleagues, both male and female, that women are most often the primary guardians of their family's health. The women come to my office dragging in their husbands, fathers, brothers, and grown sons (often by their earlobes) because these men have been in denial regarding their health. So it's not surprising to me to discover that it is primarily the Super Moms who have educated themselves about what's best for their kids, particularly when it comes to successfully providing their children with nutrient-rich food.

Today, people from all walks of life, from the White House on down, are trying to combat our obesity and diabetes epidemics and turn our toxic lifestyle around. In March 2010, Michelle Obama—the nation's First Super Mom—launched the *Let's Move!* campaign to promote a healthier, more active lifestyle as a way to combat the obesity epidemic in this country. Her work, and the spotlight she shines on the issue, is hugely refreshing and desperately needed. Around the country, groups like Urban Farming in downtown Detroit are planting vegetable gardens in abandoned lots so that the residents have access to fresh food. Today, many thousands of people support the 6,100-plus farmers' markets cropping up in cities and suburbs. And concerned citizens across the United States are beginning to take the school lunch bureaucracy to task, fighting for high-quality school meals for all children. My own work with our Healthier Options for Public Schoolchildren (HOPS) program, in which we provided nutrition and healthy lifestyle education programming to more than 50,000 elementary school children nationally, has taught me that kids will not only eat better food but will also become advocates for doing so once they understand the principles of good nutrition and how food impacts their lives. When children grasp why nutritious whole foods are good for them, and how they make you healthy and strong, they will bring this message back home to their families, which can help change the mind-set of entire communities.

WAKE UP!

With my patients, I have always found that the better they understand the causes of their medical issues and the rationale for their treatment, the better they do. I also believe that for Americans today, the better we understand the real impact our lifestyle choices are having on our health, the better the chance we can turn things around.

We are at the critical juncture where, if we do not wake up and turn the tide on our unhealthy lifestyle, we are going to increase the human and economic costs to the point that our very way of life will be severely threatened. And this is the high-altitude overview. Up close and personal, if we don't commit to leading a healthier and more active life, we will find ourselves old before our time and riddled with chronic health problems. Even worse, if we don't commit to making sure our children are eating nutritious foods and are physically active, we may well be sentencing them to a future of poor health and a shorter life span.

In Part 2 of this book, you will find the South Beach Diet Wake-Up Program, a series of seven strategies for individuals and families who want to transform a toxic lifestyle into a healthy one. I understand that change is a process, that it doesn't happen overnight, and that it takes commitment, planning, and the motivation to move forward. I also understand that trying to do too much at one time can be overwhelming and eventually lead to failure. So, this program is designed to let you tackle one piece of your life at a time, so that the changes are manageable and, most important, sustainable. You will learn how to assess your lifestyle so that you know which components need to be rethought and how to evaluate your readiness for change. You will learn how to de-clutter your life (and your mind), shop and eat in a healthier way, find time for exercise and sleep, and yes, still find time to cook. No, I don't expect you or your family or anyone to be perfect—that is not how you achieve permanent change. As so many of my readers know, the South Beach ethos is about making healthier choices most of time. If you can do that, you will have made great strides toward a healthier life.

CHAPTER 2

GETTING OLD
BEFORE OUR TIME

A few years ago a patient named Dan came to my office because he felt it was time to make sure his heart was healthy. He was only 35 years old, but his father had been diabetic and had suffered a heart attack in his late forties. Dan's family history wasn't all bad: On his mother's side, there was wonderful longevity, with two grandparents still doing well and living on their own in their nineties. Although Dan himself had no heart-related symptoms, like chest pain or shortness of breath, he had recently watched a friend at work suffer a near-fatal heart attack. Badly shaken by the incident, Dan was fearful that he might turn out to be more like his father than like his mother.

From the outside, Dan looked fine, at least when he was wearing his well-tailored business suit. Once Dan was in his examination gown, however, it was a different story. While his arms and legs were thin, it looked as if a bowling ball were stuck in his abdomen. Although Dan didn't seem to be bothered by this, I was, and I'll tell you why later.

Dan did complain about his joints. He was a weekend warrior—a tennis player who noticed that his hands were stiff and slightly painful in the mornings and that his right shoulder ached until he warmed it up, especially on cold days. The stiffness improved as he played, but he was now starting his weekend mornings and often his weekdays with over-the-counter anti-inflammatory medications. To the untrained observer, the joint pain and the prominent paunch would seem to be completely unrelated. But I knew that they were signs of an underlying degenerative process in Dan's body that was causing him to age before his time.

After I asked Dan some questions about his lifestyle, the reason for his belly became clear. His executive job required a lot of travel, which frequently meant dining out with clients. And although he tried to exercise when he was home, life on the road had taken a toll on Dan's exercise routine. I was sympathetic, because I too have trouble maintaining my nutrition and exercise regimen when I travel. Fortunately, I'm not on the road nearly as much as Dan and many of my other patients, but I do appreciate the challenges they face. I knew that, for Dan, change would not be easy and that to get his attention I would have to show him how his lifestyle was aging him before his time.

A LOOK UNDER THE HOOD

First I reviewed Dan's blood tests: His cholesterol was below 200 (considered ideal by national guidelines) but his triglycerides (the form of fat we use to store excess calories) were a bit high at 170, and his good cholesterol—the HDL—was definitely low at 35 (for both sexes above 60 is optimal). Despite the belly, his weight was within normal range for his height, but as you will see, these numbers alone cannot tell us definitively what is really going on inside.

In order to evaluate what was happening inside Dan and determine how his busy lifestyle (including his poor food choices and lack of exercise) was impacting his health, I needed to look under the hood. This meant looking at his pipes, or arteries, using noninvasive imaging techniques to determine whether his vessels were aging prematurely or, as I like to call it, "rusting." We do this by first viewing the carotid vessels with ultrasound. And then, depending on age and risk factors, we may also look into the coronary arteries with a noninvasive CT heart scan to see whether cholesterol is invading the vessel walls in the form of plaques. It was the best way to tell whether Dan was headed for an early heart attack, like his dad.

The carotid arteries run through the neck, one on each side, just underneath the skin, until they divide into separate branches that supply the brain and face with blood. Aside from their importance for supplying blood to your brain, the main carotids are also the most accessible large arteries in your body. An ultrasound probe can be placed just millimeters from the carotids, allowing for exquisite images of the vessels, including their inner linings. It is in these inner linings, called the "intima," where cholesterol gradually accumulates as we age—and it is here where we start to "rust."

The lining of the main carotid artery actually begins to thicken in childhood and continues to thicken right up into our eighties. The thickness of the artery lining, called the "intima-medial thickness," is a reflection of a person's vascular age. It is not rare to see a young adult with the arteries of a retiree and a retiree with the arteries of a teenager. The age of our vessels, determined by measuring the intima-medial thickness, reflects the disease process itself, and is a much better predictor of heart attack and stroke than all the conventional risk factors—like high cholesterol, high blood pressure, and smoking—combined.

For men over the age of 40 and women over the age of 50 with a family history of heart disease or other cardiac risk factors, I recommend the CT heart scan because it's an invaluable tool for judging the age of the heart's arteries (the coronary arteries). It is a test that I developed in 1988 with my colleague and friend, radiologist Dr. Warren Janowitz, to detect small deposits of calcium in the coronary arteries that are part of the atherosclerotic plaques that can eventually lead to heart attacks. If there is disease in the carotids, a history of early heart disease in the family, or many cardiac risk factors, I will perform the scan on patients younger than age 40 or 50. If a patient is heading for a heart attack in his or her forties, fifties, or sixties, these calcified plaques can usually be detected about 20 years earlier. Fortunately, radiation is minimal for this exam when up-to-date equipment in expert hands is used.

As in the carotid arteries, plaque buildup in the coronary arteries is a gradual process that gives us a long window of opportunity to detect whether it is present, how much is there, and how fast it is progressing. The measurement of plaque detected by the scan is known as the "Calcium Score," or, as I am proud to say, the "Agatston Score." It is considered by many experts to be the best single predictor of future heart attack, much better than simply evaluating the conventional risk factors. It is used worldwide for cardiac risk assessment. Similar to our findings with carotid thickness, using the scan we see 80-year-olds with no calcified plaque and the occasional 35-year-old with extensive plaque.

As it turned out, Dan's arteries were not pretty. His left carotid artery had the thickness of that normally found in people in their eighties. He had a Calcium Score of 20, which is what you would expect to see in someone in his midfifties. It was clear that he had inherited his father's bad genes and that this was only compounded by his unhealthy lifestyle. I show slides of Dan's arteries to other patients to prove how our vessels may be getting old way before we do. Another reason I show the pictures is because Dan has responded very well to the diet plan, exercise regimen, and medications he was prescribed. While he is getting older chronologically, his arteries appear to be getting younger.

GENES AND GUARDIAN ANGELS

Fairly simple noninvasive imaging like that I used with Dan reveals how factors that can cause heart disease—along with those that can protect our vessels—are interacting differently in each of us. And while some risk factors and the genes that govern them are yet to be discovered, that does not mean they are not affecting our blood vessels and other organs today.

In my cardiology career, I have had the opportunity to witness the discovery of many new risk factors that are continually adding to our understanding of why some people have heart attacks and others don't. When I first began practicing medicine, it was quite common to see patients with heart disease and not know why it had developed. When cholesterol was introduced as one of the first risk factors for heart disease, about half of the patients cardiologists saw in the coronary care units had "normal" cholesterol levels by national guidelines (and this still holds true). Back then, I would have been satisfied with Dan's good cholesterol and sent him home with a clean bill of health. Not today.

Today we know that it's not the total cholesterol number that matters most, but rather how cholesterol interacts with other risk factors that determines whether plaques are created and how rapidly they progress to clog our arteries. Fast progression means a heart attack at a young age. This was evidenced by two women I saw recently as patients on the same day—Kate and

Debra, ages 57 and 58, respectively. Both had practically identical total cholesterol levels—in the 270 range—and similar good HDL cholesterol levels. Yet a heart scan revealed that Kate's arteries were loaded with plaque, while Debra's were squeaky clean. That meant Kate's cholesterol needed to be treated aggressively before it led to a heart attack while Debra needed nothing more than reassurance.

What we have learned through sophisticated imaging techniques like the heart scan, and also through more advanced blood testing, is that there are individuals with many cardiac risk factors who turn out to have pristine arteries. These lucky patients may have a guardian angel (an unknown factor) that is protecting their hearts. For example, the lining of their arteries might be resistant to the invasion of cholesterol, even when there are high levels in the bloodstream. It is not unusual to hear a story from a patient about his or her still-vibrant 90-year-old great-uncle Joe, who drinks, smokes, and eats fried chicken as a staple. This might be true, but until I am able to isolate Great-Uncle Joe's protective gene or genes, I certainly cannot recommend his lifestyle.

At the other extreme are those patients, usually with family histories of heart disease, whose conventional risk factors look unremarkable but whose hearts show signs of atherosclerotic changes (hardening of the arteries) at an early age. These individuals are at high risk because of a yet-to-be-discovered factor that runs in their families. Something may be allowing cholesterol to penetrate into their artery walls even though the total amount of cholesterol in their blood is low.

The bottom line: Even if your cholesterol is high, it does not mean that you are destined for a heart attack, and even if it is low, it does not mean that you are protected from having one or that you have license to eat like there's no tomorrow.

LOOKS ARE NOT ALWAYS DECEIVING

While my patient Dan looked pretty good on the outside, some of us don't hide our internal rusting so easily. When we appear older than our chronologic age, it is often an indication that we are aging quickly on the inside as well. I am always amazed by friends and patients in their eighties, and even in their nineties, who remain active both mentally and physically and who look much younger than their years. Many of these youthful seniors, like my friend Irwin, who's in his mideighties, continue to work. Irwin, a physician, practices medicine full-time and can still dance circles around me (not actually that hard to do) at parties and celebrations. His wife, who is several years his junior, also looks and acts much, much younger than her age. They are hard to keep up with. Then there are those in their fifties and even forties who simply look old and tired. In fact, what's making them look older on the outside are often the same risk factors that are rusting them on the inside. Sometimes looks can be deceiving, but often they're not.

One unfortunate bad habit that ages us quickly, both outside and in, is smoking. When I was director of noninvasive cardiology at Mount Sinai Medical Center in Miami Beach, I sometimes played an informal game of "Guess who smokes?" with the technicians. I could invariably pick out the smokers just by looking at them. My record was quite good and still is. I'm sure many of you think that you can also identify smokers. The first impression is of rapid aging. Two important clues are their prematurely wrinkled skin and their prematurely gray hair, both of which are associated with chronic tobacco use and risk of heart attack. Their raspy voices from emphysematous lungs can also be a telltale sign. What's the common thread? Two biological processes that occur inside and outside our bodies every day: inflammation and oxidation (measured as oxidative stress).

WHAT MAKES US RUST?

Inflammation and oxidation are important survival mechanisms that have helped us endure in both ancient and modern times. Without these mechanisms, we would quickly succumb to infection, and possibly even die from something as seemingly minor as a splinter.

When these survival mechanisms are triggered too often, for reasons that have little to do with "survival," they can actually accelerate aging and promote rusting. But how can a process designed to protect us end up becoming our enemy? First, let me explain how this mechanism normally works to protect us. At the initial sign of an invader, like bacteria or a splinter, local blood vessels dilate so that extra blood carrying inflammatory factors can move briskly to the threatened site. White blood cells then arrive to surround the invader and either kill the bacteria or begin to wall off and dissolve the splinter and the affected tissue. When you sustain an injury to your skin—a scrape, a cut, or a burn, for example—you experience this inflammatory process firsthand. The injured area turns red and feels warm and tender to the touch. This is due to the increased local blood flow and the infiltration of the area with white blood cells. In other words, it is inflamed. As healing progresses, the inflammation subsides.

This same inflammatory reaction also occurs inside the body in response to internal injury. For example, when bacteria invade our lungs and cause pneumonia, the infection triggers an aggressive campaign to surround, engulf, and kill the bacteria. Just like a skin wound, the injured lung tissue also becomes hot and irritated, inducing a cough. This is a good thing as long as the inflammation can kill off the invader without inflicting too much damage to the lung itself. Often, as with a cut or burn, the area affected by pneumonia heals with a local scar. Long after the pneumonia has been cured, the innocent scar remains (just like on the skin) and may be seen on a chest X-ray years later.

Under the wrong circumstances, the inflammatory process is activated inappropriately and our own protector cells unwittingly attack healthy cells as if they were foreign invaders. For example, when you inhale the smoke and toxins from a cigarette, it unleashes a diffuse inflammatory process that can cause so much scarring that it interferes with the normal function of the lungs. This is known as emphysema, and it can leave its victims gasping for their next breath. Scars like this can also set the stage for lung cancer in much the same way that sun-damaged skin can lead to skin cancer.

Over the past decade, we have learned that out-of-control inflammation is the common denominator for most chronic disease, including cancer, arthritis, Alzheimer's, macular degeneration, coronary artery disease, and even the aging process itself. What's really frightening is that because of our destructive lifestyle, our nation is now "hyperinflamed."

A SURVIVAL MECHANISM THAT IS KILLING US

To understand why we are such a hyperinflamed society and how we got to this unfortunate state, we need to look back at another survival mechanism—one that helped our ancestors store fat when food was abundant in order to ward off starvation when it inevitably became scarce. The mechanism that encourages fat accumulation in our bellies is called "insulin resistance." By "belly fat," I am referring to the fat—also known as visceral fat—that attaches to the organs inside our abdomens. This visceral fat is different from the subcutaneous fat that accumulates under our skin, often on our hips, thighs, and buttocks and as the "pinch an inch" variety known as "love handles." It is excess visceral fat that gives us the "apple" appearance, and it is the subcutaneous fat that results in the "pear" shape. Today we know that insulin resistance leads to metabolic syndrome (prediabetes) and type 2 diabetes. But throughout human history, insulin resistance was critical to helping us survive famine.

So let's go back to our ancestors who were living in the wild. Perhaps their highest priority was procuring enough food to ward off starvation, which was nearly always a threat. Because this was long before salting, drying, and refrigeration were employed to protect food from decay, not much food could be stored for extended periods in their caves or other shelters. The one safe place our ancestors could store a fuel reserve was in their bellies. Here's how that works:

Normally, after a meal, the fat and sugar we ingest is broken down in our digestive tract and absorbed into the bloodstream. In response, insulin is secreted from the pancreas (an organ located in the middle of the upper abdomen) to move this fuel from our bloodstream into our tissues, where it supports all of our bodily functions. If no insulin is secreted by the pancreas, our tissues cannot access the fuel (sugar and fat) running through our bloodstream and we essentially starve. This is actually what happens in untreated type 1 (not type 2) diabetes. The lack of insulin secretion causes type 1 diabetics to waste away as their fat and sugar is lost in their urine. (Until the discovery and use of insulin in 1922, wards of unfortunate children wasted away, went into comas, and died while doctors, nurses, and family members looked on helplessly.)

So how did resistance to the action of insulin help us survive in the wild? When food was plentiful and we naturally consumed extra calories, these calories were stored in the abdomen as visceral fat. These visceral fat cells then swelled and caused our tissues to become resistant to insulin so it could not easily "unlock" the cells to let the fat and sugar in. Thus, after a meal, when a moderate amount of insulin was appropriately secreted in response to rising blood sugar (or blood glucose), the insulin was unable to efficiently facilitate the movement of sugar and fat out of the bloodstream and into the tissues. As a result, the amount of sugar and fat in the blood rose to higher levels than normal. To overcome the tissues' resistance, the pancreas put out extra insulin, which finally unlocked the tissues, allowing the sugar to rush in. This caused the blood sugar to fall rapidly and to a lower level than usual, a condition called *reactive hypoglycemia* (low blood sugar).

It is reactive hypoglycemia that initiates food cravings in modern times, as it did in olden days. It is also what's responsible for that sinking, weak, and tired feeling that many of us feel in the midmorning, midafternoon, and sometimes in the evening, which we relieve by reaching into our kitchen cabinets for sugary and starchy infusions—usually from processed carbohydrates like cookies or chips.

For our ancestors, this fall in blood sugar meant that they would feel hungrier and devour more food when it was plentiful. They would store this extra energy as a fuel reserve in their bellies in the form of visceral fat and would then call upon it in the winter months when food was scarce. With fat predominantly stored in the belly (and thin, muscular arms and legs, just like Dan's), our ancestors could still run, hunt, and gather while expending only the extra energy needed to carry this additional fuel reserve. One could liken it to taking a reserve gas tank on a car trip into the wilderness. Eventually they would deplete their reserve, but hopefully not before springtime, when external sources of food would again become available.

TAKING A CHEMICAL BATH

Today, in our society, when there is no famine, only feast, we do not deplete the fuel reserve in our bellies. Once this visceral fat activates our insulin resistance survival genes (also known as the thrifty genes), we continue to wolf down food, adding more excess fuel reserve that only makes us sick, tired, and, for some men, impotent (see "Rusting below the Belt," opposite).

This is only exacerbated by the empty calories so common in our overly processed food. For example, when we remove nutrients and fiber from grains by processing them, the resulting starch is digested rapidly, triggering greater swings in blood sugar. This occurs both before and after insulin resistance appears. In individuals with insulin resistance, it simply amplifies the already exaggerated swings in blood sugar and so they end up walking around hungry most of the time. I believe this reactive hypoglycemia is the major reason why supersizing has become such a prominent nutrition issue. Once we are hypoglycemic, it requires a lot more calories, taken in relatively fast, to satisfy our cravings.

But how does it make us sick?

One important way is that while the fat is circulating in the blood for longer than usual, waiting for insulin to move it into our tissues, it undergoes chemical and physical changes that facilitate its penetration through the lining of our arteries, including the arteries that deliver blood to the heart and brain. This is the origin of the atherosclerotic plaques that clog blood vessels, eventually leading to a heart attack or stroke. It's one of the reasons my patient Dan ended up with atherosclerotic arteries at age 35. The other way insulin resistance makes us sick is by encouraging excessive accumulation of belly fat. The added fat becomes a source of inflammatory molecules and oxidant stress that overstep their protective roles and instead begin to damage to our normal tissues.

None of us would choose to expose our blood vessels and other organs to

Rusting below the Belt

When I tell some of my younger male patients that belly fat could lead to a heart attack, I can see their eyes glazing over as they think, "Well, that's got to be years away from now." When I tell them that it can disrupt their sex life, lower their sex drive, and age them rapidly, beginning right now, I get their attention.

There is a relationship between a toxic lifestyle, obesity, and testosterone, the male sex hormone responsible for many biologic functions, including energy level, libido, and sexual function. It turns out that belly fat cells and the inflammatory chemicals they produce are associated with low levels of testosterone. You may have noticed that men with large guts frequently have less facial hair and don't need to shave as often as their thinner peers. This is due to low testosterone, which is also associated with erectile dysfunction, poor libido, less muscle mass and strength, and reduced energy, not to mention insulin resistance, metabolic syndrome, and type 2 diabetes. And if that's not bad enough, erectile dysfunction is also a sign of general vascular dysfunction and a risk factor on its own for heart disease.

Testosterone levels naturally decrease as we age—it's called andropause. While this occurs more gradually than menopause in women, we certainly don't want to speed it up by accumulating belly fat. So if you are shaving less and your libido is down, look in the mirror. What's enlarging above your belt may be affecting you below it.

a daily toxic chemical bath, but that is exactly what is happening to the millions of Americans walking around with too much belly fat. When insulin resistance drives us to devour those processed empty-calorie fast foods in supersize portions, our bellies just keep growing, storing much more fuel than we will ever need—unless we were to get stranded on a deserted island like Tom Hanks in the movie *Cast Away*. And this extra belly fat is what leads to the chemical bath I am talking about.

Our excess belly fat has put us into a constant state of hyperinflammation, with far more inflammation than we need to protect us from viruses or to clot our blood when we are cut. In a sense, our immune systems are in chronic overdrive. It's like alternately pressing down hard on a car's accelerator, flooding the fuel lines, and then slamming on the breaks, making it hard to keep the car in good operating shape and definitely shortening its life. Hyperinflammation has turned our onetime survival mechanism against us.

What's very disturbing is that today more of us have bigger bellies than ever before. Two-thirds of American adults are overweight or obese, and more than 34 percent have metabolic syndrome (this includes more than 40 percent of those over age 40 and more than 50 percent of those over age 60)! The main characteristics of metabolic syndrome are not just a larger waist circumference due to increased visceral fat, but also high blood pressure, borderline high blood sugar levels, high levels of fat in the blood in the form of triglycerides, and low levels of the good HDL cholesterol. When the pancreas has to continually work hard to produce the extra insulin needed to overcome the insulin resistance caused by those swollen belly fat cells, it eventually tires out and can no longer completely overcome the insulin resistance. Consequently, less sugar is moved out of the bloodstream, the blood sugar rises, and the criteria for diagnosing type 2 diabetes is eventually met (the threshold for moving from metabolic syndrome to type 2 diabetes is somewhat arbitrary). But damage to our organs begins long before the diagnosis of diabetes is made. The hopeful news is that dietary and other lifestyle changes can reverse not only insulin resistance but also type 2 diabetes if they're made before the pancreas is irreparably damaged.

We have known for many years how obesity, metabolic syndrome, diabetes, and the resultant inflammation and oxidative stress can lead to the rusting of our blood vessels and to heart attack and stroke. But it is only recently that we have begun to appreciate just how harmful this chemical bath is to the rest of our organs as well. Where's the proof? We have it and it is growing.

An analysis of 97 studies that followed individuals with and without type 2 diabetes, published in 2011 in the *New England Journal of Medicine,* found that diabetes is associated with excess premature deaths from nonvascular diseases such as pneumonia and other respiratory diseases, renal disease, liver disease, endocrine disorders, neurologic diseases such as Alzheimer's, and even suicide. It is also associated with premature deaths from many forms of cancer, including liver, pancreatic, ovarian, colon, bladder, lung, and breast, among others. This was a very large study that included 820,900 participants, of whom 123,205 died after an average of 13.6 years of follow-up. The size of the study makes the results noteworthy.

Other studies—one published in 2008 in the *Journal of the American College of Cardiology* and another in 2011 in *Diabetes Care*—showed a direct relationship between the rusting of our arteries (indicated by the amount of plaque in the subjects' hearts as measured by the Calcium Score) and death from all causes, not just from heart disease. The more plaque, or rust, the study participants had, the more likely they were to suffer a premature death.

And in a 2011 study from Sweden, published in the journal *Neurology*, 8,534 twins who'd had their height and weight checked when they were in their early to midforties were evaluated for dementia when they were in their seventies to early eighties. Being overweight at midlife increased the risk of dementia—being obese, even more so. This was true even in twins where one was overweight but the other wasn't. This is a clear indication that it is not just genetics but also how we live that determines our future.

THE FIRE IN OUR BELLIES

I have talked about the role of inflammation as a common denominator in the chronic diseases of the Western world, but I am now going to expand your understanding of how this process works. You have most likely heard about antioxidants and probably have also heard the term "free radicals" thrown around in the popular press and in advertisements for various supplements, foods, and beverages. These terms are related to a very important process that is intimately involved with inflammation. It is summarized by the concept of "oxidative stress." Numerous scientists have concluded that inflammation resulting from oxidative stress is actually the cause of many diseases and a primary determinant of how fast we age. In fact, the rusting I have been writing about is due to excessive oxidative stress. Just like an old car will begin to rust if you leave it outdoors and exposed to the elements, the human body will also start to rust if it is not properly maintained and is exposed to excessive oxidative stress. The culprit in both cases is oxygen. Of course, human beings need oxygen to survive, but unless it is tightly controlled, oxygen (our friend) can turn into our enemy.

Oxidative stress is a measure of the balance between oxidants (also known as free radicals) and antioxidants, substances that combat them. Both free radicals and antioxidants can come from the environment or can be made in our bodies. Cigarette smoke, smog, chemicals such as those used in household cleaners, and the crisp, burnt edges of an overgrilled steak are examples of environmental oxidants that carry damaging free radicals. There are some useful free radicals, however, that are formed in our bodies; these act either as messengers to regulate important functions such as blood clotting or as "targeted assassins" (as when they are made by white blood cells) to kill invading bacteria.

To combat damaging free radicals, antioxidants are critical. These substances can be found in the environment and in fruits, vegetables, olive oil, and even red wine and dark chocolate, as well as in many other healthy foods and beverages. Antioxidants are also produced by the body itself; healthy behaviors such as regular exercise and a good night's sleep stimulate their production.

When we have a low level of oxidative stress (a normal balance between free radicals and antioxidants), we are healthy. When free radicals dominate and oxidative stress is increased, we are in trouble. You can think of this balance as a *controlled burn* that is employed to consume excess underbrush and dead trees that otherwise could provide the fuel for a devastating forest fire. In monitoring a controlled burn, firefighters with fire retardants play the role of antioxidants, keeping the burn in check. In our bodies, antioxidants absorb excess free radicals, allowing for a "healthy controlled burn." If the free radicals get out of control, they can literally punch holes in normal cells, in enzymes, and in our normal DNA, and in the process create more free radicals, which can cause a chain reaction akin to a forest fire burning out of control. This damages our normal tissues and organs and stimulates an inflammatory response.

Often when we talk about a fire in our bellies, it has a positive connotation—it's an internal call to action. Other times it means we are experiencing heartburn. Now we can also think of our protruding bellies as the excess fuel that ignites a pro-inflammatory, free radical–fed fire that can burn out of control. This particular fire leads to many of our daily aches and pains and is also associated with arthritis, cancer, macular degeneration, dementia, and other acute and chronic diseases. The rusting of our blood vessels is also what happens when these internal fires burn out of control, which is what occurred in Dan's case. In fact, the same process that rusted Dan's arteries also inflamed his joints and caused the stiffness and pain he experienced—the pain that caused him to reach for an over-the-counter anti-inflammatory in the mornings.

Today we know that you can prevent inappropriate inflammation and rusting and resultant disease by avoiding outside sources that contain or promote free radicals, such as smoke (primary and secondhand) and sugary, starchy, fat-laden processed foods. At the same time, you can consume antioxidants from healthy sources like fruits and vegetables and stimulate your own body's antioxidant production through regular exercise and a good night's sleep.

But what if your organs are already injured and aging prematurely? Let's take a look at one of our body's elegant healing mechanisms that could make a difference.

ADULT STEM CELLS: THE FOUNTAIN OF YOUTH?

Since most of the damage to our blood vessels and other organs occurs without any noticeable symptoms, it is fortunate that the human body has its own internal repair crew to help slow and even reverse these injuries. These are our stem cells, which not only work to maintain our tissues so that our organs can function properly, but also work to reverse inflammation and vascular damage and make our vessels "younger"—or at least age more slowly. Most of the time, our stem cells work brilliantly. However, a toxic lifestyle that promotes oxidative stress and inflammation can make these stem cells "sick," rendering them unable to function optimally, or can even kill them off.

Several years ago, I really didn't know that much about stem cells; the research was in its infancy and was not much discussed in preventive cardiology circles. I did know that stems cells are "omnipotent," meaning they can turn into new cells and tissues to repair an injury in any part of the body. I was also aware that stem cells were being taken from patients and later reinjected to grow new blood vessels. While there have been some impressive outcomes in individual patients, the reason you haven't heard about a friend getting this treatment is that, overall, the results have been discouraging. But in medicine, as in life, persistence eventually pays off.

My real stem cell education began when Professor Keith Webster, PhD, the director of the University of Miami Vascular Biology Institute, came to me a few years ago with a proposal to study the effect of a South Beach–style diet compared with that of the Western diet on stem cells in mice. It seemed like an excellent strategy to advance our understanding of the relationship between diet, lifestyle, and chronic disease.

I have learned a great deal from Dr. Webster and his research team and from the research we have pursued. In particular, I have learned about the relation of stem cells to oxidative stress and inflammation after various lifestyle interventions. I hope that after reading about our mouse studies, you too will better understand why your lifestyle is so important to your health and longevity.

OF MICE AND MEN

Our subjects were special mice that were bred to develop type 2 diabetes and atherosclerosis, similar to the way humans do. Why mice? Diet studies are notoriously difficult to conduct on humans because you can't "blind" a human to the diet he or she is eating. Mice, on the other hand, will nibble on whatever chow you put in their cage. And you don't have to worry about mice "cheating" at night when you're not looking. Moreover the biology of mice and humans is not all that different. Mice can fall prey to many of the same diseases we do, and their illnesses progress in a similar fashion. Also, mice grow old much faster than people, which means you can see the impact of a lifestyle intervention much sooner. In this study, one group of young mice was put on the mouse chow version of the standard, processed, nutrient-poor Western diet, loaded with sugar and bad fats. A second group of young mice dined on the mouse chow version of the South Beach Diet: They ate plenty of omega-3-rich fish oils, lean protein, and abundant amounts of fiber. One subset of each group got regular exercise—we installed exercise wheels in the cages of these mice or made time in their day for a recreational swim.

After four months, the mice fed the Western diet had developed athero-sclerosis and diabetes; they had bad blood lipids, weighed more than the South Beach group, and had high blood levels of inflammatory molecules. They were also sluggish and showed signs of mental deterioration. Frankly, they looked like potbellied, bloated wrecks!

What about the South Beach mice? Both the exercise and the sedentary groups were markedly trimmer than the Western diet mice, and had better blood lipids. But the real winners were the mice that ate the right food and exercised. They had the best blood lipids and the lowest levels of inflammation.

Clearly, the South Beach–type diet was beneficial when it was fed to the mice early in life. But we wanted to know its impact on those mice that had started off eating the Western diet and already had atherosclerotic plaques in their arteries. Half of the now fat and diabetic Western diet mice continued on the Western diet, and half were switched to the South Beach way of eating. In both diet groups, half were given the exercise regimen. What were the results? All the mice on the South Beach Diet lost weight and decreased their levels of inflammatory molecules, but *only those that exercised and ate the South Beach Diet showed a regression in atherosclerotic plaques.*

HEALTHY VERSUS SICK STEM CELLS

What is even more dramatic about this study, and what may eventually prove more important to our knowledge of how the body ages and rusts, are the differences we found between the South Beach mice and the Western diet mice on a cellular level.

As part of the research, we focused on one type of stem cell, called "CD34 positive, lineage negative." Think of the CD34 cells as the "repair crew" I mentioned earlier—which in this case were "assigned" to help repair damage to the endothelium, the inner lining of your arteries that I discussed earlier.

When the endothelium sustains an injury from the chemical bath of free radicals and inflammatory cells, these CD34 repair cells, which normally hang out in bone marrow, leap into action. They head straight to the site of the injury so they can make new endothelial cells to repair the damage. Other types of stem cells perform similar functions throughout the body.

To maintain a well-functioning, youthful body, you need to have a constant supply of strong, vigorous stem cells to keep the repair process going. Unfortunately, as we age, we produce fewer and less powerful stem cells, and this is one reason why our organ systems begin to function less efficiently as we get older. In other words, we rust faster.

What our mouse study confirmed is that a poor diet can have the same negative impact on stem cells as the aging process itself. We discovered that the mice that ate the typical Western diet and developed heart disease not only had fewer stem cells, but also that the ones they did have appeared sickly and unable to do their job effectively. In contrast, the mice fed the South Beach–style diet remained vigorous and robust, and had a plentiful supply of healthy stem cells. (You can readily tell the difference between healthy and unhealthy stem cells under a microscope.) Furthermore, those who developed healthy stem cells reversed their atherosclerosis and healed their blood vessels. Wow!

THE YOUNGEST VICTIMS

Thanks to our sedentary, fast-food culture, it's not surprising that I am seeing a growing number patients in their thirties and forties who, like Dan, are suffering the ravages of America's current lifestyle. As I mentioned in Chapter 1, it appears that in the young, this devastating lifestyle is trumping our advances in medical science. We know that loading up on cheeseburgers and fries will speed up aging by killing off our body's ability to heal itself. And now we are finding that this process begins earlier and earlier in life.

Perhaps most disturbing is what I have heard from so many of my patients and friends who are teachers, many of them recently retired. They all tell me that when they started teaching 30 or 40 years ago, there used to be one or, at most, two overweight students in their classes. Now a substantial percentage of their students are overweight. This is consistent with national statistics that clearly show the epidemic of obesity reaching our children. And, as in adults, obesity leads to metabolic syndrome and type 2 diabetes. Remember, type 2 diabetes was originally called "adult onset diabetes" because it was nearly always brought on by poor nutrition and sedentary living later in life. Type 1 diabetes, which is due to inadequate production of insulin and not caused by poor nutrition, was known as "juvenile diabetes" because it generally presented in children. But today, type 2 diabetes is no longer uncommon in kids, because of their sedentary habits and their intake of junk food.

My colleague Dr. Natalie Geary practiced pediatrics in Manhattan— hardly one of the fattest areas in the United States—between the mid-1990s and 2010. During her pediatric training in the early 1990s, she remembers seeing only one case of type 2 diabetes. But in her private practice, children with type 2 diabetes became more and more common from 2000 to 2010. A host of other nutrition-related problems that had been rare in pediatrics a decade earlier, including eczema, asthma, various stomach issues, and behavior problems, also became everyday occurrences in Dr. Geary's practice. Unfortunately, the problems she and other pediatricians are seeing today are planting the seeds (and the plaques) that will sprout as early chronic disease as these children grow into adulthood.

For decades we have understood that atherosclerosis is a progressive disease that begins early in life: Autopsies of young soldiers killed in the Korean and Vietnam wars revealed that about 25 percent of them had fatty plaques in the lining of their arteries. These plaques were evidence of the beginnings of this destructive process.

The percentage is surely much higher today, as we are learning from long-term studies like the ongoing Bogalusa Heart Study. This study has tracked the prevalence of overweight and obesity in children and adolescents in that primarily rural Louisiana community since 1972 (along with their impact on cardiovascular health). The researchers found signs of blood vessel injury in children as young as 5 years old. Alarmingly, since the Bogalusa Heart Study began, the number of overweight and obese children in that town has more than tripled from 14.2 percent to 48.4 percent!

Observational Diet Studies

I am often asked why there have never been any long-term, interventional studies on diet and human beings. The answer is simple: It would be impossible, not to mention prohibitively expensive. In contrast, it is simple to study a pill like a vitamin E tablet by dividing subjects (randomization) into two groups and giving half a placebo (the control group) and half the real vitamin E (the intervention group). The placebo and the real pills are made to look identical so the subjects and the investigators don't know who got what until the code is broken at the end of the study. This is called a double-blind (neither the patient nor the investigator knows which group a patient is in) placebo-controlled clinical trial, and it is considered the gold standard for research.

Unfortunately, this approach is not always feasible and not always the optimal way to resolve a clinical dilemma. For instance, researchers never performed a placebo-controlled study to determine that smoking kills. This was because there were already so many observational studies clearly showing that smoking was dangerous that it would have been unethical to randomize patients to a smoking group. Also, it has been impossible to create a placebo (though companies are still trying) that doesn't clue the study subjects in to which group they have been assigned.

For this reason, we have to look at the "totality of evidence," which usually comes from several different investigative approaches in order to arrive

Because we now have the ability to look "under the hood," even in young-sters, utilizing the imaging techniques I discussed earlier, it's not surprising that more and more studies are finding early vascular disease. In one such study, doctors at the University of Missouri–Kansas City School of Medicine examined the carotid arteries of 70 children and teenagers, on average 13 years of age, who were overweight and already had atherosclerosis-promoting

at a conclusion. For diet, this is particularly important to understand. People cannot be blinded to what they are eating. And while you could control intake over a short period of time in a controlled situation (such as an isolated camp in the wilderness or a residential treatment center), in the real world, for the longer term, this is just not feasible. Therefore, when it comes to diet and nutrition, we have to depend a great deal on observational studies.

The best-known such study in the field of nutrition is the Nurses' Health Study from the Harvard School of Public Health, which was begun in 1976 and is now in its second phase. Directed by Walter Willett, MD, the current study has been observing the habits of more than 100,000 registered nurses who have been filling out extensive lifestyle questionnaires (nurses are likely to do this reliably) since 1989. Much of what we have learned in recent years about nutrition has come from this study and other similar, though not as large, observational studies.

Animal studies, particularly mouse studies, are helpful when it comes to nutrition because they can be so well controlled and long-term changes can be easily determined in a short time period at a fraction of the cost. In fact, today, just as with performing a smoking study, it would be unethical to place a placebo group on the typical Western diet (even though most Americans are already on it) because there is simply too much evidence that it is unhealthy. While it would be perfectly ethical and interesting to conduct a study of a vegetarian diet versus a nonvegetarian good-fats, good-carbs diet, to do so long term would, again, just not be feasible.

risk factors (such as abnormal blood fats, high blood pressure, and insulin resistance) or a family history of abnormal blood fats. The researchers used the same noninvasive ultrasound imaging test that I used for Dan. They found that when compared with those of normal-weight children, the arteries of overweight children showed signs of premature aging (rusting), and in some cases, children as young as 10 years old had arteries with the thickness of 45-year-olds.

You can just imagine what these kids' arteries are going to look like when they actually reach 45—that is, if they get there. Meanwhile, because of a lack of exercise and a poor diet, these children are vulnerable not just to heart disease and diabetes but also to the many other ailments common in obese adults, including sleep apnea, arthritis, gallstones, high blood pressure, high cholesterol, constipation, and even hormonal problems that can lead to infertility and headaches. They are more likely to get asthma and have learning and behavior problems, which may in part be caused by their inability to get a good night's sleep. And there is convincing evidence that the problems we are seeing in teens, preteens, and children far younger do indeed lead to the unfortunate health outcomes we would expect many years later.

It is these discouraging observations that make me pin my hopes on the Super Moms and on making elementary school lifestyle interventions and community programs a high priority. It is increasingly clear that the earlier we address childhood obesity, the easier it will be to stop this epidemic and give these kids a brighter future.

A FINAL THOUGHT

It's now absolutely clear that a healthy lifestyle—eating a proper diet, losing weight if necessary, and getting plenty of exercise and a good night's sleep—is the surest, safest, best way to prevent the downward spiral that is manifested by diseases like diabetes, heart disease, cancer, dementia, and the many other degenerative diseases of aging. We know how to "rust-proof" our bodies. So let's do it.

A Chat with David Ludwig, MD, PhD

Dr. David Ludwig is director of the Optimal Weight for Life (OWL) Program in the Division of Endocrinology at Children's Hospital Boston and associate professor of pediatrics at Harvard Medical School. He is author of *Ending the Food Fight: Guide Your Child to a Healthy Weight in a Fast Food/Fake Food World*, which I consider to be an excellent resource for combating childhood obesity. When I first became fascinated with the new nutrition science in the early 1990s, I kept coming across Dr. Ludwig's work. His papers on the role of the glycemic index were enlightening and had an important influence on my thinking, even before I had the pleasure of meeting him in person. Later, when we began our Healthy Options for Public Schoolchildren (HOPS) program, I sought his advice. Today, his clinic at Children's Hospital is cutting-edge, and I am delighted that he agreed to contribute his expertise to this book.

In an article in the New England Journal of Medicine, *you noted that we are just beginning to feel the impact of the childhood obesity epidemic. How bad is it going to get?*

One can think of the childhood obesity epidemic as evolving in three phases. The first phase was the rapid increase in prevalence. And although we are now seeing what looks like a plateau in the incidence of childhood obesity, it is no cause to celebrate. There will come a point when basically anybody who is biologically able to become obese will—though we know that there are some people who are protected against that for genetic reasons. The second phase is when this high prevalence—and the prevalence for childhood obesity is now higher than ever before in history—translates into weight-related complications, like type 2 diabetes, fatty liver disease, sleep apnea, and a whole host of other health problems. The third phase is when these weight-related problems translate into life-threatening complications, like a heart attack, or stroke, or kidney failure. But it takes many years or even decades between each of these phases. For example, somebody who is gaining too much weight in their thirties and forties might develop type 2 diabetes in their fifties and then get a heart attack in their sixties. But if the clock starts ticking at age 10, it's a profoundly different prospect from a public health perspective.

So, if the worst is yet to come, does that mean that our already high health-care costs for obesity-related problems will continue to skyrocket?

We have only seen the tip of the iceberg in terms of future health-care costs. They're estimated today at over $150 billion annually and within the next decade could approach half a trillion dollars a year. You know, we will not only be paying directly to care for what will be a third of the country with diabetes, and for those with associated heart disease and kidney disease and other problems, but also for lost productivity due to obesity-related illness. Workers who are too sick to come to work or who come to work with disabilities simply can't be as productive.

Parents often complain that they feel that outside forces, like TV advertisements for junk food and fast food, and peer pressure from other kids, make it difficult to control what their children are eating. What can they do to reassert their influence in the home?

Ultimately we need to re-create a society that is a more supportive place for everybody, and especially for children, to live in. This would be a place with healthy foods in the corner store, a place where there is no junk food advertising, a place where there's high-quality food in the school cafeteria, and opportunities for physical education both in school and after school.

We all need to work together to create such a society. But until that day comes, parents can create a "bubble of protection" for children in the home, so that whenever their children are at home they're in a micro-environment of good health. Home should be the place where children are naturally eating healthful foods (because there is no junk food) and where they're being more physically active, and where they're being less tempted by TV and other sedentary pursuits. So if kids eat half of their meals in the home, it lays a firm foundation. If parents can do nothing else but control the home environment, half the battle is already won. And if we can improve the schools on top of that, with better foods in the cafeteria and a little more phys ed, we've then covered three-quarters of it. That way, even if the kids have some unhealthy influences when they're at the mall or elsewhere, those will be relatively balanced by the healthful influences in the home and in the school.

If parents are reading this and they're feeling absolutely desperate about improving their home situation, what's the one thing they can do?

Get rid of all the unhealthy foods in your kitchen. Throw them out! Then ban junk food. It's the parents' responsibility to set appropriate house rules, and that includes not bringing any junk food into the house. Next, go shopping. Fill your refrigerator and pantry with nutritious and delicious whole foods that are the basis not only for healthy meals but also for healthy snacking. After you've done all this, go out and celebrate with your family. Do something special that doesn't involve fast food. Go play miniature golf or go to a water park. Make it a fun outing.

What about desserts and other treats?

I'm not saying that people can't have treats like ice cream anymore. I recommend that we all have splurges once in a while. Just do it outside of the house. It's easier to say no to children when they're asking you for the carton of ice cream in the supermarket than it is to say no every night when they're begging for a cone from the freezer. If the family goes out for an ice cream celebration once a week, it's a real treat. Everyone pays more attention to it and everyone gets more enjoyment from it.

How did we get so far afield when it comes to eating right?

Well, I think we've really forgotten some basic parenting techniques, especially when it comes to teaching kids about food. Many parents have abdicated that responsibility to the food industry, and kids have instead learned about what to eat from advertisements, which of course aren't for fruits and vegetables, but for junk food. Parents need to reclaim their rights and responsibilities in this area.

There's no question that the food industry has made a lousy surrogate parent. What should the food industry be doing right now?

The food industry has made a terrible surrogate parent. It's motivated by profit, not love for the child, and that's why it's up to parents to protect their children from this unhealthy environment, just like they would protect their children from fast car traffic on a busy street. Young children are not capable of understanding the risks of modern society. As parents, we help them understand those risks when it comes to physical dangers. We need to do the same when it comes to nutritional dangers.

Are you against advertisements directed to children?

Yes, there needs to be a ban on advertising products to young children. Professional societies like the American Academy of Pediatrics and the American Psychological Association agree that advertisements to young children are manipulative and unethical. As to exactly where to draw the line, we can let the regulatory agencies and the professional societies weigh in on the exact age, but when you see advertisements for sugary cereals attached to Saturday-morning cartoons, we know that they're not being directed to adults.

Ultimately, you believe that parents can steer their children in the right direction despite outside influences. Right?

Yes, but it requires active parental involvement. If both parents are united and committed, it can be done, especially with younger kids. For adolescents, if there's conflict in the home, or if there's depression or other behavioral issues, it becomes much more complicated. For older kids, we need to take the long view, rather than trying to win individual battles by forcing them to do something they don't want, whether it's eating right, exercising more, or avoiding the TV. Forcing issues like this will only turn them off completely. It's best to set small goals and then wait for the right opportunity to make your points.

CHAPTER 3

THE PERILS OF PROGRESS

Over the past century—and especially over the past two decades—rapid advances in technology have led to radical changes in lifestyle, changes that we never anticipated. These developments have had some very positive effects on our health; in fact, longevity doubled from the beginning to the end of the 20th century. But not all of what technology has wrought has been good, as our current obesity epidemic and the resultant chronic diseases clearly show.

Thinking about these changes reminds me of a book that my parents gave me in the early 1970s called *Future Shock,* by sociologist and futurist Alvin Toffler. In his book, which was written before the days of personal computers, smart phones, Twitter, and 24/7 news coverage on cable TV, Toffler described how future technology could impact our everyday lives. It was a huge best-seller and has since become a classic. Toffler predicted that "in the three short decades between now and the twenty-first century, millions of ordinary, psychologically normal people will face an abrupt collision with the future." Boy was Toffler prescient.

On the pages that follow, I will explore the origins of the fast-food, sedentary culture that is responsible for our failing health. I admit that I am a history buff, but there's another, more compelling reason why I believe that looking to the past is useful. I have always found with my patients that the better they understand the causes of their medical problems and the rationale for their treatment, the better they do. I also believe that, for our country, the better we understand the origins of our toxic lifestyle, the better the chance that we can turn things around. I have found that looking at the history of our current nutrition problems has been a big help in putting today's health challenges into perspective. As my hero Winston Churchill said, "Those who fail to learn from history are doomed to repeat it."

In order to fully understand why we are now experiencing an epidemic of obesity, diabetes, and other chronic diseases, it is useful to take a look back—all the way back—to the time when man roamed the earth in small tribes as hunter-gatherers. Back then, before the advent of agriculture, we gathered a wide variety of fruits and vegetables because they satisfied our sweet taste buds as well as our hunger. We risked our lives hunting game—often big game—because it provided succulent, satisfying fat and more sustenance for less effort than gathering food with a similar amount of calories. Back then, little or no grain was consumed, because, unlike fruits and vegetables, it required processing before it was edible. There were no domesticated animals, so no milk or other dairy products were consumed once a baby was weaned from a mother's breast milk.

The hunter-gatherers spent most of their days finding the next meal. The penalty for not maintaining their food supply was starvation and death. How does this impact us today? Remember, we lived as hunter-gatherers for more than two million years! Our DNA is therefore designed to survive in the wild environment, not in our modern technology-driven culture.

THE FIRST FAST FOOD: FIELDS OF GRAIN

The evolution of food production throughout human history has been motivated by the goal of producing the necessities of life more efficiently—in less time and with less physical and mental effort. We have come a long way from the hunter-gatherer period, when it took almost all of our time and energy just to acquire enough food (and shelter) to survive. Today, it is possible to manage our entire lives—working, playing, shopping, and even socializing—without ever getting up from our computers. Food gathering? Just have it delivered.

But the first step toward a more efficient food supply really began about 10,000 years ago, after the second Ice Age, which heralded the first agricultural revolution. Most populations moved from hunter-gatherer societies to agrarian societies, growing their food instead of foraging for it. For the first time, humans learned how to cultivate fields of grain. This produced more food per acre of land than the less-efficient hunting-and-gathering approach. It also meant that not everyone had to spend their entire day focused primarily on acquiring food and shelter. Since a larger population could live off less land, and since fewer people were needed to produce the required quantity of food, some members of these early agricultural societies could spend time on other activities. This led to our first inventors, engineers, thinkers, merchants, artisans, traders, soldiers, and even our first politicians. We also learned to domesticate animals and use them for food production, work, and travel. Among other efficiencies, the domesticated animals provided dairy products such as milk and cheese.

For all these benefits, there was a trade-off. Our health began to suffer. Anthropologists who have studied the remains of early agriculturists found that they were shorter in stature than the hunter-gatherers (5 foot 3 inches versus 5 foot 9 inches) and showed evidence of nutritional deficiencies, such as tooth decay and osteopenia (thinning bones), not common in hunter-gatherers. These changes are believed to have been caused by the switch to one predominant source of calories—grains like wheat and rice—which meant less variety and fewer nutrients than the plant- and game-based diet of the hunter-gatherers.

Another unfortunate consequence of larger, more concentrated populations and the domestication of animals was the birth of contagious infectious disease. As explained beautifully in Jared Diamond's compelling book *Guns, Germs, and Steel: The Fates of Human Societies,* even though these early agriculturists were not individually as strong and healthy as the hunter-gatherers, their societies ultimately predominated because they had armies (with steel weapons and, later, guns) and they had germs. Both were devastating to hunter-gatherer societies.

Because the primary goal of food production has always been to feed the most people most efficiently, when there was *enough* food to prevent starvation, secondary issues like developing fruits and vegetables that also looked and tasted good, and that were more affordable, became important considerations.

Furthermore, new cultivation techniques meant that more people could be fed with fewer varieties of fruits and vegetables than were consumed by the hunter-gatherers. It also led to the breeding of fruits and vegetables that were and still are individually larger and plumper than the wild varieties— meaning they have relatively more sugary pulp and less antioxidant- and fiber-rich skin.

Cultivation for size, appearance, and efficiency continues right up to the present day. This is illustrated by a story I heard from a retired produce executive whom I met while flying out West. He had worked for a company that grew tomatoes primarily for sale in supermarkets. He told me that laborers got paid by the amount of tomatoes they picked, so naturally they picked pretty fast. If a stem happened to stay on the tomato, then the tomato could not be sold. If the tomato got bruised when thrown into a basket, it could not be sold. The company eventually came up with a tomato that easily came off the vine without the stem and that could be picked well before it was ripe, so it was harder and did not bruise easily when thrown into a basket. It then ripened on the way to the supermarket or on the kitchen counter. While these tomatoes looked round and tasty, my plane mate confessed, the taste wasn't so great. I asked him about their nutritional value, and he answered that he didn't know, because nutrition wasn't a consideration. In defense of my new acquaintance and farmers throughout history, growers have always selected for yield, looks, and hardiness, and it probably didn't occur to them that they were breeding out much of the nutritional value from their produce.

Unfortunately, in our desire for hardier and better-looking (and ideally better-tasting) food, delivered in less time and for less cost, we've ended up making our food sources less diverse and less nutritious, and many varieties have become extinct. We have actually been deselecting our food for variety and good nutrition for centuries. Luckily, many farmers today are preserving heirloom varieties of plants (like Brandywine tomatoes and Early Snowball cauliflower), which may not look cookie-cutter perfect (and may cost a little more) but typically have more nutrients and, frequently, better taste.

THE INTRODUCTION OF EMPTY-CALORIE FOODS

Wheat is a prime example of how technology and economics combined to take nutrients out of an important food in order to make it cheaper and better tasting. It all started in 1873 at the Vienna World's Fair, where a dazzling new invention called the steel roller mill was debuted. Though no one realized it at the time, this machine would herald the age of "refined grains."

Up until the invention of the roller mill, wheat and other grains were ground into flour using millstones. Like some of our better whole-grain products today, these stone-ground grains retained all three parts of the grain kernel: the germ (the embryonic sprouting section), the endosperm (the innermost part), and the bran (the outer shell). The germ, the most nutrient-rich part of the grain kernel, contains B vitamins, vitamin E and other antioxidants, as well as polyunsaturated fat. The endosperm, which makes up about 83 percent of the grain's weight, is starchy carbohydrate. The bran contains practically all of the fiber, as well as niacin and other B vitamins, along with some trace minerals.

People touted the roller mill because it produced a lighter, finer, powdery white flour, but that's because the flour included only the white, pulpy, starchy endosperm. The fiber- and nutrient-rich bran and germ were now removed, thus turning the once-healthy grain into empty calories. But no one realized it back then. What mattered was that without the germ, which contained the fat that could turn rancid, the flour had a longer shelf life and could be shipped far and wide. With cheaper production and a longer shelf life, white-flour-based products became more affordable, and this, together with the quickly acquired taste for white-flour-based baked goods, led to an explosion in white flour consumption. Back then, this was viewed as great progress. But as we later found out, while products made from white flour might be cheaper and faster to produce, they also contribute to a whole host of modern diseases.

This began to be recognized in an unintended population study of the effects of white flour at the beginning of World War II, when army physicians reported that many military recruits had not only some degree of calorie mal-nutrition but also diseases such as pellagra and beriberi. Both pellagra and beriberi are due to deficiencies of B vitamins and minerals, the very same vitamins and minerals that were being milled out of whole grains. After the soldiers' vitamin deficiencies were discovered, it led to the "enrichment" of white bread with thiamin, riboflavin, niacin, and iron. There's an important principle to remember in this regard: If a product has been "enriched," it doesn't necessarily mean that what's added compensates for the natural nutri-ents lost in processing. That's because we have not yet learned how to isolate and replace the literally thousands of micronutrients found in whole foods. While pellagra and beriberi have been eradicated, many other unfortunate health consequences of turning our foods into almost completely empty calo-ries remain, the obesity epidemic being the prime example. Moreover, buying a food that is enriched, or thinking that you can consume empty-calorie foods and make up for it by popping vitamins or supplements, is dead wrong! (This is explained in more detail in Chapter 4.)

THE SUPERMARKET AND THE STATION WAGON

While the roller mill extended the shelf life of white flour and other refined-grain products, most other foods still spoiled quickly until the widespread implementation of home refrigerators in the early 1900s. Food could also be transported long distances in refrigerated railway cars (later in trucks), though nutrients might be lost along the way. Refrigeration was introduced in food stores as well, meaning that people didn't need to shop locally and that fresh food could be purchased less often. Consequently, small corner markets were replaced by large grocery stores. The first A&P Economy Store opened in 1912, and by 1925 there were 13,961. And once the family car became com-monplace in the 1950s, people shopped even less often and no longer needed to walk to the grocery store. A mother could drive to one of the many super-markets in the now rapidly growing suburbs and pack the family station wagon with enough food for the next week or beyond—food that, thanks to long-haul shipping, was no longer that fresh to begin with.

And technology continued to have an effect on our diet. The shelf life of already bad-for-you baked goods became further extended, first with the addition of tropical oils (coconut and palm) and later with the hydrogenated and partially hydrogenated oils known today as trans fats. (I go into both of these in Chapter 5.) Canned goods, packaged goods, and the frozen TV dinner became available. And it wasn't long before the quality of the family dinner table began to change dramatically thanks to the advent of the fast-food restaurant.

FAST FOOD: LESS WORK FOR MOTHER

From the beginning of our story, right up to the supermarket era, meals were a family affair. Because it took time to gather and prepare food, whether on the veldt or the farm, in the city or the suburbs, "dinner" (whether served at noon or in the evening) was the main meal of the day. It was only natural for everyone to sit down together and eat the food straight from the fire or the oven, while it was hot. It was inefficient and unreasonable to serve multiple dinners at multiple times. I still remember the call of my mom, often when I was outdoors playing ball: "Arthur, come in right now or your dinner will get cold!"

As fast-food franchises and TV dinners became ubiquitous, the family dinner really began to deteriorate. Why cook when you could bring food home from the drive-thru or convenience store or, better yet, have it delivered and simply reheat it in the microwave. (The first microwave oven made for restaurant use appeared in 1947; believe it or not, it was almost 6 feet tall and weighed 750 pounds.) These days, microwave ovens substitute for, rather than complement, conventional ovens in far too many homes.

This easy access to fast food is a great temptation for busy working moms, dads, and singles. It requires little or no preparation time. Each child or adult can eat something different. And there doesn't need to be a set dinnertime (also thanks to the microwave). The number of meals that involve fast food, both eaten outside the home and brought in, has skyrocketed. In some communities, almost no one cooks dinner anymore.

The effects of the fast-food culture have become clear. In fact, it has been disturbing to observe how this fast-food, sedentary lifestyle has penetrated into other regions around the world, and how its harmful health effects have quickly followed. Even the Greek island of Crete, studied so extensively in the past as the healthy model for the Mediterranean Diet, has succumbed to the spread of fast food.

Today pediatricians on Crete are seeing children with high blood pressure, high cholesterol, and obesity, conditions that simply weren't present in youths in pre-fast-food generations. On the Japanese island of Okinawa, famous for its record number of centenarians and its residents having the greatest longevity in the world, there is also trouble. Once fast food arrived to cater to the personnel living on the American military bases there, things started to go downhill. And while the older traditional Okinawans (who wouldn't dream of eating fast food) still have excellent longevity, an increasing number of youngsters (who are not so good at skipping those burgers and fries) have obesity, diabetes, and all the other problems associated with our debilitating lifestyle. Regrettably, there will be fewer centenarians on Okinawa in the future. And this unfortunate situation is being replicated all over the world—from Europe to Dubai, New Delhi to Beijing.

MAKING TECHNOLOGY WORK FOR US, NOT AGAINST US

So, what does all this bad news about technology's unintended health consequences mean for our future? Your conclusion at this point may be that I am about to recommend that we all return to the forest and live like hunter-gatherers. Actually, nothing could be further from the truth. First of all, I enjoy living in my air-conditioned comfortable home, watching football games on my high-definition TV, finding my way in any city in the world using my handheld GPS, surfing the Web, and doing almost all my shopping online. In fact, I am something of a digital junky. I love being able to locate my misplaced iPhone by using the Find My iPhone app on my iPad and telling it to send out a beeping signal—or using my iPhone to find my iPad. If I misplace both, I can still find them from my computer! Anyway, I digress. The point is that we are not heading back to the forest and that we all live better—and, in general, longer—thanks to technology.

Technology has been used to create unhealthy foods because, as they say in the computer world, it's garbage in, garbage out. The technology itself isn't the problem. It is what we ask of it. And until recently, in the area of nutrition, we didn't know what to ask for. All we wanted for many decades was cheaper, faster, no-prep food, which technology delivered in spades—as starchy, sugary, salty, high-fat, empty-calorie junk. There is no doubt that when the public demands healthier food choices, businesses and human ingenuity will deliver, whether it's heirloom tomatoes or cauliflower or the organic food Maria Rodale describes on the following pages. No, we will not move back to the wild, but with more awareness and greater demand, healthy food will become less expensive, more widely available, and convenient. Even fast food will be made healthier.

We have to create change through education and leading by example. In a growing number of urban areas, it is easy to buy locally grown fresh produce and healthy prepared foods because there is a demand for them. Already in New York City, for example, urban farmers are growing food on the roofs of apartment buildings and warehouses, and I have no doubt that eventually there will be entire "farm skyscrapers" devoted to growing the healthy produce that people will be clamoring for.

The good news is that hundreds of groups across the country are already working to bring healthier foods into our schools and our neighborhoods (see Online Resources, page 314, for links to just a few of them). The bad news is that despite these efforts, most school lunches haven't changed much and thousands of people in urban and rural areas across the country are still living in food deserts, where access to fresh food is limited. And even when healthy food is available, it is not always people's first choice, often because they mistakenly think that they can't afford it or that they don't have time to cook.

The hard truth is that we can't afford not to change. When it comes to nutrition, if we continue to take the easy way out, the toll on our health and our pocketbooks will be devastating.

A Conversation with Maria Rodale

Maria Rodale is the CEO and chairman of Rodale Inc., the publisher of this book, and the author of *Organic Manifesto: How Organic Food Can Heal Our Planet, Feed the World, and Keep Us Safe*. You can read more about her passions and family life on her blog: Maria's Farm Country Kitchen (mariasfarmcountrykitchen.com). I have to admit that I used to be a skeptic about the value of organic food, partly because it was hard for shoppers to find it and even more difficult to be confident that what was advertised as "organic" was the real thing. Recently, I had a change of heart, for several reasons. First, I read Maria's book, which gave me a new appreciation for how organic foods promote a healthy lifestyle and underscored the importance of knowing where our food comes from. Her thinking fits perfectly into the paradigm that I have explored in depth in this book: that thanks to our DNA, we are designed to eat, exercise, and sleep like our ancestors did. Then I visited her family's organic farm in Emmaus, Pennsylvania, which was an eye-opening educational and culinary experience. Since the fertilizers and pesticides they use are all natural (Maria showed me beetles protecting the plants), I could just pick a mint or lettuce leaf and eat it without washing it first. Breakfast was from their chickens' freshly laid eggs. In fact, all the food I ate that morning came from the family farm. I was ready to move in.

Thanks to Maria, I am more confident regarding the sources and value of organic food, and I am honored that she agreed to add her valuable perspective on the subject to our "wake-up call."

First things first: How do you define "organic"?

"Organic" means that a product is free of toxic *synthetic* chemicals. If you see a food labeled "organic," it is assurance that it has been grown in a safe environment using tried-and-true techniques like biological pest control instead of poisonous pesticides, or that livestock is raised without hormones, antibiotics, or pesticide-laced food. It also means that a product has been manufactured without adding dangerous chemicals.

How do you know if the food you are buying is organic?

If you want to keep these chemicals out of your home, only buy organic food that has the little green or black logo on the label that says "USDA Organic." You'll find this symbol on fruits, vegetables, meats, dairy, and processed foods. The symbol means that 95 to 100 percent of the ingredients in the product are organic and have been independently certified by a third party. So far there is no USDA label for detergents and beauty products.

Why are pesticides so dangerous?

Pesticides are designed to kill living things, and they do it in different ways. For example, some commonly used pesticides are known as endocrine disruptors. These not only disrupt hormone systems within the targeted organisms that they are meant to kill, but may also interfere with the normal hormonal balance within human bodies.

Studies have linked endocrine disruptors to an increased risk for diabetes, obesity, infertility, sterility, miscarriage, and birth defects. There is even research that suggests that these chemicals could increase the risk of autism and attention deficit/hyperactivity disorder (ADHD). There is also a link between environmental toxins, hormones, and cancer. And that's just looking at one category of synthetic single chemicals, not the combination of chemicals that are found in virtually every product and that also find their way into our bodies every time we drink a glass of nonorganic milk, or eat a nonorganic piece of fruit, or wash our clothes in chemical-laden detergents. No one knows the cumulative effect of being exposed to all of these synthetic chemicals, and especially how they are affecting our children. In fact, children today are being born with a heavy load of toxic chemicals that are being passed to them through their mother's amniotic fluid. We have no idea of what this will mean for their future, since these chemicals either alone or in combination have never been tested for safety on human health.

In your book, you alert people to the fact that their homes are filled with products—from produce to cosmetics and cleaning supplies—that contain potentially dangerous ingredients that aren't banned by the FDA. How can you identify the toxins in your environment so that you can get rid of them?

You can't really trust your eyes when it comes to toxins because so many of them are invisible. So you have to use your mind to "see" the toxins, which is not something most people are used to doing. Basically, you have to learn about what those toxins are. People may not realize it, but a lot of toxins are "sneaking" into our homes on flame retardants on clothing and mattresses, for example. They're coming in ways that you wouldn't necessarily think of in terms of organic or nonorganic. Avoid anything that has "parfum" or "triclosan" on the label, as both of these chemicals in particular are known to cause many health problems. I think the reason why they're so prevalent is because companies can sneak them into things and you don't even know it. It's a quiet danger.

If people could do just one thing to clean up their home environment, what would you tell them to do?

Obviously, with my background, I would simply say, "Don't buy anything that isn't organic." Period. If you want to do this in small steps, I would recommend not buying anything with an artificial fragrance, whether it's an air freshener, a laundry detergent, or a cosmetic. It's bringing an unnecessary toxin into your home. If you want something to smell clean, then clean it! You don't need harsh chemicals to clean either. For most things, you can use baking soda and plain soap and water. I hate it when I walk into people's homes and I'm physically attacked by all kinds of conflicting scents. I instantly get an allergic reaction.

Many people agree that organic food is better for them, but say that they can't afford the added cost of many organic products, and therefore buy cheaper nonorganic items. How do you respond to that concern?

My initial response is that the true cost of not buying organic is never factored into charts that compare, for example, the price of organic versus nonorganic apples. That price needs to factor in the toll that all these toxins exact on your health and the health of your children. Moreover, the commercial agricultural techniques that are used for nonorganics are very damaging to the environment, so we end up paying in other ways.

Applying chemical fertilizers to soil is a very short-term solution that creates long-term devastation to the soil: The soil not only loses its ability to hold moisture in rain and drought, but it also loses its nutrient density and its microbial life. So, you basically are accelerating the desertification of our planet, whereas organic agricultural practices actually improve the soil over time. Organic production also requires 20 percent less fossil fuel than chemical production. That's another bonus for the environment.

Having said that, there are ways to eat organic without blowing your budget. For example, farmers' markets are a great place to find locally grown, often more reasonably priced organic food, and they are fun to visit. If you haven't looked recently, you may be surprised by the variety of organic produce at local supermarkets, and even the well-known,, pricier chains that sell organic often have sales. Many communities have thriving food co-ops that purchase organic produce at significant discounts and community-supported agriculture programs that help sustain local farms.

You can also grow your own organic produce right in your own backyard, if you have one. Go to organicgardening.com for all the information you need to get started. If you are an apartment dweller, join or organize a neighborhood organic garden. Many communities, especially underserved urban areas, have extremely thriving community garden projects where people can get together and share information and, ultimately, food.

I always remind people: If you only buy organic, you won't be buying any processed or junk food, which will save you money. In reality, once you start removing toxins—like air fresheners—from your shopping cart, you start eliminating a lot of unnecessary and expensive products from your life.

Buying organic also means that you will be cooking more of your meals from scratch, which is often more economical, certainly better for your health, and definitely better for your quality of life.

What about the "I don't have time to cook" excuse?

It's true that when you commit to cooking your meals at home, it's not the same as pulling out two bucks and buying a fast-food hamburger. It requires work and effort, but you get so much more than just nutrition. You satisfy a deeper hunger for independence and self-sufficiency, and it is far better for your health and the health of your family.

I am CEO of a major company, I have three kids, and, if I am home, 5 out of 7 nights a week I make dinner. It requires planning, and I don't live near a Whole Foods Market. I buy almost everything I can't get out of my garden once a week on the weekend, when I go to the supermarket. Everybody in the family pitches in: My 4-year-old helps set the table, the older kids help cut the vegetables, and my husband does the dishes. When you work as a team, it can be done.

In your book, you urge the government to reconsider policies that you assert favor big, commercial agriculture over local farms and organic farmers. What would you like to see done?

Through policies that favor specific sectors of agriculture, notably corn and soybean producers, the government has become an enabler. These policies provide cheap feed for cattle, hogs, and chickens so that fast-food restaurants can sell inexpensive fast food all over the world, and this has clearly contributed to the obesity epidemic. I'm not anti-business by any means, but I think that businesses need to pay their own way and that we need to reconsider these policies.

Are you optimistic about the future?

It depends on the day. Some days I'm dismally depressed about the way things are going, but most days I'm quite optimistic. I think back to when my grandfather started talking about organic farming almost 70 years ago, and while a lot of things have gotten worse, there have been vast improvements in terms of the openness of the discussion and the accessibility to organic foods and products. So the fact that I can go to my local supermarket and buy a whole week's worth of organic groceries that have the USDA Organic label would have been beyond my grandfather's comprehension, beyond his wildest dreams.

So I think it's up to us, this generation, to ask, "How can we take this all the way?" Because, the truth is, we're still not very far along.

CHAPTER 4

WHAT'S WRONG
(AND RIGHT) WITH "DIETS"

While, as evidenced from its title, this book is intended to be a "wake-up call," I don't want you to wake up confused and bleary-eyed, but rather alert, educated, and aware. The good news is that our knowledge of nutrition has increased exponentially over the past decade or so. The bad news is that this has not yet translated into better nutrition for the great majority of Americans.

You can find good evidence of our continuing confusion and ignorance regarding nutrition at the checkout counter of your local supermarket. How the same collection of tabloids can make the same false claims on their covers week after week and still sell is a great question for the sociologists. It certainly does prove that Abe Lincoln was right when he said, "You can fool some of the people all the time." But you should no longer be fooled into wasting your time, money, and energy on bad nutrition advice. The purpose of this chapter and Chapter 5 is to cut through the deluge of diet and nutrition advice you face daily and teach you how to make better sense of it all. There are still legitimate areas of confusion among experts, but these pale in comparison with the areas upon which we agree.

TOO GOOD TO BE TRUE

Even though my patients are well aware that I created the South Beach Diet and that I believe in a long-term healthy lifestyle approach, some are neverthe-less seduced by cleverly marketed, seemingly "magical" ways to effortlessly lose weight. Recently, my patient and friend Jim came into my office for a routine follow-up of his cholesterol and blood pressure. Jim had clearly lost weight—10 pounds over 2 weeks, it turned out—and I naturally asked him how he had lost so much weight in such a short time. I was hoping he would report that he had been on Phase 1 of the South Beach Diet and had recommitted to a long-term healthy lifestyle. No such luck. What Jim told me is a very common story, often recounted in various iterations by other patients and friends both in and out of the office. "Haven't you heard about the 'hormone diet'?" Jim said. He had learned about it from a friend on the golf course, where a great deal of "medical information" is exchanged. He then went online and ordered a hormone (which will go unmentioned), which supposedly "ate fat." "Very interesting," I commented. "And what have you been eating while taking this magic hormone?"

Jim went on to explain that a strict diet was part of the program. He then proceeded to describe a 500-calorie, very restrictive regimen. He stopped drinking alcohol (which heretofore had been a nightly activity) and ate essentially the same prescribed foods daily. This consisted of two eggs for breakfast, a salad in the late afternoon, and a chicken breast and a vegetable for dinner. Amazing that he lost weight, huh? Jim attributed his weight loss not to the restrictive diet or to giving up alcohol, but to the fat-eating hormone. Also amazing that I had never read an article in the medical literature about such a miraculous hormone. How could Big Pharma have passed up such a sure winner? Actually, as I later discovered, the hormone *was* reported in the medical literature, only it didn't eat fat or anything like that. In fact, the few journal articles I found concluded that it was as "good as a placebo."

A few days after my visit with Jim, a new patient, Sally (age 52 and postmenopausal), who had just moved to South Florida, came in and reported that she had lost 40 pounds over the past 10 months. I was naturally anxious to hear her story, assuming she had been on the South Beach Diet. But nope. Though she had apparently missed out on Jim's Internet hormone, Sally's story sounded eerily similar. She had gone to a diet guru up north who had put together a concoction of herbs suited to her "special" body chemistry (I've heard that one before). Her cocktail included ginseng, something derived from deer antlers—it might have been the bone marrow—and other stuff either she'd forgotten or I'd never heard of. In any case, she was otherwise advised to eat lean protein and vegetables. She even told me about her first real cheat—a bakery roll—which, she said, made her feel bloated and sick. If eating lean protein and vegetables sounds like Phase 1 of the South Beach Diet (except for the magic concoction), I agree. More on that later.

Sally and Jim happen to be very intelligent people. Losing weight "instantly and effortlessly" represents such a strong desire in a society that wants everything and wants it now, that it is understandable how people succumb to trying anything that promises a quick fix. In fact, their stories sounded so good at first that I was almost ready to sign up. But every time I hear a similar tale of a magical diet, it has the same ending. The diet ends, the magic ends, and the weight returns.

LOSE WEIGHT FAST WITH DR. AGATSTON'S ICE CREAM DIET

The signature diet that exemplifies "fad diets" to me, and the one I use most often to illustrate their problems, is the famous Cabbage Soup Diet. By consuming nothing but cabbage soup for three meals a day, of course you will lose weight quickly, because you are on such a severely calorie-restricted diet.

Patients often tell me about diets that instruct them to eat the same foods day after day. There are usually rules about types of foods or individual foods that must or must not be combined in a meal. Whether it involves protein shakes, cookies, or chicken breasts, the common thread of these diets is that they are all severely restrictive as well as extremely low calorie and very boring. There is usually a "hook" as well—something like Jim's hormone pill or Sally's antler extract or the promise of how a particular additive will stave off hunger and burn fat. In fact, a woman recently told me that mixing vodka and grapefruit juice would "eat away the calories in any meal."

This brings me to my idea for a new, very restrictive, low-calorie but tasty diet—the Dark Chocolate Ice Cream Diet (yes, I am an admitted chocoholic). Since a half cup of chocolate ice cream averages between 150 and 200 calories, you could have a nice little bowl at breakfast, lunch, and dinner and still end up eating just 450 to 600 calories a day. You would lose weight quite rapidly eating such limited calories, and dark chocolate has some real nutritional benefits, thanks to its heart-healthy polyphenols.

As good for you as dark chocolate can be, please don't take me seriously here. You'd be missing out on so many other important nutrients, which can only be found in a wholesome diet.

THE TWINKIE DIET

I must admit that my new ice cream diet has had some recent competition. Some of you may have read, as I did, about a Kansas State University nutrition professor, Mark Haub, who in 2010 set out to prove that he could eat a steady diet of junk food and still lose weight as long as he sharply reduced his caloric intake. His eating plan became known as the Twinkie Diet, and it attracted a lot of media attention. Dr. Haub's diet consisted of foods never found on a healthy weight-loss plan, like Hostess Twinkies, frozen pizza, Little Debbie Star Crunch cookies, Doritos Cool Ranch corn chips, Kellogg's Corn Pops cereal, and, for dessert, some Duncan Hines brownies. Strangely, he washed it all down with *diet* Mountain Dew. Dr. Haub did eat some vegetables daily, like an occasional portion of baby carrots or a can of string beans, but what was totally missing from his regimen were whole grains, meat, seafood, and fruit. To compensate for the lack of protein in his diet, he drank one protein shake daily along with an occasional glass of milk. He also took a daily multivitamin pill and exercised about 60 minutes a week.

Dr. Haub had been struggling with his weight for years and had bounced from diet to diet. Before inventing the Twinkie Diet, he had consumed about 2,600 calories a day. On this new diet, he ate about 1,800 calories a day, with about two-thirds of them coming from junk food. At the end of 8 weeks, he had lost 27 pounds. Dr. Haub certainly demonstrated that you can lose weight if you restrict calories, but he also acknowledged that his was not a diet you would want to stay on—you'd be missing too many essential nutrients (even with the vitamin pill, which adds few). I would also argue that most people couldn't stay on a diet like this, even if they wanted to. That is because the swings in blood sugar caused by the processed carbohydrates found in all these sugary and starchy foods cause cravings and ultimately defeat the best of intentions to limit calories.

A similar scenario was demonstrated in the popular 2004 documentary *Super Size Me*. Morgan Spurlock, the creator and star, only ate food from McDonald's for an entire month. After enjoying this fast-food diet for the first week or so, he developed insatiable cravings that resulted in rapid weight gain and a host of unpleasant physical and psychological symptoms.

So, unfortunately, I must warn you: As soon as you stop my Dark Chocolate Ice Cream Diet or the Twinkie Diet, the weight will predictably return and will probably exceed its baseline level. And, while on these diets, you will be depriving yourself of important nutrients. That's the problem with these severe calorie-restricted strategies. They are not a lifestyle, they are unhealthy because they are nutrient-poor, and ultimately, the weight nearly always rebounds. This also holds true when you severely restrict calories by taking pills that suppress your appetite. Though for sustained weight loss the hopelessness of short-term, severe calorie restriction is well known, the marketing of such miracle diets continues unabated, and patients and friends like Jim will continue to be disappointed.

THE TWO IMPORTANT DIET COMPONENTS

Every diet, good or bad, consists of calories (the energy supplied by the foods we eat) and nutrients. Unfortunately, when it comes to diet, Americans tend to focus almost exclusively on calories. For our distant ancestors, and right up to about 50 years ago, concern with diet and nutrition mostly revolved around people not getting enough total calories, which translated into not getting enough nutrients as well. And there was good reason for this concern: Famine due to drought, pestilence, war, and natural disasters has recurred from time immemorial as a fact of life.

There are, however, exceptions where nutrition problems have not been the result of insufficient caloric intake. Take the example of the "limey," a slang term for British sailors of the 1700s. These sailors were otherwise adequately nourished but suffered from scurvy, a disease caused by vitamin C deficiency. At the time, scurvy had killed many more sailors than were ever lost in battle. The reason: Perishable fruits and vegetables could not be kept edible on long voyages and the sailors had to subsist on cured or salted meats and dried grains alone, meaning they had no source of vitamin C. Scurvy ceased to be a problem in 1747, when British Royal Navy surgeon Joseph Lind demonstrated that citrus fruits prevented this condition. Thereafter, the British sailors always kept limes on their ships to provide vitamin C and prevent scurvy—hence the name "limey."

In the United States, insufficient food intake was a major problem in many areas until after World War II. In fact, it was because many World War II army recruits were found to be calorie and vitamin malnourished that white bread was fortified and government guidelines were created mandating minimum calorie criteria for school lunches. Remarkably, these caloric guidelines have existed in more or less the same form until the latest incarnation of the Childhood Nutrition Reauthorization Act (now renamed the Healthy, Hunger-Free Kids Act), which was signed into law in December 2010.

With the intake of enough or too many calories, nutrients are not usually a problem (the limeys being one notable exception), so they are generally ignored. We also frankly didn't know a lot about essential nutrients until relatively recently. That's why our misguided focus on calories, not nutrients, has persisted in this country, even though excess calories have become our predominant problem, even for the poor.

EMPTY CALORIES AND MALNUTRITION

As I said before and will say again because it is so important, Americans are consuming a huge number of empty calories. By "empty calories," I mean foods that contain plenty of calories but are devoid of nutrients. The most common example is white bread, which is made up almost exclusively of starch (basically chains of sugar molecules) with almost no vitamins or minerals.

Now, if you happen to be an endurance athlete, then you need a great deal of extra fuel to burn on your long runs, swims, or cycling races and during your training. Cyclists racing in the Tour de France, for example, burn between 7,000 and 10,000 calories per day. Not all of this needs to be nutrient-rich foods like fruits and vegetables, and frankly, couldn't be. This is a situation where some pure starch—extra fuel that is simply burned—is appropriate, because that's what these athletes need. But for the rest of us, those of us not training for the Tour de France or a marathon, who are burning many fewer calories with our daily activities, our calories need to be nutrient-rich. The more empty calories we consume, the fewer health-promoting nutrients we take in, resulting in our becoming overweight but undernourished.

In fact, today, malnutrition in children is resurfacing as a major problem. But this time it's not due to the traditional cause of not taking in enough calories; today's children are often nutrient deprived. Our children—rich and poor alike (though the problem is greatest among the urban and rural poor)—are frequently *overfed* but literally *undernourished*. They may get plenty of calories in the form of sugary, starchy, and fatty foods, but they lack the fruits, vegetables, whole grains, fiber, and good fats that are essential to their optimal health and a long life free from chronic disease. I'll say it again: These kids are overweight but malnourished! As I will talk about in Chapter 7, this is one of the reasons why it is critical to change the food served in school cafeterias.

So, how does all this relate to modern diets? Because of the emphasis on calories and quick weight loss rather than on nutrients and lifestyle, our society has simply been on the wrong track. Patients and friends are always asking for a pill "just to get them started." They think that if they could simply take a pill that would suppress their appetite for a few weeks, they would be able to sustain that initial weight loss.

Unfortunately, my clinical experience and that of my colleagues, as well as the medical literature, does not bear this out. Our infatuation with calories and quick weight loss has sent us down the road to disaster. We now know that the only solution is to eat right. Not so many years ago, we believed that it wasn't a problem if our diet wasn't nutritionally sound—we'd just pop a handful of vitamins and supplements. Several large and impressive studies—the Heart Protection Study, the Heart Outcomes Prevention Evaluation (HOPE) Study, and the GISSI Heart Failure project—have proven that this is a losing strategy.

In fact, the only thing popping such pills accomplishes is creating expensive urine—where most of the vitamin supplements end up. (That said, I do recommend some supplements, such as omega-3 fish oils and vitamin D.)

What we have learned just in the past decade or so is that our fruits and vegetables are chock-full of literally thousands of phytonutrients that work in combination to keep us healthy in ways that we cannot replicate in a pill; maybe someday in the future we'll be able to, but not anytime soon. Many of these nutrients are antioxidants, such as polyphenols (there are thousands of phytonutrients like this that are ubiquitous in the plant kingdom), which were designed to protect the vegetable and fruit plants from exposure to the natural toxins in the environment. When we eat these fruits and vegetables, we protect ourselves from the same environmental toxins.

The same antioxidants contained in these fruits and vegetables also protect us from oxidation and its associated cell-damaging inflammation. In fact, as I explained in Chapter 2, it is oxidation that causes us to age faster, or "rust." Junk foods tend to be pro-oxidant and tend to promote the aging process. In order to maintain good health, we need a wide variety of fruits and vegetables (in many colors) and any diet that does not emphasize this is dangerous. Yes, this does eliminate just about all the quick-weight-loss schemes.

THE MAGIC OF ANTIOXIDANTS

Along with fad diets, today we are also seeing a lot of advertising for miracle antioxidant drinks and potions. Some of this information is absolutely true. Foods like berries and pomegranates, for example, are rich sources of antioxidants. The problem comes when you depend primarily on just one or two of these superfoods. I have seen patients who drank a high-antioxidant juice for breakfast daily and ate no other servings of fruits and vegetables the rest of the day. I was glad they were getting some antioxidants for breakfast, but, as I told them, simply drinking juice once a day isn't enough.

The best evidence today encourages us to eat a rainbow of fruits and vegetables. That's because each color—red, yellow, orange, green, blue, purple, and others—represents a healthful array of phytonutrients with benefits that

(continued on page 66)

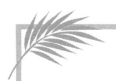

Sandy's Story
A Real-Life Turnaround

I have always had a weight problem, but it really escalated when I started college, and it kept getting worse throughout my adulthood. By my 54th birthday, I weighed 285 pounds and was seeing a cardiologist. I was a physical wreck. I had high blood pressure, bad angina, and daily acid reflux, as well as irritable bowel syndrome, and my feet hurt all the time. I couldn't stand for more than 5 minutes before I had to find a chair. My left knee ached so badly that on many nights it even woke me out of a deep sleep. On top of all this, I had developed back pain. When my angina got worse, I was afraid to go back to the doctor because I was worried that I would be diagnosed with diabetes or kidney problems.

When I finally did see him again, it wasn't because I was worried about myself, but because I had a roommate with diabetes who relied on me. I knew that if I got sicker, I would not be able to do anything for her or for myself. I had long ago given up believing that I could ever lose weight, but I could see the writing on the wall. If I did not stop this progression, I'd be the one who had diabetes, or heart disease, or worse.

The cardiologist suggested that I read *The South Beach Diet* and follow the program. I bought the book the next day and began my adventure, starting on Phase 1 of the diet. I joined a gym and began a moderate exercise program. Almost immediately, I began to feel better. In the first 6 months, I lost 40 pounds and slowly another 30 pounds. On the next visit to the doctor, we were able to cut my blood pressure meds in half! (Today, I don't have to take any because my blood pressure is normal.) The angina had also disappeared. The irritable bowel syndrome was gone too. My back had stopped hurting and so had my knee. All my other blood readings were within the excellent range. I was able to participate in things like volunteer work that required 8 hours on my feet.

As I lost weight, I not only felt better about my health but I felt more physically fit than I ever thought I could feel. In fact, I felt so good that I decided I would take a second job. I also became active in a local program to help improve the quality of kids' school meals. I became a farmers' market shopper and started buying almost all my produce there. I also resumed doing things that I once loved, like writing poetry. And the woman who couldn't stand up for more than 5 minutes at a time began going on long hikes with friends. I even bought my first bike.

In short, I stopped seeing myself as a "fat girl" with limitations.

I have never thought of South Beach as just a "diet." I think of it as the way I need to eat to stay well. Sure, it is sometimes hard to keep up the motivation, especially when my weight loss plateaus. But when I remember all the things I am able to do now compared with not that long ago, well, it's what keeps me going. I realize I don't have to be perfect. If I mess up one day, I get right back to eating correctly at the next meal. If I skip my exercise routine one day, I go back to it the next. I now know I can never use "I've blown it" as an excuse for not exercising or for eating everything that isn't nailed down.

I often look back and see how my journey has also influenced the others in my life. Members of my family followed my lead and now participate in a Sunday family baseball game, because we all need the exercise. My nieces and nephews come over for healthy pizza parties, where they choose their own veggie toppings. Now, more than ever, I understand the impact of my choices. And because most of the time I make the choices that are good for me, I don't have to worry when I sometimes falter.

South Beach has become a way of life for me. It helped me bring myself back into the land of the living.

are only beginning to be appreciated. And that's why the best strategy is to consume a wide variety of fruits and vegetables and include some from each color grouping. You don't want to miss out on a nutrient that in 5 years will be found to be the key to preventing lung cancer. Actually, this is very unlikely because it is highly doubtful that any one nutrient, no matter how good, will equal the health benefits of consuming many varieties. Remember our ancestors, the hunter-gatherers. They naturally made a broader selection of the fruits and vegetables they had available than we do today. And the fruits and vegetables they ate were also more nutrient-dense than those we have cultivated over centuries with a focus on size and appearance rather than on nutrition.

On page 254, we include a list of 15 "MegaFoods," rich in antioxidants and other vital nutrients. We also offer a variety of MegaRecipes, starting on page 259, in which several of these foods are used together. We are simply trying to help your effort to eat more nutrient-rich foods. While these foods are an important component of any healthy diet, don't forget that the greater and more diverse your selection of such foods, the healthier your diet will be.

WHAT ABOUT PHASE 1?

I've just reviewed the futility of "too good to be true" weight-loss plans. And yet, people often ask me, "Don't you promise quick weight loss on Phase 1 of the South Beach Diet?" The answer is yes; people do tend to lose weight quickly during this 2-week phase. But it's important to understand that Phase 1 is healthy because it includes a wide variety of unlimited vegetables, lean protein, low-fat dairy, and good fats. It does eliminate grains, even whole grains. But while whole grains are great sources of fiber and B vitamins, they are not the only sources and can safely be eliminated—especially over the short term. Fruits are also eliminated initially because of their sugar content. This helps people detox from their sugar cravings and it works very well. After a couple of weeks, however, once those cravings are under control, it's important to add fruits back into your diet because they contain such a vast array of nutrients and add variety and enjoyment to your meals and snacks, which is essential if a healthy diet is to become a lifelong habit. Whole grains and root vegetables are also added back into your diet on Phase 2.

So the purpose of Phase 1 is to get rid of the cravings caused by exaggerated swings in blood sugar in order to gain control of your appetite and progress to Phases 2 and 3—a healthy lifestyle. If you don't have cravings or substantial weight to lose, then you can start on Phase 2. We have seen a common problem with individuals who do so well with weight loss on Phase 1 (and who are feeling so good) that they do not want to progress to Phase 2. This is a mistake that hinders long-term success. For continuing health and happiness and for maintaining an optimal weight, a diet must be transformed into a way of life.

THE SOUTH BEACH DIET *IS NOT JUST A DIET*

I've repeated over and over that the South Beach Diet is not just a diet—it's a lifestyle. What do I mean by that? Allow me to return to a conversation I've often engaged in both in and out of my office that further illustrates America's complicated relationship with diets.

I will commonly be told, "The South Beach Diet was great. I lost a lot of weight and got off my blood pressure medication, but now I do my own diet."

"Wonderful," I'll say. "What's your own diet?"

"I just watch the bad stuff as much as I can—the starches and sugars and bad fats, but otherwise, I do my own thing. I just don't go overboard," he or she will say.

My immediate reply: "What you are describing *is* the South Beach Diet. It's Phase 3."

It is amazing that when people think of diet, they think only of a circumscribed weight-loss program. In fact, diet can be defined as the kinds of foods that a person habitually eats. Think of the Mediterranean diet, which has been followed for hundreds of years. I think that qualifies as a lifestyle. When people have lost weight and improved their blood chemistries and have learned the South Beach principles—choose good carbs, good fats, lean sources of protein, and plenty of fiber—and are making healthy choices most of the time, then whether they know it or not, they are on the maintenance phase (Phase 3) of the South Beach Diet and have adopted it as a lifestyle.

WHO NEEDS A WEIGHT-LOSS DIET?

When it comes to evaluating a person's overall health, I emphasize blood chemistry and waist circumference rather than weight. This is because

The South Beach Diet: A Crash Course

Because I have written so much about our eating principles in my previous books, I won't go into great depth about the diet in this book. Nevertheless, I am often asked about our three-phase approach. Here's a crash course:

Phase 1: This is the shortest and strictest phase of the South Beach Diet, lasting only 2 weeks. Phase 1 is for people who have a substantial amount of weight to lose or experience significant cravings for sugary foods and refined starches. During this phase, you'll jump-start your weight loss and stabilize your blood sugar levels to minimize cravings. You'll be eating a diet consisting of unlimited vegetables, including plenty of salads; healthy lean protein (fish and shellfish, chicken and turkey, lean cuts of meat, soy); loads of beans and other legumes; reduced-fat cheeses; eggs; low-fat dairy; and nuts and good unsaturated fats, such as extra-virgin olive oil and canola oil. You'll enjoy three satisfying meals a day plus two snacks, and you'll even be able to have some dessert. What you won't be eating are starches (bread, pasta, rice) or sugars (including fruits and fruit juices). While this may be hard at first, your cravings will soon disappear, and in just 2 weeks, you'll be able to add many of these foods back into your life. Also keep in mind that exercise during this and all of the phases of the diet is important to your overall health and will improve your results. Phase 1 gives you positive reinforcement because you lose weight fairly rapidly over the 2-week period, but the main purpose of this phase is to stabilize blood sugar and eliminate cravings. You'll then have much better control over what you eat. And while the rapid weight loss is exciting and gives you the incentive to keep on losing, it's important to move on to Phase 2 to begin more gradual weight loss and the evolution from diet to lifestyle.

healthy individuals with optimal blood chemistries come in all different sizes and shapes. You can be "fat and fit," a term used to describe a person with a slow metabolism who is a bit chunky yet has the blood chemistry of a health-food-addicted endurance athlete. In fact, that person might *be a*

Phase 2: Those individuals who have 10 pounds or less to lose, who don't have problems with cravings, or who simply want to improve their health can start the South Beach Diet with Phase 2. If you're moving on to Phase 2 from Phase 1, you'll find that your weight will continue to drop steadily (although more slowly) and that your cravings will have subsided. You'll gradually reintroduce many of the foods that were off-limits on Phase 1, including more good carbohydrates, such as whole fruits, whole-grain breads, whole-wheat pasta, and brown rice, as well as some root vegetables (like sweet potatoes). You'll also be able to have a glass of red or white wine with meals if you like. Don't be discouraged by your slower weight loss during this phase. Your goal is to gradually reach a weight that's healthy for you and that you can maintain while developing a healthy lifestyle. Otherwise, it's just a quick fix.

Phase 3: You'll enter this phase of the South Beach Diet once you reach your healthy weight. At this point in the diet, you'll easily be able to monitor your body's response to particular foods, and you'll find yourself naturally making the right food choices most of the time. You will know to choose a higher-fiber, nutrient-rich baked sweet potato over a baked white potato. You'll know to choose brown or wild rice over white rice, and blueberries or raspberries over watermelon, and overall you'll maximize your consumption of healthy fruits, vegetables, and whole grains. You can also enjoy a decadent dessert on occasion, and when you do, you will probably find that you've satisfied your sweet tooth after just a few bites. By the time you enter Phase 3, the South Beach Diet will have become a way of life, and its sound eating principles should keep the weight off while you stay fit and healthy.

health-food-addicted endurance athlete. Such individuals are at low risk for chronic disease. They characteristically do not have cravings and do not overeat. Even if they manage to lose a few pounds, it will be almost impossible for them to sustain that weight loss if they eat normally, because they are already at a healthy weight.

Then there are the "normal weight obesity" individuals, people who have normal body mass indexes (BMIs) but have extra fat that is often well hidden (typically as visceral fat in their bellies). They are at a normal weight but at high risk for chronic disease because of that visceral fat and their abnormal blood chemistries.

The problem is that too many Americans think of diet and nutrition in terms of aesthetics rather than as a healthy way of life. A diet is something you "go on" when you are trying to lose weight—usually as rapidly as possible— and go off when you meet your goal. The South Beach Diet was not developed as a short-term weight-loss plan, but rather as a method for changing lifestyle and eating attitudes long-term. In fact, I originally started recommending the diet to my heart patients to improve their blood chemistries so they wouldn't suffer an initial or a recurrent heart attack. Their dietary changes had to be sustained for years—in fact, forever—not just for weeks or months, because weeks or months do not result in the prolonged changes in cholesterol, blood sugar, blood pressure, and other factors required to prevent a heart attack.

Ultimately, as expected, these patients' waist circumferences and total weights dropped significantly, at which point they were not at risk for a heart attack. As delighted as they were with their newly svelte profiles, for me their real success was reflected in their blood chemistries, rather than by their BMI, the scale, or how they thought they looked in the mirror. Unfortunately, our culture has a deeply misguided view of nutrition, healthy eating, and what a healthy body should look like, and that has to change. I want you to help lead the way, and I need your assistance in this endeavor.

It has been very gratifying to hear so many stories over the years from those who have made the South Beach Diet a way of life. There is nothing better than meeting someone who has been on the diet who tells me, "Dr. Agatston, it's not really a *diet*—it's a lifestyle."

CHAPTER 5

EAT TO LIVE . . . WELL

Back in the mid-1970s, on one of my visits home from medical school, I remember preparing a sugar-laden breakfast for myself (frosted cereal and cinnamon toast) on a day when my uncle happened to be visiting. Uncle Abby, a math professor (not a medical professional), watched me in the kitchen and advised, "Arthur, you should eat a more balanced meal, something with some protein and vegetables, maybe." Being the confident medical student, I quickly answered that while a cause of cavities, there was actually no other reason to be concerned about my sugar consumption. That's what I had learned in medical school and what I believed. Even a decade or so later, my refined-flour, high-sugar breakfast would actually be touted as "heart healthy," simply because it was "low fat." You might be surprised to hear how little medical professionals knew about nutrition just a few decades ago. Our ignorance certainly contributed to our current sorry state of affairs.

In the 1980s, after finishing my medical training, I began attending the annual meetings of the American Heart Association and the American College of Cardiology. More than 30,000 researchers, clinicians, and others in the cardiac health-care field would descend on a city to learn about the latest advances in fighting heart disease. I occasionally went to the nutrition updates, hoping to discover something new to help me treat my patients. It was always easy to find a seat because these sessions were usually three-quarters empty. I guess it was felt that lip service had to be paid to the field of nutrition, even though very little new information was presented. I always left disappointed.

The lectures were always the same, advocating the traditional approach of calculating calories in, calories out, and limiting *total* fat calories without any distinction between good fats and bad fats or good carbohydrates and bad carbohydrates. This traditional approach didn't resonate with cardiologists, because it did not work for our patients. The message in the 1980s and '90s was "eat whatever carbohydrates you want, as long as they don't have fat." Dietary fat was viewed as the sole nutritional culprit when it came to heart disease. The focus was on weight loss and cholesterol, with almost no mention of the role nutrition plays in our general health. I could have even packaged my high-sugar med school breakfast, slapped a "no cholesterol" sticker on it, and sold it as heart-healthy.

That's not so far from what actually happened back then, and I know, because carbohydrates were not even on the radar at the time and I too was seduced by the incredible array of "zero cholesterol, no fat" products lining the grocery shelves—products that epitomized empty calories. I watched as my belly and the bellies of my patients and friends grew accordingly. This was a sad chapter in the history of our nation's eating habits and contributed to exponential weight gain across the country.

In the years following this "all the low fat you can eat" messaging, processed foods and fast foods became easier and easier to access, "thanks" to advances in food technology, and people cooked at home less and less. Add the digital revolution's negative impact on our daily energy output and we find our nation in the midst of the obesity and health crisis we have today.

Fortunately, the basic principles for a healthy lifestyle are no longer controversial. Unfortunately, the majority of Americans have not adopted these healthy eating principles. From the American Heart Association and the USDA to government and professional associations in Canada, Europe, and Australia, the latest nutritional guidelines send a clear and consistent message: A healthy diet must include good carbohydrates (vegetables, including legumes, fruits, and whole grains), lean protein, and good fats. While our knowledge of the qualities and benefits of various foods and nutrients will continue to grow because of ongoing research, the fundamentals of a healthy diet are not likely to change. That's why it's so important to understand the basics of good nutrition. Good nutrition is not just about weight loss. It is about feeding your body what it needs in order to feel great day in and day out and to help prevent acute and chronic disease. The good news is that a healthy weight is a natural by-product of healthy eating. We frankly did not know this years ago when the emphasis was on weight loss alone. But we do now.

Even though we've come a long way since those calories-in, calories-out lectures, many people still count total calories without considering the *quality* of those calories. While calories clearly do count, I have never felt that counting calories, grams of fat, or carbohydrates or weighing your food is compatible with a pleasurable and natural lifestyle. This type of constant calculating and measuring was certainly not done in any of the traditional societies that have been studied. In our experience, we have always found that when you are making good food choices, you are satisfied with reasonable food quantities and counting calories becomes superfluous. But it's critical that you understand the qualities of foods and learn how to make the right food choices. So let's take a look at what these good food choices are.

GOOD CARBS, BAD CARBS

Although the first sentence of my first book, *The South Beach Diet,* clearly states, "The South Beach Diet is not low-carb," there is still a lot of confusion out there, particularly regarding carbohydrates. To this day, some people think of the South Beach Diet as low carb when it is anything but. In fact, our diet has always recommended eating the *right* carbohydrates—vegetables, fruits, and whole grains—and plenty of them. I think the confusion exists because many people thfink of carbohydrates only as sugars and starches (the bad carbs), which we restrict on our diet. (See page 68 for a summary of the three phases of the South Beach Diet.)

In reality, carbohydrates include a vast array of foods. Good carbohydrates are considered good because they are nutrient-dense and fiber-rich. Bad carbs are the sugars, starches, and highly processed foods that are largely devoid of nutrients and fiber, such as sodas, cakes, cookies, and breads and other baked goods made with white flour, as well as white pasta, white potatoes, and low-fiber cereals.

A very nice illustration of the real-world difference between good and bad carbs was demonstrated in a study performed by researchers at Tufts University. The researchers gave one group of 9- to 11-year-olds one of three types of breakfast once a week for 3 weeks: a sugary commercial breakfast cereal (a bad carb), a bowl of oatmeal (a good carb), or no breakfast at all. (Don't worry: After the experiment was over, the children in the no-breakfast group for that week were immediately fed!) The researchers then tested the children's cognitive functions by administering specific mental tasks, like memorizing the names of fictitious countries on a map and repeating back numbers presented in a series. Both groups of breakfast-eaters generally did better than the nonbreakfast-eaters, and overall the oatmeal-eaters outperformed the sugary-cereal-eaters. When the researchers did the same experiment with 6- to 8-year olds, they found the effects were even more pronounced in the younger children. So, one way to help your child do better in school is to make sure he or she has a nutritious breakfast based on a good carb like oatmeal.

The researchers attributed the better cognitive performance to the higher amounts of fiber and protein in the oatmeal. Both slowed down the digestion of the carbohydrates into the bloodstream, providing a steady infusion of energy and helping the children feel fuller for a longer period of time. This study not only reinforces how important it is to give kids a good breakfast, it also underscores how good carbohydrates contribute to better performance throughout the day.

THE IMPORTANCE OF WHOLE GRAINS

I'm sure it won't surprise you to hear that grains are the most widely consumed carbohydrate in the United States. While rice consumption predominates elsewhere in the world, in this country we eat mainly wheat. It was some time after the advent of the steel roller mill in 1873, that the majority of wheat that Americans consumed took the form of white-flour-derived products. Since white flour is made from the starchy endosperm part of the grain (with the fiber-rich bran and nutritious germ removed), it is easily broken down into simple sugars in the mouth, stomach, and small intestine and absorbed rapidly. This plays havoc with our blood sugar, resulting in hunger and cravings. Just think of it this way: *Simple sugars with no nutrients digested rapidly equal empty calories that make us hungry for more.*

Whole grains and true whole-grain products, on the other hand, include the fiber and nutrients—particularly B vitamins and minerals—and are turned into simple sugars more slowly than refined grains. Consequently, they do not cause exaggerated swings in blood sugar. While more whole-grain products are continually appearing in supermarkets, there are still plenty of products that masquerade as whole grain. That's why you need to read labels when buying bread, crackers, cereal, pasta, or any other grain product.

Today many supermarkets offer a wide range of whole-grain flours, as well as raw whole grains (both packaged and in bulk), including barley, oats, bulgur, and brown rice. You may be surprised to learn that the nutrition considerations for rice are much the same as for wheat. In white rice, as in white bread, the fiber and the germ that contain the nutrients have been removed. That's why people who depend on white rice as their primary source of calories can develop vitamin deficiencies such as beriberi (just like the army recruits who had vitamin and mineral deficiencies before white bread was enriched with B vitamins). Because brown rice retains more fiber and nutrients than white, it is preferable. One of my favorite grains, quinoa, has become popular recently because of its high nutrient content. It is particularly high in protein and is a very good source of the essential amino acid lysine (a building block of protein), which is often missing from other grains and plant foods.

So whole grains have the advantage of more nutrients and more fiber. Furthermore, studies consistently bear out that regularly eating whole grains translates into real-world better-health outcomes. In fact, one study showed that those who reported eating at least three servings of whole grains daily had 10 percent less visceral (belly) fat than those who reported eating whole grains infrequently. Interestingly, the same study also showed that the fat-busting benefits of whole grains were lost when people ate them along with four or more servings of refined grains daily.

THE IMPORTANCE OF FRUITS AND VEGETABLES

When it comes to enjoying good carbs on a healthy diet, I cannot stress enough the importance of eating a variety of fruits and vegetables in many colors. As a group, these foods are the most nutrient-dense and are generally high in fiber. While we've always known that fruits and vegetables contained important nutrients, it is only recently that we have begun to discover just how many. Thousands of phytonutrients have already been discovered in these foods, and more are being found daily. And we are only just beginning to understand their enormous contributions to our health and well-being.

Today we know, for example, that cruciferous vegetables like broccoli, cabbage, brussels sprouts, cauliflower, kale, and bok choy are antioxidant, vitamin, and mineral powerhouses that can help lower our chances of developing cardiovascular disease. These vegetables have also been found to reduce age-related memory loss, combat certain forms of cancer, and help prevent a host of other diseases. Carotenoid-rich sweet potatoes, carrots, and other orange vegetables can help reduce low-density lipoprotein (LDL) cholesterol, lower high blood pressure, and protect against inflammatory conditions like asthma and arthritis. And lycopene-rich tomatoes can help protect against prostate cancer.

The benefits continue when it comes to fruits. Take blueberries, raspberries, and strawberries, to name just a few of my favorites. They are excellent sources of phytonutrients and antioxidants including vitamin C. Other fruits, like bananas and citrus fruits, provide potassium, which helps maintain a healthy blood pressure. And the dietary fiber from all fruits is important for health in general (see "Facts about Fiber" on page 78).

While most fruits and vegetables are excellent sources of good carbohydrates, not all are created equal. Some starchy vegetables, mainly root vegetables such as beets and potatoes, should be limited. Even here there are significant differences in their health profiles. They can be graded on the amount of nutrients and fiber versus the amount of starch (and sugar) they contain. The starches in these vegetables, like those in refined grains, are chains of glucose molecules that can cause exaggerated swings in blood sugar.

Of our commonly eaten vegetables, many types of white potatoes contain a great deal of starch and little fiber (especially when eaten without the skin). The sweet potato, on the other hand, is particularly nutrient-rich, with vitamins A, C, and B$_6$, and has considerably more fiber than the white potato, which is why it's a Phase 2 favorite on the South Beach Diet. It's interesting to note that the long-living Okinawans regularly eat sweet potatoes.

As with vegetables, there is a difference in the nutritional quality of fruits, depending on the amount of natural sugar they contain relative to their fiber and other nutrients. Generally, berries such as blueberries, raspberries, and strawberries have favorable fiber and nutrient-to-sugar ratios. Apples also have plenty of fiber and nutrients. On the other end of the spectrum are certain tropical fruits, such as pineapple and watermelon, which are particularly high in sugar and have relatively less fiber. For the most part, whole fruits are great nutrient sources, which is why I have always recommended eating whole fruits versus drinking their juice. That's because in many fruits most of the nutrients are found in their brightly colored skin, which also contains a good deal of fiber. (In the case of citrus fruits or fruits with rinds, the fiber and nutrients are in the pulp or flesh.)

Fruit juices certainly contain some good nutrients, including antioxidants, but when a fruit's skin is removed during processing, much of the fiber and some of the antioxidants can be lost with it. Additionally, the removal of fiber results in the faster absorption of the natural sugar (fructose) from the juice. When it comes to fruits, think of it this way: The whole fruit is better than fresh squeezed, which is better than concentrated juice. In fact, concentrated fruit juices can adversely affect blood sugar in diabetics, much like sugary soft drinks.

So, in summary, the good carbs are the nutrient-dense, fiber-rich whole grains, vegetables, and fruits that are essential to maintaining good health. Bad carbs are the sugary and starchy, highly processed foods that lack fiber and add nothing to your diet but empty calories. Remember, it is not about low carb or high carb; it is about the *right* carbs.

There is no question that if you want to get more whole grains, fruits, and vegetables into your diet, the best place to start is at home. Introducing your children to these foods early in life can be a major factor in their health and wellness as the years progress. I know how parents struggle with getting their kids to try these foods. That's why in our South Beach Diet Wake-Up Program, we give you tips on expanding your children's food repertoire. It's also why I urge you to read the stories of our Super Moms included in the book. I was impressed by how successful they have been in making vegetables and fruits a well-received part of their children's diets.

FACTS ABOUT FIBER

When it comes to fiber, I have always admired the work of Dr. Denis Burkitt, a British Army surgeon in World War II, who recognized and popularized its importance. His expertise came during and after the war when he lived and worked in Africa, where processed food was unheard of and fiber intake was high. During his 25 years in Africa, Burkitt simply never saw cases of appendicitis, diverticulitis, or colon cancer. He famously commented, "America is a constipated nation. . . . If you pass small stools, you have to have large hospitals." Based on his observations, Burkitt became the first physician to publicize the role fiber plays in our health. We now know that Americans are indeed fiber deficient—most of us consume only about 12 to 18 grams a day, when we should be consuming between 20 and 35 grams. That's why I encourage my patients to get more dietary fiber, particularly from vegetables, fruits, and whole grains.

Soluble fiber (so called because it dissolves in water) is found mainly in vegetables like peas and carrots; fruits like apples and citrus; legumes; and barley, oats, and oat bran. This type of fiber slows the absorption of sugar from the intestines, which helps control insulin secretion and swings in blood sugar. It also binds with bile acids in the intestine to block the absorption of cholesterol by the body. Legumes, in particular, have been shown to lower bad LDL cholesterol levels without reducing those of good HDL cholesterol.

Insoluble fiber, found in most whole grains but mainly in wheat, doesn't dissolve in water; rather, it absorbs many times its own weight in water. This water adds bulk and softness to the stools and thereby *speeds up* the movement of food through the intestines, helping to prevent constipation. Insoluble fiber is also thought to protect against diverticulosis, in which small out-pouches develop in weak spots of the wall of the large bowel, and also against diverticulitis, in which these pouches become inflamed. Insoluble fiber, like soluble fiber, also slows digestion of starches and helps prevent swings in blood sugar.

In addition to fiber's positive impact on our gastrointestinal system, we also know that by slowing down the digestion of carbohydrates, fiber helps prevent type 2 diabetes and a litany of other diseases associated with our poor Western diet. In 2011, results of the very large National Institutes of Heath–AARP population study were reported in the *Archives of Internal Medicine*. The researchers looked at death rates from all causes in 219,123 men and 168,999 women between the ages of 50 and 71, who were followed for an average of 9 years. They found that participants who had the greatest fiber intake had the lowest death rates over the course of the study. They emphasized that their findings were consistent with so many of the positive effects known to be associated with fiber, including its ability to (1) increase bulk and reduce the transit time of feces moving through the bowel; (2) increase excretion of cholesterol-containing bile along with known fecal pro-carcinogens (substances that promote cancer); (3) lower cholesterol levels; (4) improve insulin sensitivity; (5) lower blood pressure; (6) promote weight loss; (7) reduce the harmful effects of bad LDL cholesterol; and (8) help reduce inflammation. One surprising finding from the study was that those who consumed more fiber were less likely to have died from infectious and respiratory diseases. This is all consistent with an important theme of this book: Good nutrition is not just about preventing heart disease but about preventing most chronic diseases. So, getting sufficient fiber through healthful carbohydrates and, if necessary, a fiber supplement should be a high priority.

FATS: THE GOOD, THE BAD, AND THE UGLY

As I said earlier, as recently as the 1980s and '90s, the conventional wisdom was that all fats were bad. Now we know that there are good fats, bad fats, and *really* bad fats. Two major studies done in the 1990s helped increase our under-

(continued on page 82)

Alcohol: To Your Health?

Alcohol itself is not a true carbohydrate, although spirits like whiskey, bourbon, vodka, and beer are derived from the fermentation of grains (rye, malted barley, and wheat). Fermented grapes are the primary ingredient in wine and champagne. Alcoholic beverages are often labeled "low carb" or "no carb," but don't let that language fool you into believing you can drink alcohol without consequences. Alcohol is high in calories, and largely empty calories at that. These really add up when alcohol is consumed with mixers like sugary fruit juice, soda, or flavored syrups. Labeling alcohol as "low carb" is like labeling white bread as "low cholesterol"—technically true but nutritionally misleading.

Alcohol is not broken down into sugar in the intestine or liver, but is directly burned for fuel. So if you are drinking several alcoholic beverages along with your meal, your body will first burn the alcohol before accessing its own stores of carbohydrates and fat for energy. Over time, this can really pack on the pounds, which is a common occurrence in both men and women. To add insult to injury, alcohol can also be an appetite stimulant. If you've had one too many, you may have less self-control when it comes to rejecting the rich chocolate cake in favor of that bowl of mixed berries.

In addition, the list of medical problems heavy drinkers encounter is very long and touches just about every organ system. Heart disease, dementia, cirrhosis of the liver, and ulcers are just a few conditions at the top of the list. Cardiologists commonly see heart arrhythmias (abnormal heart rhythms) known as "holiday heart" after only slightly excessive alcohol intake (often during holiday party season). And although this condition is usually benign, it can be quite serious and demand immediate medical attention, especially if it is the result of binge drinking. Furthermore, oncologists have seen an association between alcohol intake and breast cancer, colon cancers, liver cancer, and head and neck cancers. (*Note:* For smokers who drink, the risk of these cancers is considerably greater.)

Drinking more than moderately (moderate alcohol intake is generally defined as one alcoholic beverage daily for women and two for men) can also increase the bad fat known as triglycerides in the bloodstream. High triglycerides are usually associated with low levels of good high-density lipoprotein (HDL) cholesterol, especially in people with belly fat. When I see elevated triglycerides with a normal to high HDL, I suspect excess alcohol intake and I am usually right.

However, there's another way that I can tell heavy drinkers apart from moderate drinkers and teetotalers. You may have noticed the telltale ruddy complexion of chronic drinkers and even observe how many turn a bit red when they imbibe. This is because the alcohol is dilating their blood vessels, which it is thought to do via the stimulation of nitric oxide production. Nitric oxide is actually a "good health molecule" that helps keep our blood vessels smooth and open. Studies have consistently shown that moderate (not excessive) alcohol intake does decrease the rate of heart attack and possibly diabetes, which could in part be attributed to the action of nitric oxide. Moderate alcohol intake can also increase your good HDL cholesterol.

For years, we have heard about the "French paradox," referring to the fact that the French seem to be thinner and have less heart disease than you would expect from their diet, which often includes high amounts of butter and other forms of saturated fat, frequently washed down with a glass of red wine. Through the years, scientists have hypothesized that there must be something in red wine that is protective, and recent research has pinpointed the antioxidant resveratrol, a type of polyphenol (a healthful phytonutrient), as a likely candidate.

How red wine affects the body remains unclear, but recent studies show that sipping a glass of red wine with a meal can decrease the amount of inflammation-producing free radicals found in the blood after a meal.

My final word on the subject: Overall, a *little* red wine or a moderate amount of alcohol (without a sugary mixer) with dinner has been looking pretty healthy, along with being pretty tasty. Just don't go overboard.

standing of fats, and the results of this research are still important today. The one that first woke me up to the benefits of good fats was the famous Lyon Diet Heart Study, first reported in 1994. In it, researchers tested the effect of a Mediterranean-style diet on 605 patients who had survived a first heart attack. Half the group (302 patients) was asked to eat more omega-3-rich oils (primarily in the form of a canola oil spread), more olive oil, and more fiber. The 303 patients in the control group were given no specific dietary advice but told to eat a prudent diet. The results: After just 27 months, the patients who followed the Mediterranean-style diet had a dramatic 73 percent decrease in either death from heart disease or a nonfatal second heart attack as opposed to those in the control group. This was quite a remarkable result, and it was the beginning of the end for the low-fat diet as a panacea.

Three years later, the Harvard School of Public Health Nurses' Health Study demonstrated the benefits of good fats and the deleterious effects of bad fats in more than 80,000 participants. In the November 20, 1997, issue of the *New England Journal of Medicine,* the researchers concluded: "Our findings suggest that replacing saturated and trans unsaturated fats with unhydrogenated monounsaturated and polyunsaturated fats is more effective in preventing coronary heart disease in women than reducing overall fat intake."

The Good

The good fats are the polyunsaturated omega-3s and the monounsaturated omega-9s. Omega-3 fatty acids can be found in good amounts in sunflower seeds, walnuts, and flaxseeds, and in their oils, and in fish (particularly oily fish like salmon and herring). Because omega-3s cannot be produced by the body, they are considered an essential fatty acid.

Omega-9 fatty acids (also known as oleic acid) are found in canola, peanut, and olive oils; in avocados; in nuts such as almonds, hazelnuts, peanuts, pistachios, and pecans; and in seeds like pumpkin and sesame. Omega-9s are not technically essential fatty acids because they are produced by the body in small amounts. Numerous studies have documented a link between the consumption of anti-inflammatory omega-9-rich foods and a decreased risk for developing heart disease, asthma, breast cancer, and other cancers, as well as various autoimmune and neurodegenerative diseases believed to be associated with inflammation in the body.

The three major types of omega-3 fatty acids found in foods are alpha-linolenic acid (ALA), from plants such as flaxseed and walnuts; and eicosapentaenoic acid (EPA) and docosahexaenoic acid (DHA), gotten primarily from fish. Once ingested, the ALA is converted to EPA and DHA, the types that are more readily used by the body. Unfortunately, it is estimated that the average American consumes only about 23 milligrams of omega-3 fatty acids per day. This is far lower than the National Institutes of Health recommendation that adults get at least 650 milligrams of EPA and DHA daily. And, for adults with coronary heart disease, the American Heart Association recommends getting 1 gram daily of EPA and DHA, preferably from oily fish—although it also says that an omega-3 fatty acid supplement could be considered in consultation with a physician. I agree with these recommendations. For patients with markedly elevated triglycerides, higher doses of fish oil are quite effective. Look for fish oil supplements from reputable manufacturers; they are safe and do not contain mercury because the oil has been distilled to ensure no contaminants are present.

Omega-6s: America's Worst Balancing Act

Another type of essential polyunsaturated fat are omega-6 fatty acids, found in vegetable oils such as corn oil and soybean oil, as well as in grains and grain-fed beef and poultry. Oils high in omega-6s are also found in a lot of our processed foods.

Omega-6 fatty acids are a precursor for hormones necessary for the *inflammatory* responses that are essential for survival. Our ancestors naturally consumed them in balance with omega-3s, a precursor for many *anti-inflammatory* hormones. The meat they ate from the wild game they hunted contained a fraction of the omega-6s found in today's grain-fed meat sources. In fact, in the hunter-gatherers' diet, omega-6s accounted for 0.5 to 1 percent of the calories they consumed, which resulted in a ratio of omega-6s to omega-3s between 2:1 and 4:1 in their tissues. Today omega-6s constitute 8 to 9 percent of our calories, and our ratio of omega-6s to omega-3s is between 10:1 and 20:1. Wow—no wonder we are a hyperin-flamed society.

In fact, according to well-known lipid researcher Joseph Hibbeln, MD, this out-of-balance ratio may be a major reason for Americans' huge spending on over-the-counter anti-inflammatory drugs (aspirin, ibuprofen, and other nonsteroidal anti-inflammatory drugs) in an effort to combat inflammatory problems like arthritis, muscle pains, and headaches. This, in turn, can lead to high costs for hospitalizations from the resulting stomach problems (particularly major bleeding) and for the drugs used to treat these stomach problems.

We know that inflammation is the common denominator in many of the chronic diseases of the Western world. In fact, societies that consume more omega-3s than Americans have lower rates of obesity, diabetes, vascular disease, and depression than we do. We would do much better by decreasing our intake of omega-6s and adding more sources of omega-3s to our diet. The bottom line: Omega-6s are not always a bad fat, since they can produce good inflammatory responses, but they turn into one when they are overconsumed. Today we are unfortunately doing just that.

The Bad

The bad fats are the saturated fats, found predominantly in meats and dairy. Saturated fat raises our bad LDL cholesterol and is associated with heart disease, diabetes, and several forms of cancer. Some saturated fat has always been a natural part of our diet, but the wild game and even the cows and sheep of a century ago ate grasses and were much leaner than today's meat sources, which are typically fed grain and fattened up in pens. While saturated fat is not nearly as bad as trans fat (described opposite), when consumed in excess, calories from saturated fat will crowd out the healthier calories from good fats and good carbs from your diet. This is similar to what has happened with the omega-6s. We are simply getting too much saturated fat in the American diet today.

Saturated fat is also found in plant sources, such as coconut oil and palm oil. Coconut and palm oil are very stable oils (meaning they don't go rancid easily, even at high temperatures) and have been the traditional fat staple in tropical regions, where heart disease has been rare. Up until about 1980, imported palm and coconut oil were commonly used in this country to prolong the shelf life of baked goods. But once saturated fat was generally recognized as unhealthy (and the vegetable oil industry began a powerful negative lobbying campaign against the tropical oils), they were virtually banned in the United States, only to be replaced by another shelf-stable fat—trans fat— which turned out to be far worse for our health.

While the jury is still out on the health benefits of these tropical oils, palm oil in particular is looking good, thanks to its high levels of the antioxidants beta-carotene and vitamin E. Virgin coconut oil is also looking better in the latest medical literature. Just remember that if either of these oils is hydrogenated or partially hydrogenated, they then become dangerous trans fats. Like all oils, both should be used in moderation.

Stearic acid (found in the cacao seeds from which chocolate is made) is another plant source of saturated fat. The good news is that the stearic acid contained in chocolate does not increase blood levels of total and LDL cholesterol. And studies show that dark chocolate—not white chocolate or milk chocolate—increases the body's production of nitric oxide. Interestingly, the blood pressure-lowering effects of chocolate appear to be related to the amount of flavonoids present. Look for dark chocolate containing at least 70 percent cacao and the least amount of added sugar to reap the most heart benefits. Enjoy it—in moderation.

The Ugly

Remember the principle that if we deviate too far from what our forefathers ate, we do so at our own peril? This peril has reared its ugly head in the history of trans fats, which are found naturally in food sources in extremely small amounts and have never been an important component in any population's diet. Trans fats are made by adding hydrogen molecules to liquid vegetable oil to make it solid and shelf-stable. This affects their molecular structure, causing them to act more like saturated fats in the body. Trans fats can be found in stick margarines (but not in most soft tub margarines, now more commonly known as vegetable oil spreads), in foods fried in hydrogenated oils, and in many packaged snack foods containing hydrogenated or partially hydrogenated oils. Trans fats were chosen to replace the tropical oils because they were made from polyunsaturated fats, but *adulterated*. Unfortunately, these

Helen R.

Super Mom, South Jordan, Utah

"I'm raising children who know where their milk and eggs come from."

After the birth of my twins 10 years ago—a boy and a girl—I put on a lot of weight and my cholesterol was creeping up. I wanted to make sure that I would be around to raise my children and see my grandchildren, so I went on the South Beach Diet. Once I learned about healthy food and began to eat better, I wanted to feed my family better too, and so I began cooking for them following the diet's basic principles (but without actually putting them on a diet, of course). My cholesterol is now normal, I am at a healthy weight, and, to be frank, I think the diet literally saved my life.

We live in a small subdivision outside of a city on less than a half acre of land, but we still have enough room to keep a flock of chickens for eggs, and goats for milk and dairy. We joined a farmers' co-op where we buy fresh produce and meat. I also buy wheat and other grains in bulk there, and I grind them in a countertop grain mill to make my own flour. I always have whole flax, buckwheat, oats, and red and white wheat at home. I make my own bread, since I am very fussy about the kind of bread that I serve to my family. If I bought it at the supermarket, it would cost about $4 a loaf. I can make one that is as good or better for 50 cents a loaf. We don't ever use any white rice or white potatoes, but we do use brown and wild rice, sweet potatoes, winter squash, all foods that, I learned from my time on South Beach, are fine on a healthy diet.

fats have turned out to be the worst kind for our health, far worse than satu-rated fats, and that's why I call them "the ugliest fats of all."

Like saturated fats, trans fats raise bad LDL cholesterol levels. But worse than saturated fats, they can also lower the levels of good HDL cholesterol. In

I also buy whole oat groats, and when we want a bowl of cereal, we stick them in the grain mill and we roll them ourselves. The kids would rather eat what I make them for breakfast than sugary store-bought cereal. That's because they know what I give them tastes better. I had to fight really hard to get the perfect work shift, so I start at 8:30 a.m. every day, which gives me time to get up and actually have breakfast with the kids (my husband leaves the house before 6 a.m.). The kids and I always make breakfast together. One of them does the grinding, the other the cooking. We set the table together and then we sit down and eat together. Since my husband works a different shift, he picks them up from school, but the minute I get home from work, about 5:30, I take my coat off and head to the kitchen to make dinner. We all start cooking together, then my husband sets the table for us and we all sit down and have a family meal—every single night. I love that. The TV is always turned off during dinner. That's a family rule. No cell phones are allowed either.

My kids do their homework when they come home from school, and they also have their "farm" chores. I also make sure that they have plenty of time to run around and play in the afternoon. Kids need to be kids. If a teacher loads them down with too much homework, I go in and complain. They need some time to exercise too.

I'm raising children who know where their milk and eggs come from because they know how to milk a goat and collect eggs from the hens. We treat all of our animals very well. My children have been taught that the more love you give to your animals, the more they give back to you. They feel very lucky that we are able to eat as well as we do.

a 2006 review article published in the *New England Journal of Medicine,* researchers concluded that trans fats increase the risk of heart disease more than any other nutrient on a per-calorie basis, even when consumed in small amounts. Other studies have shown that trans fats may also increase the risk for obesity, diabetes, Alzheimer's, and cancer.

Since 2006, the US Food and Drug Administration has required that all food labels include the amount of trans fat in a product. And many states and cities have already passed legislation, or have pending legislation, banning the use of trans fats in restaurant cooking and other commercial food facilities. This is excellent news.

While much of the research on good fats and bad fats has focused on their impact on cardiovascular disease and cancer, new studies are continually shedding light on how "good" unsaturated fats may also have a beneficial effect on conditions such as osteoporosis, macular degeneration, multiple sclerosis, age-related memory loss, infertility, and other chronic ailments. This exciting research is in its earliest stages, and we will continue to follow these studies with great interest. But what's important to remember is that these studies don't mean you should run out and start consuming unsaturated fats with abandon. All fats, even the good ones, are calorie-dense and should be consumed in moderation.

LEAN PROTEIN

Almost as often as I am asked about good carbs and good fats, I am also asked about the best sources of protein for a healthy diet. After author Michael Pollan caught America's attention with his *In Defense of Food* mantra, "Eat food. Not too much. Mostly plants," and the 2008 movie *Food, Inc.* showed the conditions in which livestock were often raised and slaughtered—making many people think twice about ever having another steak or hamburger or piece of chicken—these questions only increased.

Not surprisingly, most of us associate protein with muscle. We always hear about bodybuilders consuming protein shakes and supplements. It is true that our muscles and organs are largely composed of protein and that protein is also the main component of the structural connective tissues found in and between all of our organs. But protein is also an important building block of enzymes, which are responsible for most of the communications that regulate all of our body's functions.

Whether you get your protein from meat- or plant-based sources, it is essential for maintaining a healthy body. The inclusion of lean healthy protein in your daily diet is also helpful for weight loss. Protein foods are digested slowly, and it takes a lot of energy to fuel their metabolism. Protein also keeps us feeling fuller longer and doesn't cause spikes in blood sugar that can stimulate overeating.

The basic units of protein are called amino acids. Those that the body can make on its own are the nonessential amino acids. Those that the body cannot produce are called essential amino acids, because they must come from our diet. Foods that contain all the essential amino acids are complete proteins; those that are missing one or more are incomplete. All animal protein— meats, poultry, seafood, dairy, and eggs—is complete. All plant protein is incomplete, with the exception of soybeans and soyfoods and the grain quinoa, which are complete.

Among the questions I hear most often when it comes to protein are: How much protein should I eat? Can it hurt my kidneys? Can it hurt my bones? The answers depend on how healthy you are and your age and activity level. (If you are pregnant or breast-feeding, this requires a separate discussion with your doctor or pediatrician.) For young athletes, protein is especially important for building muscle and bone and will also help them maintain a healthy weight. If you have a teenager involved in sports, be sure that he or she eats ample amounts of lean protein, including low-fat dairy products. (One of my favorites, nonfat Greek yogurt, has 15 grams per 6-ounce serving.) In older folks, and those with kidney problems, diabetes, high blood pressure, or liver disease, protein is not broken down efficiently, and too much protein can cause problems.

For healthy people not suffering from these conditions, however, sufficient protein is necessary to maintain good bone health and will not hurt your kidneys. That said, unlike fats and carbohydrates, there is an upper limit of protein that our livers and kidneys can handle. This is about 35 to 40 percent of our daily calories; beyond that, we can get sick. This illness was seen in American pioneers who sometimes found themselves subsisting *only* on the meat from small critters such as rabbits, which had virtually no fat. It was even called "rabbit starvation," a condition rarely heard of today.

So what sources of protein are best? The fact is, all whole foods contain some protein, including grains, vegetables, fruits, legumes, nuts, and seeds. That's why if you're a vegetarian or a vegan, you can get plenty of protein without eating meat, dairy, or eggs. You simply need to enjoy a wide variety of plant-based protein-rich foods, since we know that the body will automatically combine amino acids to create complete protein from the foods that you eat over the course of a day. But you must eat a varied diet.

Quantity is not the only consideration when it comes to protein; quality must be factored in as well. Even with a specific protein food such as steak or salmon, there can be very significant nutritional differences depending on the source of these foods.

"YOU ARE WHAT YOU EAT ATE"

You've undoubtedly heard the phrase "You are what you eat." With what we know about nutrition today, I think that we should amend the statement to "You are what you eat ate." That's because the nutrient value of the animal protein that ends up on your plate varies widely depending on what food was available for that cow, pig, lamb, chicken, or fish to eat.

There are important health implications in eating a cut of meat from an animal that was grass-fed and that roamed pastures, as opposed to one that was grain-fed, kept in pens, and injected with antibiotics and hormones. Grass-fed livestock is leaner and has higher amounts of good omega-3 fats and lower amounts of bad fats than grain-fed livestock, which has high amounts of omega-6 fats and potentially harmful chemicals. Similarly, the wild salmon that eats ocean plants, plankton, and small fish is filled with plenty of omega-3s and is preferable to farm-raised salmon that was fattened on grains—and who knows what else—and that has fewer omega-3s. (Unfortunately, more than half the salmon we get in this country today is farmed, though some fish farms are better than others.) The same is true when it comes to poultry. An organic pastured chicken raised without antibiotics, synthetic hormones, or pesticides and fed organic feed is the chicken you want to buy.

We can certainly extend this concept to the plant universe and include the importance of knowing where and how your plant-derived foods were grown. Were they raised on nutrient-depleted soil and sprayed with pesticides? Or were they grown using sustainable agriculture techniques and biological pest control?

Our pioneer ancestors—the early American farmers—knew where everything they ate came from, since it was the livestock they raised, the game they hunted, or the produce they grew. Today, most of us have no idea where our food comes from. This is, however, beginning to change. Savvy consumers are seeking out products that clearly state where and how they were grown and manufactured; they are looking for the organic seal and buying grass-fed beef, wild-caught salmon, and pastured chickens.

In time, and with intensified consumer demand, we should be able to know the lineage of almost every morsel of food we put into our mouths.

A WORD ABOUT SODIUM

Whether sodium should be regulated, like trans fats and cigarettes, has been a hot issue lately. My concern, however, is that there isn't enough focus on the processed, fast, unhealthy foods that are really the primary source of sodium in our diets.

In January 2011, the American Heart Association issued an advisory recommending that *all* Americans consume no more than 1,500 milligrams of sodium a day. This is the equivalent of just over half a teaspoon of salt. (The new USDA dietary guidelines call for a daily sodium intake of less than 2,300 milligrams, and recommend only 1,500 milligrams for people 51 and older, African Americans, and people who have hypertension, diabetes, or chronic kidney disease.)

(continued on page 94)

Consider Vegetarian?

If you are worried about the sources of animal protein found in your super-market today, about how the animals were raised and fed, or have ethical concerns about eating meat, this could push you toward a simple solution. Become a vegetarian.

There are three major types of vegetarians. *Vegans* are the strictest and eat nothing from animals, including meat, poultry, seafood, dairy products, and eggs—not even honey. *Lacto-vegetarians* eat dairy products like milk, cheese, yogurt, and butter, but not eggs. *Lacto-ovo vegetarians* eat dairy products and eggs. Others are semi-vegetarian, in that they eat only fish or white meat like poultry and avoid beef, pork, and other "red" meats; or they simply restrict their meat consumption to small amounts on rare occasions.

The challenge for vegetarians comes in finding quality sources of protein and, if you are a vegan, in making sure you get enough of the nutrients you could be missing by not eating any animal-derived protein. The stricter the diet, the tougher the challenge, but it is certainly doable. So if you get enough protein, omega-3s, calcium, iron, zinc, vitamin B_{12}, vitamin D, and other essential nutrients, taking a vegetarian approach to nutrition can be very healthy. Since vegetarians can easily embrace the South Beach Diet's basic principles of eating good carbohydrates, good fats, and lean (nonmeat) sources of protein, we have always supported this way of eating with a wide variety of appropriate recipes. The health problems I observed in the past were mainly in vegetarians who filled up on white-flour-based baked goods and pasta and other refined carbohydrates, which often led to elevated tri-glycerides, weight gain, obesity, and even diabetes. Because becoming a vegetarian requires being nutritionally literate, most vegetarians I meet today have learned to emphasize good carbs in their diets and are healthier than the vegetarians I treated years ago.

Studies show that a vegetarian diet can reduce the risk of chronic disease; this is likely because of the lower intake of saturated fat and the higher intake of fruits, vegetables, whole grains, nuts, soy products, fiber, magnesium, potassium, vitamins C and E, folate, and carotenoids, flavonoids, and other phytonutrients. A carefully planned vegetarian diet is appropriate for nearly all life situations, including pregnancy, lactation, infancy, childhood, and adolescence, and for athletes, as well. Other research has documented that a vegetarian diet is associated with a lower risk of death from ischemic heart disease and that vegetarians also appear to have lower LDL cholesterol levels, lower blood pressure, and lower overall rates of type 2 diabetes and cancer than nonvegetarians. While I am certainly not recommending a vegetarian diet for everybody, it's hard to ignore such compelling data. I frankly believe that the good health results in vegetarians are due, in large part, to the wide variety of nutritious foods they eat and their avoidance of fast foods and unhealthy fats. I also believe that vegetarians, as a group, tend to lead a healthier lifestyle in general than nonvegetarians.

For the majority of Americans who do eat meat, remember that it is not your only source of protein and that you don't need to eat it every day. If you're already eating good carbs and fats, like nuts, seeds, legumes, and soy, you're getting high-quality protein from these foods. The short answer when it comes to animal protein is this: Eat lean. That means giving up the marbled steaks, prime rib, bacon, and brisket, which contain artery-clogging saturated fat along with inflammatory omega-6s, and replacing these foods with seafood, white-meat chicken and turkey, and lean cuts of beef, lamb, and pork.

Eating less sodium certainly seems reasonable and easy to do, but the problem is that the average American currently consumes at least *twice the recommended amount of sodium every day,* primarily from the salt found in processed and fast foods. Consider this: The typical quarter-pound cheeseburger and large portion of fries from a fast-food restaurant may contain more than 1,600 milligrams of sodium, and that's just for one meal! A can of commercial soup purchased from a supermarket may have between 500 and 800 milligrams of sodium per serving, and usually the serving size listed on the label is a lot smaller than the amount someone would actually eat. And the soup may be just the first course!

So, is it time to throw out the saltshaker? Not so fast. While high amounts of dietary sodium consumption have been linked to an increased risk of high blood pressure, stroke, heart attack, and kidney disease, the risk is not the same for everyone. In reality, only half of the people with hypertension are salt-sensitive, which is defined as experiencing a greater than 10 percent increase in blood pressure after eating a salty meal, and only one-third of those with normal blood pressure are. As far as I'm concerned, the real problem is with the tremendous amount of sodium already added to processed foods, not the small amount of salt you sprinkle on your grilled vegetables. (Of course, this assumes moderation in your own home-cooked recipes.)

Whether or not you are sodium-sensitive, I urge you (and everyone) to avoid processed and fast foods because they are bad for you in so many ways. If you are sodium-sensitive, you need to be extra careful about adding salt to your meals. If you aren't, then a small amount of salt added to taste should not be a problem.

THE ESSENTIAL PRINCIPLES OF HEALTHY EATING

The point of this entire chapter has been to reinforce the fact that variety and quality are essential when it comes to making the food choices that will allow us all to eat well and live free of the chronic diseases that are plaguing the Western world.

When it comes down to it, the principles of healthy eating are actually quite simple. The future health and welfare of this nation lie in more of us adopting them and ultimately making them our way of life.

Please keep these essential principles of healthy eating in mind:

- Evaluate the *quality* of the fats, carbohydrates, and protein you eat—not just the quantity. *Corollary:* Eat whole foods.

- Consume a wide variety of healthy foods, especially vegetables and fruits. *Corollary:* Don't depend predominantly on one food or just a few foods; in other words, don't eat the same foods every day.

- Avoid empty-calorie foods. *Corollary:* Taking supplements does not compensate for empty calories.

- Know what you eat ate. *Corollary:* Learn about how your food was produced and processed. Skip the fast food.

- Remember that calories count, but stop counting calories, grams of fat, carbohydrates, protein, or anything else; it doesn't work in the real world. *Corollary:* When you make healthy food choices most of the time (and get regular exercise), your body will find its healthy weight.

- Don't deviate from the diets of your forefathers; you do so at your own peril. *Corollary:* As Michael Pollan so aptly put it, "Don't eat what your great-great-grandmother wouldn't recognize as food."

CHAPTER 6

NEW CONCERNS
ABOUT GLUTEN

Let me emphasize again the final point I made at the end of the last chapter. We should eat like our ancestors. If we fail to, we do so at our own peril.

I am referring to the lessons of past generations—from those who roamed the earth 100,000 years ago to our great-grandparents. Some researchers argue that since our DNA was originally designed for us to live in the wild as hunter-gatherers, that's the diet we should return to today. It's certainly worth considering.

For one thing, the hunter-gatherer diet was free of all processed carbohydrates. In fact, the diet was completely grain free, since grains had to be dehusked, cracked, milled, or ground, and ultimately cooked before they could be eaten.

In contrast to our typical Western diet, the hunter-gatherers' diet tended to be high in protein and cholesterol—though not in saturated fat. They consumed a variety of nutrient-rich fruits and vegetables and thereby got plenty of vitamins and minerals when food was available (except for the mineral sodium, which was never abundant in natural foods). The hunter-gatherers did not consume dairy once they were weaned from their mothers' milk, because there were no domesticated animals to milk.

One criticism of the hunter-gatherers' diet is that it relied too much on animal protein—particularly meat—and is therefore a poor model to emulate today. It is important to recognize, however, that the game meat our ancestors hunted was much lower in saturated fat and pro-inflammatory omega-6 fats and much higher in anti-inflammatory omega-3s than today's meat and poultry.

Fortunately, naturally lean range- and pasture-fed meats and poultry, as well as game meats with a healthier balance of fats, are becoming more widely available today. And with our increasing knowledge and concern about understanding "what we eat ate," these and other healthier sources of protein should continue to become more accessible and less expensive. Meanwhile, look for lean cuts of meat, and don't forget about wild-caught seafood and vegetable sources of protein, like soy and quinoa.

BECOME GLUTEN AWARE

Not having the know-how to grow crops meant that the hunter-gatherers had to keep moving to find their next meal. This made life difficult, but ironically it spared them from some of our modern-day nutritional disasters. Today, we eat what we grow, and we process our food in ways that are both unnatural and unhealthy. In contrast to the hunter-gatherers, most Americans eat carbohydrates that are highly processed, with the bulk of them coming from wheat. Thanks to our ever-increasing intake of white-wheat-flour-based products, we have been receiving a huge dose of a protein component in wheat called "gluten."

Gluten is found in all forms of wheat, whether processed or whole grain (including bulgur, durum, semolina, spelt, and farro) as well as in barley, rye, and triticale. It is also often used as an additive in products, including soy sauce, candy, malt vinegar, and yogurt, to name just a few. So you could easily be ingesting gluten without realizing it, even if you are avoiding wheat. In addition, it appears that modern methods of growing and processing wheat have drastically increased our consumption of gluten.

The most severe manifestation of a gluten problem is celiac disease, a condition affecting approximately 1 percent of Americans, although incredibly, *about 97 percent of cases go undiagnosed.*

Three disturbing facts make it particularly important to raise awareness about gluten-related health problems. First, in those with known celiac disease, it has taken on average 9 years to make the diagnosis. These patients often go from doctor to doctor, unsuccessfully looking for help to feel better. Second, the incidence of celiac disease is rising dramatically. A Mayo Clinic study has shown that the incidence of celiac disease has quadrupled in recent decades. Third, our intake of gluten has been markedly increasing. If gluten is impacting so many more lives, we had better become aware of its manifestations and learn what to look for.

What is celiac disease? Why has it been so hard to diagnose? Why is it increasing so dramatically? And what does it have to do with your own health and happiness?

When people eat foods containing gluten, the digestive enzymes in their small intestines are unable to break down the gluten protein into chains of amino acids small enough to be readily absorbed into the bloodstream. Amino acids are the building blocks of protein, just as glucose is the building block of starch. We just do not digest gluten as well as we do protein from other food sources. In patients with celiac disease, the undigested protein triggers an immune-inflammatory response in the intestinal wall that damages its lining. This can cause a spectrum of gastrointestinal symptoms, including abdominal pain, cramping, gas, diarrhea and/or constipation, which are often misdiagnosed as irritable bowel syndrome or some form of colitis. But intestinal damage from gluten can and often does occur *without these symptoms.*

Because of the inflammation and consequent intestinal damage in those with celiac disease, important nutrients and minerals may not be absorbed normally through the intestinal wall into the bloodstream. This can lead to a spectrum of other signs and symptoms including fatigue, neuropathy, iron deficiency anemia, vitamin D deficiency, osteoporosis, infertility, migraine headaches, and depression. In addition, because the damaged intestinal barrier can also be breached by proteins that normally would not enter the wall, this can initiate autoimmune reactions that can damage otherwise normal tissue. When this happens, it can result in conditions such as thyroiditis, arthritis, fibromyalgia, psoriasis, and even type 1 diabetes, all of which have been associated with celiac disease.

This incredibly wide spectrum of seemingly unrelated problems and presentations explains why celiac disease and other gluten-related problems have been so hard to diagnose. Doctors have been chasing the individual disorders without putting together the big picture. It has also been suggested that one reason for the doctors' and the public's low level of awareness is that since the treatment of gluten problems is with nutrition rather than with medication, Big Pharma has not come up with research funds and educational programs.

Although celiac disease cannot be cured, it can be managed very effectively by eliminating all foods containing gluten. That's because the ingestion of even very small quantities of gluten (often inadvertently from packaged foods and even from certain medications and supplements) can set off the troublesome symptoms for those with the disease. Luckily, celiac disease can be tested for, first with blood tests and then with an intestinal biopsy for a definitive diagnosis.

But gluten doesn't just trouble Americans with celiac disease. Many others have what is known as a gluten intolerance, which some experts think may actually affect a *majority* of people in this country. Its manifestations are wide-ranging and similar to those of celiac disease. In contrast to celiac patients, however, gluten-intolerant individuals can consume small to moderate amounts of wheat products without adverse effects. Unfortunately, unlike celiac disease, there is no reliable test for making a definitive diagnosis of gluten intolerance.

PHASE I: IT'S GLUTEN FREE

My interest in gluten intolerance being a player in some of what ails us grew largely out of my experience with my own patients on Phase 1 of the South Beach Diet. As many of you know, the first phase of the South Beach Diet is free of grains and is therefore gluten free (see the "South Beach Diet: A Crash Course," page 68).

Over the years, I have witnessed and been reliably told of many cases where conditions such as juvenile arthritis, irritable bowel syndrome, depression, migraines, and even psoriasis and other skin problems either improved

(continued on page 102)

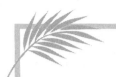

Angela W.
Super Mom, Miami, Florida

"We wanted to give our daughter the best start in life that we could."

When we first got married, my husband and I became vegetarian primarily because we thought it was the healthiest way to eat. For a while, he was a raw vegan, which meant that he ate only raw fruits and vegetables. I tried it for a while too, and I felt great, but it was very hard to keep doing it. Through that journey together we learned a great deal about how food is grown and the effects of pesticides on fruits and vegetables. Believe it or not, I can actually taste the pesticides now. Although my husband and I are no longer vegetarians, we still eat a lot of organic produce, and we eat only organic eggs and meat as well.

Even before we became parents, we were horrified by what we saw happening to the children in this country. I can't believe the garbage that kids today are eating! I can only wonder what is going to be happening to these kids 20 or 30 years from now. And just look at the incidence of disease among my peer group—there is so much obesity and diabetes. When I learned I was pregnant with a girl, my husband and I decided that we wanted to give our daughter the best start in life that we could.

Most of our friends are all very nutrition-conscious. They don't buy commercial baby food; they make their own. My husband and I decided that we would do the same. That way, we'd have more control over what our daughter eats. We try to avoid foods that we believe contribute to childhood allergies, ear infections, and other health problems that are rampant among children today. For example, our friends with older children had kids who developed gluten allergies and lactose intolerance, so we decided not to give our daughter foods with gluten from the start and to introduce dairy products very carefully.

It doesn't take me more than an hour or so on a Saturday to make Jenna's meals for the week. Basically, we steam or boil the raw food (mostly fruits and vegetables), puree it with a food processor or hand mixer or mash it with a fork, divide it into individual servings, and freeze it in an ice tray. We take it out of the freezer and heat up individual portions as needed. We haven't given her meat yet, but we've tried every kind of vegetable, like sweet potato, chard, spinach, and kale. She didn't like spinach at first, but I mixed it up with some mashed banana and she loved it. Since we are not giving her any grains with gluten, we feed her rice cereal, and she likes that too. Her pediatrician says she is doing fine on what we are giving her.

We belong to an organic co-op, a buying club organized by other families in our neighborhood. We pay a set fee on a weekly basis and we get a box of organic products: fruits, vegetables, eggs, organic chicken, and goat's milk, which is easier to digest than cow's milk. We pick up our box at one of the member's homes on Monday nights after work. You can ask for specific items if you like, but basically the club buys whatever is in season and divides it up among the members. It's a good deal: It costs us about $45 a week, and if I tried to buy all that produce in a natural foods store, it could easily be over $100.

Members of the co-op who have older children tell me that when they bring their box of produce home every week, the kids love going through it. They discover all kinds of new fruits and vegetables that they didn't know existed and are eager to try them. Then together, the family goes online and looks for recipes to make using the new produce. I can't wait until my daughter is old enough so that we can cook together.

or resolved completely during Phase 1 of our diet. I have also commonly seen individuals who did not want to move on from Phase 1, not just because of the rapidity of weight loss but because they felt so well. I had always attributed this good feeling to the reversal of metabolic syndrome, with its unpleasant swings in blood sugar, and also to the placebo effect from watching the numbers go down on the scale. But I have come to believe that many of these dramatic improvements were due to the removal of gluten from the diets of subjects who were gluten-intolerant and didn't know it. Some of these people even turned out to have celiac disease. It is logical that if at least one in a 100 Americans has celiac disease, and a great majority of them remain undiagnosed (along with many others who have a gluten intolerance), then the Phase 1 gluten-free experience would bring awareness of any gluten-related illness to many of these individuals.

Let me tell you about one such case.

Richard, a 50-year-old orthopedic surgeon, had suffered from gastrointestinal problems since childhood, and they had often made his life miserable. He recalled that back in medical school, his symptoms were so unpredictable that he refrained from eating for hours before exams or public events out of fear that he would be stricken with painful cramps, gas, or diarrhea.

As time went on, Richard added esophageal reflux to his list of woes. By his midforties, he had an elevated blood sugar and a middle-age paunch. A mutual friend, a physician who had trained with Richard, urged him to go on the South Beach Diet to shed his excess weight. And he did. Richard lost weight (and belly fat) quickly during his 2 weeks on Phase 1, but what surprised him was the dramatic reversal in his gastrointestinal symptoms. They resolved! His cramps, reflux, and diarrhea vanished.

Richard proceeded to Phase 2 of the diet, but when he added back whole-grain bread, his symptoms returned. He found he was able to tolerate fruits but not bread. This was a major "aha moment" for him. He realized for the first time that wheat products might be the source of his misery. His research led him to Dr. Peter H.R. Green, the director of the Celiac Disease Center at Columbia University in New York City, who confirmed that he did indeed have a gluten problem; Richard was eventually diagnosed with celiac disease.

It's important to note that celiac disease does run in families, and Dr. Green discovered that Richard's mother had been a lifelong, previously undiagnosed celiac disease sufferer. Remarkably, even as a physician with a history of many consultations with gastroenterologists, Richard had gone undiagnosed for more than 20 years!

Richard's experience and many similar stories from other South Beach patients on Phase 1 led me to my own "aha moment." Their stories prompted me to look at processed refined carbohydrates—and those made from wheat, in particular—as the potential culprit that was causing some of their myriad complaints. It was eerily similar to the way I had looked at refined carbohydrates as a cause of the increased incidence of weight gain and metabolic syndrome years ago. Just as it can lead to metabolic syndrome, our consumption of highly processed carbohydrates may also be responsible for the increased incidence of celiac disease and gluten intolerance in this country. Remember, metabolic syndrome wasn't discovered until 1989, and now it is epidemic. Gluten intolerance appears to be growing in a similarly rapid way. Our current intake of gluten from our massive consumption of white-flour-based processed foods is unprecedented.

Another fact that piqued my interest in gluten is that our hunter-gatherer ancestors were grain free and therefore gluten free. Grain did not become an important part of our diet until the first agricultural revolution 10,000 years ago. But back then, grain did not contain nearly the amount of gluten protein that today's wheat does. It would seem that our DNA was not designed for us to digest large amounts of grain and gluten. And in more recent times, our great-grandparents, though they consumed grains, would not have been exposed to the enormous number of gluten-containing packaged goods and fast foods we are consuming today.

THE SOUTH BEACH GLUTEN SOLUTION

At this time, I don't know, and I don't think anyone knows, the full extent to which gluten intolerance is affecting our health. So, when patients report having nonspecific symptoms consistent with gluten intolerance, I carefully review their diet history and proceed accordingly with blood tests for celiac disease, including genetic testing. For example, one recent symptomatic patient reported that when she visited her son in Greece and consumed local, healthy Mediterranean food for a few weeks, she had "never felt so great." Another patient with a fairly classic presentation of gluten-related problems (including several autoimmune disorders) recalled that when she went on Phase 1 of the South Beach Diet to lose weight before her son's wedding, she

The Lactose-Intolerance Connection

Remember that the hunter-gatherers did not consume dairy products once they were weaned from their mother's milk. Today, many people around the world are intolerant to lactose (the sugar found in milk), which causes them to experience uncomfortable symptoms like gas, stomach cramps, nausea, and diarrhea. Lactose intolerance has several interesting parallels with gluten intolerance.

Like grain, dairy has been around for thousands of years, and much of the world's population is lactose intolerant. This means that these individuals are lacking lactase, the enzyme in the small intestine that breaks down lactose into the simple sugars glucose and galactose, which are then easily absorbed into the bloodstream. Without enough lactase, lactose cannot be broken down and absorbed, and consequently proceeds down the intestine, where it often results in the unpleasant symptoms described above.

Lactose intolerance increases with age as our lactase production decreases. Depending on the amount of lactase they produce, individuals will tolerate various amounts of dairy, but if they consume more than their threshold, watch out. This is different from a milk allergy, which causes an immediate reaction to even a small amount of milk. An allergic reaction to milk can be likened to celiac disease because even a small amount of the offending substance precipitates an immediate reaction. Lactose intolerance, felt "fantastic" but assumed it was just the weight loss. Both patients had a favorable response when their gluten intake lessened or disappeared. Remember, even if the celiac tests are negative, a person may still be gluten intolerant, and unfortunately there are no reliable tests to diagnose this. That's when I prescribe what I call the "South Beach Diet Gluten Solution."

This "prescription" is a 1-month (at least) trial of not eating wheat and other gluten-containing grains, as well as any foods with added ingredients

on the other hand, is like gluten intolerance because the offending substance causes problems when not digested properly, but without the acute and immediate insult associated with celiac disease or an allergic reaction. Our individual ability to digest these substances is what determines the threshold amount of gluten or lactose that will induce an adverse reaction. People with lactose intolerance are usually able to tolerate some milk in their coffee, but an ice cream milkshake spells trouble.

Let's imagine what would happen to our population if we suddenly increased our dairy consumption severalfold. And what if the dairy was often hidden in products so that we were not even aware of how much we were consuming? And what if the condition of lactose intolerance was not on our radar screens and usually went undiagnosed? A substantial percentage of Americans would be quite uncomfortable a lot of the time.

I believe that this has in fact happened with gluten. It appears that a very significant increase in our consumption of gluten has occurred over the past 30 to 40 years, and we are just beginning to appreciate its impact on our health. The apparent similarities of the two conditions end when we realize the myriad serious health problems associated with gluten compared with the unpleasant but limited symptoms of lactose intolerance.

Oh, and by the way, the inflamed intestines of those with celiac disease destroy the enzyme lactase and therefore commonly cause lactose intolerance.

where gluten may be lurking. In effect, this "gluten solution" is really Phase 1 of the South Beach Diet, with the addition of fruits, alcohol in moderation, sweet potatoes, and brown rice and other nonglutenous grains. Or, put another way, it's Phase 2 without any foods containing gluten. Going gluten free with this approach can be a useful exercise to see whether symptoms improve and energy levels increase. It certainly doesn't hurt, because there are still plenty of good carbohydrates, including plenty of gluten-free grains, left to consume. I have found this trial to be very helpful for many of my patients and have seen quite a number of positive results, including the symptom improvement in the two women described above.

Fortunately, many healthy gluten-free products are on the market today, including many varieties of good-carb breads, pastas, and crackers made from brown rice flour, bean flour, and buckwheat flour. Don't make the mistake of going overboard with these products though. Look carefully at the ingredient list on gluten-free products. Many are made from white rice flour with little or no fiber, and many have added sugar and fat. Such products (like the low-fat and no-fat refined wheat-flour products that are laden with sugar and starch) can cause swings in blood sugar that can lead to hunger and cravings.

Keep in mind that both celiac disease and gluten intolerance are not just adult disorders. These problems are often seen in children, from infancy on. So if your child has stomach issues, skin problems, or allergies, talk with your pediatrician and ask about doing a trial of wheat-free or gluten-free eating. You may be surprised at the results.

As an aside, I also want to point out that athletes are taking an ever-increasing interest in a gluten-free approach to eating. As I write this, Novak Djokovic has just defeated Rafael Nadal in the 2011 Wimbledon final. Many who were impressed with Djokovic's game in the past also noted that his fitness level seemed to let him down in long matches. This all changed over the 2011 season, when (seemingly out of the blue) he began to dominate the professional tennis tour. What produced the change? The *Wall Street Journal* reported that his adoption of a gluten-free diet seemed to charge him up both physically and mentally.

Djokovic now consistently wins long matches (as well as short ones) and demonstrates outstanding fitness and concentration. He does not suffer from celiac disease but appears to be gluten intolerant. While anecdotal, there have been several reports of other professional athletes adopting a gluten-free diet and improving their performance. Hopefully, studies will be conducted to confirm these observations.

In the meantime, whether you are young, old, sedentary, or athletic, avoiding processed carbohydrates is likely to improve your health. Extending this recommendation to avoiding *all* wheat products for at least 1 month is a trial worth undertaking, especially if you have some of the potential gluten-related issues described above. I do, however, recommend that you see your physician first to get advice and baseline blood tests.

There is no question that our modern society has introduced too many foods that have not stood the test of time. It is reasonable to begin turning back our nutritional clock to help reverse the ill effects of our devastating fast-food lifestyle. The sooner, the better.

CHAPTER 7

THE POWER OF
THE DINING TABLE

Years ago, my wife and I were having dinner at a local restaurant when we saw something I remember to this day. A boy around 12 years old was sitting at a nearby table having dinner with his parents—to all appearances a happy family occasion. But when we looked closer, we noticed the preteen was wearing headphones and apparently listening to music, clearly oblivious to anything else going on at the table. We really didn't know or care if he was listening to rap or Mozart; we simply couldn't imagine ever allowing our own then-young sons to behave this way. We vowed that our family dinners, whether out or at home, would never look like that.

Unfortunately, the disconnected (or should I say, connected) youngster and his less-than-concerned parents represent a cultural problem that has gotten much worse in the past 20 years. As a society, we never planned to eliminate the family dinner. It just happened. Today families rarely sit down together for meals, and when they do, there is often very little communicating going on. Additionally, far too many children are "dining" on the grab-and-go junk food that has been made all too convenient, and the food they get at school is often not any better. *This has to change.*

As I will discuss later in this chapter, there is plenty of evidence that nutritious meals, eaten at an actual dining table, are good not only for our physical health but also for our mental health, and that includes both adults' and children's. In fact, it is equally important for empty nesters and for those who live alone to engage in dining rituals like setting the table and sitting down to a healthy home-cooked meal. All too often, people who live on their own or who no longer have children living under the same roof end up mindlessly eating whatever is most convenient wherever they happen to be. Unfortunately, this behavior often piles on unwanted pounds and also prevents people from actually enjoying what should be one of the most pleasant times of the day: mealtime.

Fortunately, change is possible. I saw this firsthand when I visited an inner-city high school in Philadelphia. It is one of 20 public schools participating in an ongoing educational health and nutrition program being conducted by the Agatston Urban Nutrition Initiative (AUNI) through the Netter Center for Community Partnerships at the University of Pennsylvania. While at the school, I watched Jazmin, a high school junior, conduct a healthy-cooking demonstration for her peers. With ease, the young chef whipped up a stir-fry of sliced red and green bell peppers, broccoli, and carrots. As she tossed the vegetables around in a large skillet, she described how she prepared the ingredients and explained their nutritional value. She was clearly enjoying herself, and I thoroughly enjoyed her presentation.

After the cooking class, I asked Jazmin who in her family cooks meals like this. I expected her to say "my grandmother" or "my great-aunt" or something like that. I was surprised when she replied, "Well, no one." She told me that fresh food is hard to come by in her neighborhood and that for most of her life she has eaten processed foods, usually take-out from fast-food joints. In fact, Jazmin said, almost nobody in her community cooked. But what seemed to bother her more was that even her family celebrations were built around going out to a fast-food restaurant or bringing fast food home. The school-run program was her first exposure to "home" cooking.

Recently I was back in Philadelphia to meet with the AUNI program directors, and I observed another cooking class. There was Jazmin again, only this time in a different role: She was teaching fourth and fifth graders how to cook and encouraging them to share their experience with their families. The kids did an amazing job, expertly preparing a tasty and healthy meal and having a great time doing it. This was an after-school elective program, and I remarked to the principal that it would be wonderful if nutrition education and cooking classes could be part of the standard curriculum rather than just an after-school option.

I asked Jazmin what else she had been doing since I had last seen her, and she said she was also volunteering at a seniors' center in her neighborhood. When I first met her, she told me that no one in her family had taught her to cook, and now here she was, determined to change the future for others by teaching many grandmothers to cook.

Jazmin's experience cooking in school illustrates that such programs not only present a wonderful opportunity to teach children about good nutrition but also encourage them to bring this learning home. We've seen this approach work with smoking, where kids who were taught the dangers of smoking in school then went home and begged their parents to quit. I remember kids who were so motivated that they threw away their parents' cigarettes. Similarly, in the schools where we've worked to establish healthy nutrition programs, we've heard from parents who say that they're now buying more fruits and vegetables because their kids are asking them to.

Jazmin's observations about her West Philadelphia neighborhood are not unusual: Nationally, it is estimated that one in three meals today is eaten out of the home, mainly at fast-food restaurants. This figure is corroborated by others from the Bureau of Labor Statistics, which show that the average household spends $2,189 at restaurants and take-out establishments, or 58 percent of the $3,753 it spends on groceries. The percentage is even higher for some demographic segments, such as householders ages 25 to 34 (67 percent) and people who live alone (67 percent). As I have already noted, this trend is taking a terrible toll on our health, which is the primary reason it is so important to reverse it among the younger generation.

DINING OUT: THE CHALLENGE

Eating out frequently is, in itself, a recipe for disaster. I see the results in many of my patients who travel and entertain clients for work. Although they are not eating in fast-food restaurants, they still have a very hard time keeping their weight, blood pressure, and cholesterol levels under control. Just recently, a patient in his late twenties provided an excellent explanation of why restaurant eating can be a challenge.

John came to see me during a school break because his previously mild hypertension had gotten out of control. It turned out his school was a prestigious culinary academy on the West Coast. John told me that I wouldn't believe the amount of salt, butter, and sugar that was poured into the epicurean dishes he was learning to prepare. When he commented to his instructor that the ingredients in a particular recipe weren't very healthy, the answer was, "Whoever said anything about healthy?" Since that conversation with John, I have never looked at a restaurant meal in quite the same way. It was clear that John's rich gourmet meals, which had caused him to pack on the weight, had also put his blood pressure over the top.

Studies confirm what I have observed so often in my practice and have experienced myself. The more meals you eat outside the home, the more likely you are to be overweight and suffer from obesity-related ailments. Although you can order sensibly from most restaurant menus, the fact is, when you are not in control of how the food is prepared, you are likely to consume far more bad fats, bad carbs, excess calories, and sodium than you would if you ate a home-cooked meal. In addition, when large plates of food are left in front of you for long periods of time, it promotes mindless eating, often beyond appetite satisfaction. (No need to waste the food you've paid for; ask for a doggie bag.)

A case in point regarding the hazards of eating out is the counterintuitive story of my friend Michael, a noncompliant patient with coronary artery disease and type 2 diabetes. His high-powered job requires him to travel a lot and entertain at upscale restaurants. Michael often has difficulty sticking to a healthy diet when he is tempted by great food. He once called me from California's Napa Valley, and when I asked what he was up to, he said, "I'm on my way to the French Laundry. It's the best restaurant in the world." Wonderful place to go, I thought, when you're supposed to be trying to lose weight. So I told him, "Great. Just don't eat anything."

The tale continues. While on one of his many business trips, Michael unfortunately—at least I thought it was unfortunate at the time—slipped and broke his ankle. He was required to stay housebound for 6 weeks while it healed—his longest stretch at home in years. I thought, "Uh oh, more trouble."

People who experience orthopedic injuries and become immobile almost inevitably gain weight because they're forced to become sedentary and often use food as an antidepressant. Not Michael. He's an excellent cook who knows how to make healthy food that tastes good, and so does his wife. He proceeded to *lose* 28 pounds in 6 weeks and his diabetes completely resolved. His blood tests looked great and so did he. Once healed, Michael hit the road again for a long West Coast swing. My message to him before he left: "As your doctor, I am obligated to tell you that if you gain the weight back, my therapeutic approach will be clear—I'll have to break your other leg!"

"A CHICKEN IN EVERY POT, A CHEF IN EVERY KITCHEN"

There is no doubt that eating home-cooked meals is better both nutritionally and psychologically. The sad reality, however, is that from a time perspective, it has become much easier to feed a family quickly with processed, mass-prepared food than by cooking at home. And many families erroneously think fast food is cheaper as well.

Yes, cooking healthy meals at home does take more time and planning. But that doesn't mean it isn't worth doing. To the contrary: With knowledge, some forethought, and practice, it can become a manageable, enjoyable, and affordable experience. We give you tips on shopping for and cooking family meals on pages 192–215.

A wealthy patient of mine provides an unusual illustration of the benefits of well-planned home-cooked meals. She lost weight, normalized her blood chemistries, and has maintained her good health. How did she do it? Simple. She hired a five-star chef, gave him her guidelines for healthy eating (and some South Beach Diet cookbooks), and told him, "If I gain weight, you're fired!" After 3 years, he is still cooking for her family and she still looks great, as do her husband and two sons.

The fact is, in reality, most people don't need a five-star chef to make healthy meals at home or to help them lose weight while following the South Beach Diet lifestyle. But I was thinking this could be an innovative government program: "A chicken in every pot, a chef in every kitchen." It might be beneficial for the national nutritional debt I talked about in Chapter 1, but obviously not too good for the national monetary debt. The story of my lucky patient with a personal chef demonstrates the potential for turning our nutrition and health around if we could just make it easier for everyone to have access to healthy food.

With greater demand from educated consumers, there will be farmers' markets, food co-ops, and natural foods supermarkets in more and more neighborhoods. It is already happening in many areas, just not nearly fast enough. So for now, for those of us without a personal chef or a food co-op down the street, eating healthy requires a commitment and we can afford to do it. When we understand the ultimate nutritional, psychological, and economic costs of not having healthy family dinners, we will understand the absolute necessity of making this commitment.

Once you start cooking healthy meals at home, their many benefits will provide plenty of incentive to continue and they will become much easier to plan and prepare. We can all learn to make nourishing family dinners (as well as breakfasts and lunches). I know this because there are so many Super Moms and Dads from all walks of life out there who are doing this right now. They've experienced the payoff and know it is worth it.

THE PERKS OF FAMILY MEALS

Let's review some compelling research that shows the importance of family meals not only for children's health but also for their emotional well-being.

Children who routinely eat meals with their families are more likely to maintain a healthy weight, eat a healthier diet, and have a lower risk of developing abnormal eating patterns (like bingeing or purging, fasting, or taking diet pills), according to an article published in 2011 in the journal *Pediatrics*. Researchers at the Family Resiliency Center of the University of Illinois analyzed 17 studies on the impact of family meals that included 182,836 children and adolescents between the ages of 3 and 17. Children who ate three or more meals a week with their families were 12 percent less likely to be overweight, 20 percent less likely to eat unhealthy foods, 24 percent more likely to eat healthy foods like fruits and vegetables, and 35 percent less likely to engage in disordered eating behaviors.

A study published in *Circulation* in November 2010 documented the sig-

Nicole S.

Super Mom, Katonah, New York

"I've worked really hard to get my kids to try new foods."

I have a 6-year-old and a 3-year-old. Both girls. My friends marvel at the fact that both my kids eat vegetables. They love asparagus, they ask for brussels sprouts, they eat cauliflower, broccoli—they gobble up pretty much any vegetable that I serve them. They even eat edamame! In fact, that's a staple in our house.

I've worked really hard to get my kids to try new foods. I can pretty much get them to try any new food that is within reason. I'm not going to pick something like caviar that's going to look yucky to a child, but my younger girl tried salmon with balsamic vinegar the other day. Now, she didn't like it, but she tried it. I let her spit it out if she hates it, but at least I get her to give it a try.

How do I do it? We have a family ritual around trying new foods, and it works for us. It started when I read my first child the book *Green Eggs and Ham,* by Dr. Seuss. Remember that book? In it, a character named Sam tries to get another Seuss character to eat green eggs and ham in all sorts of places—in a house with a mouse, in a box with a fox, and so on—until, at the very end, he does try the green eggs and ham and discovers that he actually likes them! That's one of my kids' favorite books, so I read it to them a lot. Every once in a while, while we're reading it, I ask them, "How does he know that he doesn't like green eggs and ham if he never actually tried them?" When I want my kids to try a new food, I remind them of the book. I tell them, "If you don't try it, you don't know if you'll like it, and if you try it, you may like it."

nificance of fruit and vegetable consumption for children's future cardiovascular health. Since 1980, the Cardiovascular Risk in Young Finns Study has followed 4,320 children ranging in age from 3 to 18 years, focusing on diet

They will usually try it. Then, after we've found one they do like, we do a little food dance. We all put our hands in the air and we literally dance around, going "OOOOOHHHH, new food!" Again, it's all about making food fun.

What I've also discovered is that when I find a new food that the kids like, it doesn't necessarily mean that they'll eat it every time. Kids get bored, and if you give them the same thing every day, they're not going to eat it. Incorporating the new foods about once a week is what I've found works best.

I don't let them eat junk, but I've learned that if they get too hungry, they will grab anything. So I put out small plates of healthy snacks all day, especially colorful fruits and vegetables, like berries and carrots. I also give them nuts, cheese, and whole-grain crackers. They don't ask for sugary stuff. I give them fresh fruit or a squeezable yogurt pop for dessert. I don't give them chips or juice; they drink water and organic milk. I only serve them organic meat, dairy, eggs, and poultry. I worked for Planned Parenthood as a nurse before I had children, and I saw girls coming in who had gotten their periods as early as 9 and 10 years old, and I came to believe it's from all the hormones and antibiotics in our food. So I try to avoid giving my kids anything that is loaded with chemicals.

We can't keep them away from fast food entirely—that's not realistic. We did celebrate a couple of their friends' birthday parties recently at McDonald's. We taught them that this is a special treat. My husband was with them at the party and he didn't get them the french fries, because he told them we don't eat this kind of food. They didn't even question him. They ate the apple slices instead and were happy.

and lifestyle. A 27-year follow-up of 1,622 of the study participants found that the now-grown men and women who had consistently eaten the most fruits and vegetables from childhood on had more flexible, healthier arteries, compared with those who ate the least amount of these foods. So if kids eat more fruits and vegetables at family dinners today, it appears they will have healthier arteries as adults.

Family meals go well beyond nourishing young bodies. They also seem to play a significant role in producing happier, better-adjusted kids who are less likely to fall prey to problems like substance abuse. Numerous studies confirm that children who are raised in homes where they frequently eat meals with at least one parent do better in every aspect of their lives than children from homes where family meals are rare. A 2010 report, "The Importance of Family Dinners VI," issued by the National Center on Addiction and Substance Abuse at Columbia University, concluded that teenagers who ate dinner with their parents three or fewer times a week were twice as likely to use tobacco, nearly twice as likely to use alcohol, and 1.5 times as likely to use marijuana, compared with teens who ate dinner with their parents five or more times a week. Not surprisingly, those teens who rarely had meals with their parents were also more likely to have friends that dabbled in illegal drugs and alcohol.

What is interesting about this report, which was based on a survey of 1,055 teens and 456 of their parents via the Internet and 1,000 more teens on the phone, is that the teenagers themselves understood the value of family dinners. In fact, 72 percent of them agreed that eating dinner frequently as a family is very or fairly important. Perhaps even more telling, three out of four teens surveyed said that they actually talked to their parents about what was going on in their lives over dinner. And they said that the more often they ate dinner with their parents, the more they talked!

Still other studies have shown that teens who routinely ate meals with their parents or who "felt close" to their parents not only had higher grade point averages at school and intended to go on to college, but also were less likely to engage in early sexual activity, use drugs, have suicidal thoughts, or be in a serious fight. Overall they were happier and healthier and led more productive lives.

So maybe I have my own mom and dad to thank for my healthy adulthood and that of my three siblings. I grew up in a family of four children in the 1950s and '60s, and I remember our family dinners very well. I certainly didn't think about the emotional benefits at the time—dinnertime was just dinnertime. But I do recall great discussions about politics, medicine (my father was a doctor and my mom thought she was), school, and other issues of the day, such as recent Yankee trades. I have fond memories of our family dinners, and I wish that today's children could reap the benefits I and many others of my generation experienced from this important cultural tradition.

GEORGE WASHINGTON ATE HERE

The importance of eating together extends beyond the family dinner table. In Ron Chernow's superb chronicle of our first president, *Washington: A Life*, he recounts that even during the horrible winter at Valley Forge, Washington and his staff still took the time to sit down daily for a formal lunch.

That lunch table was a social hub where ideas were exchanged, strategies were brainstormed, and relationships were built. Young officers could soak in the knowledge of those older and more experienced and could comfortably express their own ideas as well. Sharing a meal was important for team building then, and this has not changed. In fact, communal meals have become potentially more important for solidifying relationships in our overscheduled, social-networking, virtual world, where actual face time has diminished.

THE WASTED OPPORTUNITY OF THE SCHOOL LUNCH

If, in the middle of the winter at Valley Forge, George Washington could make time for lunch with his colleagues, why can't we schedule sufficient time for our kids to enjoy a sociable lunch at school? Sadly, speeding through meals has become a way of life for most of today's schoolchildren, and not by their own choice. According to a comprehensive report, "The State of Nutrition and Physical Activity in Our Schools," 34 percent of US schools give the last student in the lunch line as little as 10 minutes to finish eating. And if that's not enough to ruin an appetite and encourage bad eating habits, the report also notes that some schools are so overcrowded that they have to schedule lunch breaks starting as early as 9:25 a.m. to accommodate the entire student body. This is discouraging. How are we ever going to teach our kids to sit down and enjoy a meal if their adult role models don't think it's important to incorporate this concept into the very place where kids spend so much of their time?

A few years ago, Alice Waters, one of the foremost advocates for school lunch reform, came to Miami Beach to participate at a symposium the Agatston Research Foundation sponsored on childhood obesity. I had been influenced by her Edible Schoolyard project, which she established in 1995 at Berkeley, California's Martin Luther King Jr. Middle School. At the symposium, however, I was particularly fascinated when she described how, as part of the program, students sat down to eat lunch at round tables with tablecloths and real utensils. The students were joined by an adult who engaged them in conversation. Boy, what an opportunity for acculturation, socialization, healthy eating, and relaxation during the school day. Schools, especially elementary schools, are the best place to begin to change our toxic lifestyle. It is in schools that we can teach kids to appreciate and enjoy healthy food while they learn the importance of good nutrition and good manners for a happy, productive life.

How do I know this can be done? Because we have done it and are currently doing it.

IF YOU SERVE IT, THEY WILL EAT IT . . . EVENTUALLY

My experience with school lunches began back in 2004 with the development of the Healthier Options for Public Schoolchildren (HOPS) program. When I first decided that an important focus of our foundation should be childhood nutrition, I naively thought we could just march into a high school, change the cafeteria food, and prove that healthy food was good for kids. When I consulted a patient and friend, Melanie Fox, a well-respected elementary school principal in Miami, I was quickly set straight. She told me that high school students prefer to eat off campus rather than in the school cafeteria.

Melanie became a consultant for HOPS and quickly convinced me that our program would be much more effective in elementary schools, because elementary school children would be much more amenable to a transition to healthy breakfasts, lunches, and snacks. Melanie turned out to be absolutely right.

Led by Danielle Hollar, PhD, and Marie Almon, MS, RD, the Agatston Research Foundation took on the school meals program in four of six elementary schools in Osceola County, Florida (two of the schools participated as control schools and operated as usual). Our goal was to perform a cafeteria makeover and engage the administration, faculty, cafeteria workers, and, most important, the students in the process. This turned out to be quite challenging, but surprisingly, the biggest obstacle we faced was not the attitude of the kids—which was great—it was that of the adults.

While there were plenty of hurdles, we learned that, with some flexibility and a willingness to make adjustments, things could be changed. Dr. Hollar engaged an educational products company called OrganWise Guys, headed up by Michelle Lombardo, to organize schoolwide assemblies and provide nutrition education materials. Lessons were integrated into the classroom, and Dr. Hollar and Marie Almon taught cafeteria personnel how to select the most nutritious foods from local vendors and from those listed on the USDA commodities fact sheets. Posters depicting a healthy fruit or vegetable of the month (often one the kids may not have tried before) were put up in the schools' hallways. School gardens were started so the children could see where their food came from. Through food tastings and nutrition education showing food's relation to a strong and healthy body, the kids gradually accepted and became excited about the new, nutritious foods they were being served. One third grader so enjoyed her first taste of grapes that she asked whether her mother could get these at the market so she could enjoy them at home.

Our healthy nutrition approach benefited all kids, thin and heavy alike. We learned this because HOPS began as a study, where we tracked the weights, blood pressures, and standardized test scores of about 4,700 kids for 2 years in all six schools. In the HOPS intervention schools, we found that both the heavy and thin kids achieved a healthier weight, and they also tended to have lower blood pressures. Perhaps most gratifying, the students in the HOPS intervention schools received significantly better math scores on Florida's standardized tests. Good nutrition made for better grades.

This was all very reassuring. For me, however, the most important finding was that, given the right setting, elementary school children will embrace healthy food and often take the message home. One of my most moving stories is about Johnny, a fourth grader whose mother called the school principal when Johnny refused to eat what he correctly perceived to be the less-than-healthy dinner his mother was serving him at home. Johnny's mother pleaded with the principal to ask Johnny to eat the food because she had already spent her food budget for that week. She promised to provide healthier dishes the next week. Johnny was bringing the lessons of good nutrition back to his family.

The fact is, nutrition education should not be a contest between home and school. Good habits established in the home need to be reinforced at school. And perhaps more important, the schools must provide healthy meals and nutrition education for those kids who aren't given healthy meals at home. Our children are our most important resource, and such cooperation is essential to ensure their welfare.

GOOD DIET *AND* EXERCISE IMPROVE BRAINPOWER

As part of our HOPS program we encouraged more exercise, though accomplishing this during the 2 years of the study was difficult because of the restricted time schools allow for physical education and recess. The importance of a rigorous physical education program was highlighted by one of the HOPS control schools, which did not have the benefit of the nutrition program but did have an award-winning physical education program. This school had decided that physical education was a priority, even though most public elementary schools in Florida were sacrificing phys ed in favor of additional preparation time for the statewide standardized tests. Because of the state's curriculum guidelines at the time, the "exercise" school was unique. The rules have thankfully changed to require more physical education in schools, but not all educators seem to understand its value. Not long ago, the *Christian Science Monitor* reported that, purportedly, in some South Florida schools, walking to the cafeteria was counted toward fulfilling the exercise requirement. We found that the children in the PE-focused school tended to experience less weight gain, though they did not do as well as the kids in the HOPS intervention schools. Clearly, the best outcomes would certainly have resulted from combining vigorous exercise with good nutrition.

This finding is consistent with an ever-growing mountain of data linking exercise and brainpower (I will discuss this more in Chapter 8). One intriguing study published in the *Proceedings of the National Academy of Sciences* in 2009 showed that cardiovascular fitness changes occurring between the ages of 15 and 18 predict not only cognitive performance at age 18 but also educational achievement later in life.

I strongly believe that if we do not include physical education in schools, it will have an adverse impact on long-term as well as short-term health and achievement. The evidence indicates that extra time spent on test preparation at the expense of physical education and healthy school lunches is counter productive and even destructive. It is no substitute for the mental and physical health benefits of good nutrition and exercise. Our children deserve better.

SPREADING THE WORD:
THE UNIVERSITY-COMMUNITY STRATEGY

After our experience with the HOPS study, in which it became clear that children would welcome healthy food and that positive results could be realized, I looked for a way to spread the program to additional schools and schoolchildren and their families. This led to a collaboration with the Netter Center for Community Partnerships at the University of Pennsylvania, where my son was an undergraduate. Led by its founding director, Professor Ira Harkavy, and supported by a fabulous staff, the Netter Center integrates community service into the university curriculum.

The Agatston Urban Nutrition Initiative was established as a Netter Center program to improve community nutrition and health, with a particular focus on kids in grades K through 12. Penn students and faculty run and staff the program. Wharton business school students, for example, teach public schoolkids how to run fruit and vegetable stands in their schoolyards to raise money for their own school programs. Other Penn students work with the kids to plant school gardens and teach nutrition and cooking so high school students like Jazmin can work with younger children and bring the message of healthy eating home to their own families. Because the program is integrated into the university curriculum, it is sustainable—a very important feature.

The Netter Center and AUNI are currently developing a network of universities dedicated to building such university-community partnerships across the country. College students have an energy and enthusiasm that's well suited to community service and to providing education, guidance, and mentoring to public school children. If all goes well, not only will these students spread the word about how important good nutrition is to good health, but they'll also encourage families to once again embrace home cooking and communal dining.

The power of the dining table to influence our nation's health and well-being should not be underestimated. Every meal that is eaten on the run, in your car, or gulped down staring at a screen is a missed opportunity, whether you are dining solo, with your spouse or friends, or with your children. By design, mealtime should provide a break in your hectic schedule, a few moments of calm when you can catch your breath, or catch up on what is happening in the lives of your loved ones or friends. It is a time to enjoy and appreciate the home-cooked food on your plate. It is a time to be nourished both physically and emotionally.

So, sit down, savor your food, relax, talk, share, and reclaim the power of the dining table.

CHAPTER 8

THE HIGH COST OF INACTIVITY

Walking on South Beach, I can easily assess the amount of time various passersby are spending in the gym. The warm weather and proximity to the beach mean that the scantily clad are out and about. Lincoln Road plays host to a parade of people of all ages with fit bodies and toned muscles. The biggest beneficiary of their workouts, however, may be a vital anatomical part you can't see: their hippocampus.

The hippocampus resides deep in our brain and is considered our memory center. It is particularly vital for learning and processing new information. We have long known that as we age, our muscle mass tends to decrease and our bones tend to lose density (osteopenia or osteoporosis). It turns out that our brains also tend to atrophy with age, along with our hippocampus. This shrinking is known to be associated with mild cognitive dysfunction, which can progress to dementia and possibly to Alzheimer's. But fortunately, the hippocampus does not always atrophy, and everyone's hippocampus certainly doesn't atrophy at the same rate.

We used to believe that once a portion of the hippocampus or any other part of the brain atrophied, it was lost forever. Recently, however, neuroscientists have found that brain cells are neuroplastic; in other words, under the right circumstances, brain cells (like most cells in the body) can regenerate. Animal studies have shown that aerobic exercise can boost production of a growth factor called "brain derived neurotrophic factor," or BDNF, which increases the size of the hippocampus and in so doing improves learning and memory. This has raised the inevitable question: Could exercise have the same impact on human brains?

In a landmark study published in 2011 in the *Proceedings of the National Academy of Sciences,* researchers looked at the effect of exercise on the human hippocampus in individuals in their mid- to late sixties, a time when the hippocampus tends to get smaller (not coincidentally, about the same time as the "Where did I put my keys?" syndrome begins to hit). Using magnetic resonance imaging (MRI), they showed that a modest exercise program not only prevented atrophy in the hippocampus; it actually made it *larger.* As with the animal models, BDNF levels also increased in the exercising humans. So, if you want to be smarter and prevent dementia, use your head and start exercising.

MORE HIDDEN BENEFITS OF EXERCISE

Your memory is not the only area helped by exercise. In fact, it seems that exercise is about as close to being a panacea as anything in our medical arsenal. If you could take a magic potion to improve your overall health, protect against chronic disease, and give you more energy, you would certainly take it, right? We are coming to realize that exercise just might be that magic potion. Its benefits go well beyond stronger muscles and better endurance. You just have to learn how to exercise properly and efficiently (we have been doing a lot wrong in recent years) in a manner that fits into your life fairly seamlessly. A great attribute of exercise is that once you get into a routine, you'll never want to skip a session. This may be due to the feel-good, opiate-like hormones known as endorphins and to the more recently studied neurochemicals called endocannabinoids that exercise produces, as well as other factors. Whatever the mechanism, exercise is addictive.

Once you appreciate the benefits of exercise, I hope you'll make regular exercise a part of your life. In Chapter 2, I wrote about how our bodies are aging, or "rusting," prematurely from a "chemical bath" due to the related problems of oxidation and inflammation. I ascribed this largely to our fast-food lifestyle and failure to consume enough anti-inflammatory, antioxidant fruits, vegetables, and healthy fats. But that's not the whole story.

Exercise also plays a defining role in this equation.

As I touched on in Chapter 2, exercise is anti-inflammatory and stimulates our intrinsic production of antioxidants, helping to keep the degenerative rusting process under control. It even helps combat the "oxidant stress" that's created by eating fast food. Research shows that people who exercise regularly and have a fast-food meal have more pliant blood vessels than the couch potatoes who consume the same bad meal. It is therefore not surprising to learn that getting enough exercise has broad benefits mirroring those of eating a nutritious diet. To review quickly, regular exercise strengthens your bones, preserves your muscles, and slows the degenerative changes of aging, including arthritis. It can also boost your mood and your sex life and give you more energy in general. Aerobic exercise ("cardio") is great for your heart and lungs. It reduces the risk of high blood pressure, diabetes, and consequent heart attack and stroke. And it can even protect against many forms of cancer.

Abundant scientific research has shown that physical activity can reduce the risk of cancers of the breast, colon, endometrium (the lining of the uterus), prostate, and lung. Of these cancers, evidence is strongest for its protecting against breast and colon cancer, two of the most common. A study published in 2010 in the *Archives of Internal Medicine* analyzed data from the Nurses' Health Study gathered from 1986 to 2006. During that time, there were 4,782 cases of invasive breast cancer among the 95,396 postmenopausal women who were followed for those 20 years. Women who engaged in the highest amounts of activity after menopause were at the lowest risk for developing breast cancer. We're not talking about mountain climbers or marathoners here: The researchers cited brisk walking as one of the activities that helped protect against cancer.

While you are helping to lower your risk for breast cancer when you exercise, you are also reducing your risk for colon and rectal (colorectal) cancer. A meta-analysis (in which study results are combined and then analyzed) of 52 studies published in 2009 in the *British Journal of Cancer* found that those who were most active were 24 percent less likely to develop colon cancer than those who were the least physically active. Considering the fact that in 2010 alone there were more than 209,000 new cases of breast cancer and 142,500 new cases of colorectal cancer in men and women in the United States, simply exercising more could result in hundreds of thousands fewer cases of these cancers over time.

WHY IS SITTING SO BAD FOR US?

So it's clear that exercise is good for fighting cancer. But just how bad is the tremendous amount of time we spend sitting these days? In the very large Cancer Prevention II study, begun in 1992, American Cancer Society research-ers analyzed the effect of leisure time spent "sitting" and death rates from all causes including cancer in approximately 123,000 participants between the years 1993 to 2006. According to their findings, reported in a 2010 article in the *American Journal of Epidemiology,* time spent sitting was "independently associated" with total mortality, especially from heart disease, regardless of physical activity level. In other words, based on this study, your risk of death may be more dependent on how much you sit than on how much you exer-cise. "Chair time" was a strong risk factor for dying of a heart-related event and for many forms of cancer as well. Women who sat more than 6 hours a day had an especially high risk of death as compared with those who spent half that time sitting. This is not to say that physical activity didn't matter. People who were sedentary and the most inactive were at a greater risk of dying than those who spent a lot of time sitting but did daily activities like housework, walking, or shopping. While "exercise time" clearly does wonders for the body, it appears it cannot overcome the destructive effects of spending too much time sitting.

This raises the question, just why *is* sitting so bad for you? A research group at the University of Missouri found that in addition to deconditioning your body (if you don't use it, you lose it), sitting alters the way the body metabolizes fat. Among other things, it shuts off lipase, a pancreatic enzyme that is key for the absorption of fat into muscles. Lipase deficiency allows fat to build up in the bloodstream. This can result in elevated levels of bad LDL cholesterol and tri-glycerides, excess belly fat, and, ultimately, prediabetes, diabetes, and heart disease.

Exercise Can Help Combat Colds

There is evidence that the pain-in-the-neck common cold can be warded off by exercise. A brisk walk every day can boost your immune system and help you stay cold free, or lessen the severity of a cold if you get one. Researchers at Appalachian State University tracked the respiratory health of 1,002 adults ages 18 to 85 for 12 weeks during the winter (January to April) and the autumn (August to November) of 2008. They found that those who did moderate aerobic exercise 5 or more days per week for at least 20 minutes a day had 43 percent fewer reported sick days from colds than those who exercised for less time or not at all. Reporting their results in the *British Journal of Sports Medicine,* the researchers noted that the severity of symptoms fell by 41 percent among the participants who felt the fittest and by 32 percent in those who were the most active, regardless of age. They also noted that while the immune activity brought on by exercise only lasts for a few hours, it is the cumulative immune effect that seems to keep regular exercisers healthier.

Today, there's no question that the benefits of exercise go well beyond having stronger muscles and better endurance. And yet most Americans are doing way more sitting than exercising. According to recent statistics, about two-thirds of American adults report that they are physically inactive—that is, they are sedentary most of the time. And only about 22 percent of American adults say that they do any meaningful exercise at all. To put this in perspective, the 65 percent of the population that routinely drives instead of walks, sits instead of stands, and rides the elevator instead of taking the stairs is at an increased risk for all the chronic conditions I mentioned above and will ultimately pay a high price in terms of their physical and mental health. This has important implications for how we design the workplace in the digital era. Sitting at a computer all day can kill us.

THE HIGH COST OF INACTIVITY

Often in medicine, as in life, we can best appreciate the importance of something only when it has been taken away. In clinical practice we observe first-hand what happens to an individual's cardiac risk profile when that person has an abrupt change in lifestyle. This brings me to the story of Nancy, a patient who had always been the picture of good health. Her frequent visits to my office were mainly to accompany her husband, who had serious heart issues. Nancy had always been my role model when it came to exercise and nutrition. In her midsixties, this former professional dancer kept in wonderful shape with activities ranging from walking and biking to Pilates and kickboxing. She was doing great until she blew out her anterior cruciate ligament (ACL) in a ski accident and had to undergo surgery. Her recovery was complicated by an infection, and for the first time in her life, Nancy couldn't exercise. She became depressed, discouraged, and indulgent with her diet. She gained 25 pounds in just 4 months, and her blood chemistries suddenly reflected prediabetes, which had never been an issue for her.

Stories like Nancy's are replayed in my practice regularly when patients are involuntarily sidelined by injury or illness and forced to be sedentary. (My globe-trotting friend Michael, whom I mentioned in the last chapter, is an exception, since he used his housebound recovery time to prepare healthy meals.) Fortunately, Nancy's story has a happy ending. Once she was able to do active rehab, she lost the weight, improved her blood sugar, and began to feel better psychologically and physically.

Unfortunately, too many Americans have the exercise habits and diet of the injured Nancy, only they haven't been in a ski accident.

FROM THE HUNTER-GATHERER TO THE ROBOTIC LAWN MOWER

Before we focus on what has happened to physical activity in the modern world, let's take another quick look at the way our bodies were designed to function. In the age of the hunter-gatherer, men and women had to expend an enormous amount of calories just to provide enough food and shelter to survive. Even after the agricultural revolution, calorie expenditure remained high. Hard physical activity was still the norm on the farm and in the fields. In the early days of the industrial revolution in the 1800s, factories and mills were becoming automated but the work continued to require a great deal of exertion.

As the industrial revolution progressed, more labor-saving devices were developed, but it wasn't until the digital revolution that our calorie expenditure radically decreased. Just as Nancy's accident removed exercise from her life, technology has largely removed vigorous physical activity from our daily lives as a society. And though we might think that we have replaced its benefits with a little exercise at the beginning or end of the day, we may be deluding ourselves. You might be surprised to learn that from the early 1900s through the 1970s, there was a trend toward consuming *fewer* calories in the United States! Could this be true? Weren't we getting fatter? The answers are yes and yes. We were getting fatter. And we were consuming fewer calories. The reason for this apparent paradox is that with major migrations from the farm to the city, we were also doing less daily vigorous labor and therefore required fewer calories. We got fatter because the decrease in exertion "outweighed" the decrease in calories. Disturbingly, since the 1970s, the trend toward consuming fewer calories has reversed itself. And, as you know, this is not because we have returned to the fields. We are doing less physical activity in our workplaces and in our homes than ever before. No wonder we have an obesity epidemic.

Which brings me to the robotic lawn mower. In the past you might have worked up a sweat doing yard work, but consider how this one typical task—cutting the lawn—has evolved to the point where human beings quite literally don't have to lift a finger. Up until the past 200 years or so, when the grass had to be cut, we took out our machetes, and later our scythes, and hacked it down. It was grueling work. Once the manual cylinder lawn mower was invented in the early 19th century, it saved energy (and time) but still took a fair amount of muscle to get the job done. Next came the power mower, which practically moved itself along but still required physical exertion to achieve a manicured lawn. This was followed by the tractor mower, which allowed you to cut the grass while sitting down. Now you don't even have to walk out of your house to mow your lawn. Why go out in the hot sun when you can buy a computer-driven robotic mower that does all the work for you? If you don't believe me, just Google "robotic lawn mower." You might want to buy two in case one malfunctions.

Technology has also automated our workplaces. In my own office, we no longer have to travel the halls carrying patients' charts from room to room, because our medical records are electronic and we are paperless. I recently visited a genetics lab that had just replaced 20 full-time employees with 2 humans and a roomful of robotic arms. I watched in amazement as the robots processed blood samples from various clinical studies around the world while the sole human in the room monitored the activity on a computer (or maybe the robots were monitoring her?). The second human was giving me the tour. Today gall bladder removal, hysterectomy, and even heart surgery, which were routinely performed standing, are starting to be done by surgeons sitting at a computer. The surgeons manipulate instruments that work robotically through small incisions with the help of miniaturized cameras. The surgeons can see what they're doing more clearly than ever before. This robotic surgery even has the potential to be done remotely. In the future, surgeons may not even have to get dressed and leave their homes—scary.

Again, don't get me wrong. I am not arguing that we trash all the computers and go back to the wild or back to the field or to hacking grass. Technology is critical to our efforts to become so efficient and productive that all in our country and around the world can live better lives. It's just that we have to recognize that human beings were not designed to be sitting bent over computers all day and that doing so is taking a tremendous toll on our health. And this will only get worse with further automation.

STAND UP FOR HEALTH!

I recently came across an editorial in the journal *Diabetes* called "Health-Chair Reform," written by James A. Levine, MD, of the Mayo Clinic. In the article, Dr. Levine warns, "Modernity has imposed a Chair Sentence; work, home and play are the shackles." He references studies that show the devastating impact of "chair living" and describes how this is in direct opposition to the way the human body was designed to work: upright and mobile. "The human evolved to feed, shelter, and invent while ambulatory," he explains. "The human, simply put, was not designed to sit all day."

I have been a fan of Dr. Levine's since I met him on a visit to the Mayo Clinic many years ago, when he described what I still consider to be his ingenious approach to measuring the energy burned by our activities throughout the day—not just during exercise. To do this, he "wired" each of his subjects with special motion-tracking underwear that recorded all their daily movements. He could tell when they were lying down, sitting, standing, or moving. I often think of him as the man who explained why Don Knotts (*The Andy Griffith Show*'s Barney Fife) was so thin. He never sat still and was always in motion. He may not have exercised, but he was constantly burning calories.

Based on his motion-tracking work, Dr. Levine developed an important new concept called NEAT, an acronym for "nonexercise activity thermogenesis." NEAT includes all the calories that we burn from activities other than formal exercise (anything from a shrug of the shoulders to unconscious pacing while talking on the phone). His research found that NEAT is a key determinant of obesity or slimness, since an obese person sits 150 more minutes each day and burns 350 fewer calories than a thin person who tends to get up and move more.

According to Dr. Levine, walking is the best way to work NEAT into your life. He suggests things like taking a walk around the block before showering in the morning, marching in place every time a TV ad comes on, having walk-and-talk "meetings" during the day with your spouse or children, walking to co-workers' offices to talk to them in person instead of e-mailing, and so on.

In fact, Dr. Levine is so passionate about ending our sit-down-all-day, lounge-all-night culture that he configured his own office and those of some other Mayo Clinic staff members with treadmill desks that enable them to walk at 1 mile per hour while working at a computer (built right into the desk). At this rate, Dr. Levine found, the average person can burn about 100 more calories every hour than would be expended sitting in a chair. Thanks to Dr. Levine's work, treadmill desks are now widely available and are being used by a number of companies nationwide to keep their employees fit. While a treadmill desk may not be in your immediate future, I do offer some easy ways to get moving on pages 237–240.

Get Fit with Fido and Get Fido Fit

When it comes to getting moving, I have long been a fan of dog walking. I have two dogs myself, and believe me, my huge black Lab (who looks like a bear) can definitely get my heart rate up as we trot around the neighborhood. I like to tell patients that they should walk their dog twice a day, whether they own one or not.

As I was writing this book, a new study done at Michigan State University found that dog owners really do get more exercise than those who don't own a dog. Published in 2011 in the *Journal of Physical Activity and Health,* the study found that dog owners were 34 percent more likely to get at least 150 minutes per week of exercise than those who don't own a dog. Nearly half of the roughly 2,200 dog owners identified in the study reported that they exercised 30 minutes a day at least 5 days a week; among nonowners, only about a third exercised that consistently.

Other recent studies on the health benefits of dog ownership for both adults and children are equally interesting. Here's a quick synopsis:

- ✔ Walking with a dog has advantages over walking with a human. In a study done by the Research Center for Human-Animal Interaction in Columbia, Missouri, walkers accompanied by a dog were likely to be more consistent about their walking program and showed better improvement in their fitness levels than those accompanied by a human companion. In the human-companion walking group, participants regularly dissuaded each other with excuses like "It's too hot" or "I don't really

In the same issue of *Diabetes* that explores the perils of sitting, another article, "Physical Activity, Sedentary Behavior, and Health: Paradigm Paralysis or Paradigm Shift?" by Peter T. Katzmarzyk, PhD, notes that recommendations for 30 minutes a day of moderate-to-vigorous exercise accounts for just a mere 1.5 percent of the total 10,080 minutes in a week—or 3 percent of the

feel like going today." The researchers felt compelled to point out that none of the dogs ever discouraged someone who wanted to take them for a walk.

- ✔ Elementary school children are more active when their families own a dog. A study of 2,065 youngsters conducted by St. George's University of London and published in the *American Journal of Public Health* in 2010 found that 9- and 10-year-olds in families with dogs had higher levels of physical activity than children from families without dogs.

- ✔ Teens can benefit from dog walking too. According to a 2011 study of more than 600 adolescents by the University of West Virginia, recently published in the *American Journal of Preventive Medicine,* teens whose families owned a dog were found to be more physically active than similar adolescents whose families didn't own one.

As it happens, Fido could probably use a little more time on the leash, too. According to a survey released in February 2011 by the Association for Pet Obesity Prevention, more than half (55 percent) of US dogs are now overweight or obese. That's about 43 million pudgy pooches that, like their overweight human masters, are consequently at higher risk for arthritis, diabetes, high blood pressure, heart disease, and kidney disease.

So, if you own a dog, grab the leash and head outside. It will be good for your pet and great for you, and hopefully for everyone else in the family as well when they join you on your walk.

time we spend awake. Dr. Katzmarzyk suggests that this small amount of exertion may not be adequate to counteract the negative impact of a sedentary life, and he has a good point. Just contrast the amount of time we are supposed to spend exercising each day with the amount of time that the average US household watches television—about 32.5 hours a week! As Katzmarzyk observes, simply advising people to get a certain amount of moderate-to-vigorous exercise daily may not be enough; it may be more effective to caution people about the hazards of inactivity. In other words, maybe doctors shouldn't be telling patients to get on the treadmill but should rather be telling them, "Listen, you need to cut back on your sitting!"

THE STORY OF THE DOUBLE-DECKER (NOT THE BURGER)

Perhaps the most famous exercise study of all inadvertently addressed the dangers of too much sitting. It was performed in London a few years after World War II, when Britain was experiencing an increased rate of heart attacks. No one knew why. Insufficient exercise was not even considered to be a leading candidate at the time.

In the study, Jerry Morris, MD, and his team compared the heart attack rates of bus conductors with those of bus drivers. He published his results in the leading British medical journal *Lancet* in 1953. They showed that conductors of the famous London double-decker buses, who spent nearly their whole workday on their feet, going up and down 500 to 750 steps each day, had half as many heart attacks as the bus drivers, who sat during their work hours. This was an excellent study because the drivers and conductors were from the same socioeconomic strata and, other than their job duties, led very similar lives. In a subsequent study, Dr. Morris also found that London postmen who walked or rode bikes had a fraction of the heart attacks of the postal workers who had desk jobs.

Dr. Morris was not an exercise physiologist but an epidemiologist (a doctor who specializes in population studies). After completing these studies, he decided he'd better learn something about exercise physiology since it appeared to be so important. After tutelage from a famous exercise physiologist, he concluded, "Exercise normalizes the workings of the body." In a 2009 interview with London's *Financial Times,* at the age of 99, he attributed his longevity to his daily walks, which he had been taking since childhood. At the time of that interview, he was still making his way to his office at the London School of Hygiene and Tropical Medicine every day. (He died a few months shy of his 100th birthday.) The *Financial Times* dubbed Dr. Morris the "man who invented exercise," and I can think of no better legacy to leave for future generations.

THE BEST WAY TO EXERCISE

While Dr. Jerry Morris was not initially considering physical activity in the double-decker bus study, his findings were the first to create awareness of the consequences of sedentary work environments. Unfortunately, many of our initial exercise solutions for combating sedentary jobs were not ideal. We must be cautious when we begin to exercise in ways our ancestors never would have dreamed of.

Our hunter-gatherer ancestors didn't do bench presses or bicep curls while sitting with a backrest, and they certainly didn't run on pavement or do marathons or triathlons. Consider that the Olympic marathon commemorates the legendary run of the soldier Pheidippides, who ran from a battlefield near Marathon, Greece, to Athens in 490 BC to bring news that the Persians had been defeated. Unfortunately, he collapsed and died at the end of his run, a grim reminder that long, exhausting exercise is not always healthy. Hunter-gatherers did walk long distances regularly, but vigorous physical exertion was characteristically performed in short spurts. Physically demanding hunts were followed by restful downtime.

Today the ill effects of long-distance running, especially on pavement, have become very apparent to orthopedic surgeons treating the injuries of overzealous baby boomers. I stopped running on pavement years ago when my knees, back, and hips told me to. Back then I often woke up in the morning and got out of bed like an old man, taking baby steps to counter various aches and pains until my muscles warmed up. Now my exercise routine

(continued on page 138)

Get Your Kids Moving

Perhaps those suffering the most from the "chair sentence" described earlier in this chapter are children, who are spending less and less time engaged in the physical activity their bodies need to grow and develop normally. I believe that the overweight and obesity epidemic, and the resultant increase in diabetes and early atherosclerosis we're seeing in kids, is not just related to how much junk food they are eating but is also a direct result of too much sitting, both at home and at school.

When I was growing up, we had recess every day. We were given the opportunity to run around outside, like kids are supposed to, and burn off some energy. Today, recess is considered a luxury, and many schools have slashed the amount of free time that kids have to be kids, replacing it with prep time for standardized tests. My response is that study after study has shown that physical activity is essential for a child's brain development, and that forcing kids to sit still all day to make them "smarter" could be having just the opposite effect. We know for sure that it is making them fatter.

A 2009 study published in *Pediatrics* reaffirmed the importance of recess for improving health and also noted its effect on improving classroom behavior. In the study, researchers from Albert Einstein College of Medicine reported on about 11,000 third grade boys and girls, ages 8 to 9, who were enrolled in the national Early Childhood Longitudinal Study and whose teachers had been asked to assess their classroom behavior. The researchers compared the data of children who had less than 15 minutes of recess daily with those who had more than 15 minutes of recess daily. They found a clear and consistent trend: Children who had more than 15 minutes of daily recess were rated by their teachers as better behaved than those who had less. This supports other studies showing that children who participate in more physical activity are able to concentrate better in class, which translates into higher test scores and grade point averages. Our own Healthier

Options for Public Schoolchildren experiences, discussed in Chapter 7, showed this as well.

Inactivity among children is not just a problem in the United States; it is a growing problem throughout the world, as kids across the planet are becoming less active. In the Global School–based Student Health Survey, conducted from 2003 to 2007 and published in 2010 in the *Journal of Pediatrics,* researchers analyzed data submitted by 72,845 students from 34 countries. They looked at the amount of time students were engaged in activities like walking and riding their bikes to school—things that you automatically associate with childhood. In more than half the countries surveyed, less than 25 percent of the boys met the physical activity recommendations, and in almost all countries (except India), less than 25 percent of the girls met the recommendations. Furthermore, more than one-third of the students spent 3 or more hours a day on sedentary activities. This was in addition to the time they spent sitting in class or doing homework.

Sitting in front of screens is not only turning our children's brains to mush (as my mother used to caution would happen to me when I watched too much TV), it is turning out to be a serious health hazard as well. Consider the disturbing results of a study published in 2009 in the *Archives of Pediatric and Adolescent Medicine,* in which children between the ages of 3 and 8 wore accelerometers so that researchers could measure their physical movements over a 7-day period. On average, each child spent about 5 hours per day on sedentary activities, with an average of 1.5 hours in front of a screen, like a TV, computer, or video game. According to this study, the children who spent the least amount of time in front of a screen had significantly lower blood pressure than those who put in the most screen time, regardless of their body mass. The American Academy of Pediatrics recommends that parents restrict screen time to no more than 2 hours a day of educational, nonviolent programs for children over age 2, and recommends zero screen time for children under that age. Excellent advice.

includes not only nonimpact cardio but also Pilates, for stretching and strengthening core muscles. These muscles, which support the abdomen, lower back, pelvis, and hips, are crucial for accomplishing the activities of daily life without injury. Since I've been doing Pilates, I have been hopping out of bed in the morning and (knock on wood) am more often than not pain free. Actually, today I feel better than I did in my younger jogging days.

While running is clearly not great for the bones and joints, the conventional wisdom always held that it was good for the heart. Recently, however, this is being questioned by researchers who are observing high levels of plaque on the CT scans of some marathoners. I have anecdotally observed this in my practice as well, and while the final word is not in about whether long-distance running is bad for your heart, it appears that cross-training (which involves lower-impact exercise using a variety of muscles) is a better strategy for keeping heart disease and many other ailments at bay. As with good nutrition, variety is the key when it comes to healthful exercise. Cycling and swimming are both lower impact than pounding the pavement and have longer precedent. Just watch out for cars and sharks and remember not to overtrain.

Paul Chek, an exercise guru whose work I have followed over the years, concluded more than 20 years ago that our bodies were built to function in ways that helped the hunter-gatherers survive. Movements such as twisting (required to throw a stone or spear), pulling, pushing, squatting, bending, and lunging not only served a useful purpose in our ancestors' day-to-day lives but also helped them build fitness, core strength, and flexibility. That's why today we appropriately call this "functional" exercise.

When you deviate from the principles of functional exercise, you can run into trouble even though your muscles might look good in the mirror. Take some of those men and women with overdeveloped muscles we see on the street. I have several of these strong-looking individuals among my patients, and I have learned that they are not necessarily as strong as they appear. They have what has been referred to as "mirror muscles," which are not necessarily very functional. One such specimen who came in for an office visit told me how he had returned from his classic gym workout to his home, where he bent over to pick up his 2-year-old and immediately threw out his back. The reason: He was not in the habit of doing functional exercises to build up his core. This unfortunate patient is yet another example of how looks can be deceiving.

Fortunately, the benefits of core functional fitness are appreciated by most trainers today, many of whom include this type of exercise in their prescribed workouts. These conceptual changes are also reflected in today's gym equipment. About 2 years ago, I passed a well-known high-tech gym in New York City and couldn't resist walking in for a closer look. Through a window I witnessed a very low-tech training method: A 40-something woman was pushing a sled with weights on it from one end of the gym to the other and then pulling it back again. I thought that this was fairly primitive for such a high-tech gym. But then I realized that "primitive" is what we should be striving for. This was the type of functional exercise that Paul Chek would applaud.

MAXIMIZING EXERCISE TIME

I can hear you groaning to yourself and saying, "Does working regular exercise into my life mean that I have to get up extra early to spend 45 minutes on the treadmill, elliptical, or bike? Isn't there a way to burn more fat in less time?" Since, as you will learn in the next chapter, a full night's sleep is very important to your health, I am very happy to report that the answers are, "No, you don't have to get up earlier than usual" and "Yes, there are ways to burn fat faster."

You can accomplish this the same way the hunter-gatherers did and elite athletes do: with interval training. In my book *The South Beach Diet Supercharged,* I presented the concept of interval training for the average person with the expert assistance of exercise physiologist Joseph Signorile, PhD. Since I wrote that book, the medical literature has continued to document the benefits of intervals—big time. In interval training, you alternate between short bursts of intensive effort and easier recovery periods, as opposed to exercising at a steady, continuous pace. For example, instead of walking on a treadmill for an hour at a steady state, you alternate between walking very fast for 15 seconds up to 1 or 2 minutes (called the "work period") and then slowing down for a similar duration to recover (the "recovery period"). Once you've recovered, you pick up your pace again to start the work period, and the cycle continues. There are huge advantages to short bouts of intervals over lengthier steady-state workouts. When you work at a higher intensity doing intervals, you can burn as many calories in 20 minutes as you would in about 40 minutes of steady-state exercise. Additionally, with interval training, it appears that metabolic changes in muscle allow you to burn more fat in less time for the same amount of calorie expenditure.

This may contradict what you've been told about exercise and burning fat—specifically that the best way to burn fat is to work at a training heart rate of 60 percent of your maximum heart rate. People are often told that once they reach that target heart rate during exercise, they should maintain that level by taking their pulse or wearing a heart rate monitor. It used to be thought that you had to work hard for at least 20 minutes before you started burning fat, but we now know that's not true. If you do intervals, you can burn fat faster and have a more productive workout in less time.

Interval training has long been used by elite endurance athletes (think wind sprints) to help them achieve peak performance. It was key to the training regimen of the legendary British runner Roger Bannister and helped him break the 4-minute mile back in 1954, a feat that was believed to be impossible. Now there is good evidence that interval training can be useful for all of us, and especially for those with problems like obesity and diabetes. Even if you are a couch potato, you can start an interval exercise program. See pages 228–37 for our Wake Up and Move 2-Week Quick-Start Plan, which involves doing interval exercise and core training on alternate days. Just remember to consult with your doctor before making any sudden changes in your activity level, particularly if you've been inactive for some time or have known health problems.

WAKE UP AND MOVE

On a recent visit to New York City, I dropped in on a colleague, Tony, who had moved there from Cleveland not long ago to take a position at a Manhattan hospital. I had not seen Tony since he had resettled, and it was obvious that he had shed a considerable amount of weight—30 pounds as it turned out. When I commented on his fitter look, he kindly attributed it to the South Beach Diet. I was happy to take credit but felt there had to be more to it than that. Tony had in fact moved from a driving city, where he went everywhere by car, to a walking city, where he went nearly everywhere by foot. It turned out that he walked about 20 blocks to and from the hospital every day, which was faster than traveling by cab, car, or subway. This walk was incorporated into his day and not part of a planned workout.

Tony's experience is consistent with studies that show that people who live in cities with good walking neighborhoods (like New York and San Francisco) are thinner than those who live in driving cities. Even within these driving cities, it's been found that people who live in areas amenable to walking (usually those with good sidewalks) are thinner and healthier than people who live in areas where driving is necessary to fulfill their daily needs. This is all good news, but it can get even better when communities make a concerted effort to promote good health. A study published in the *Archives of Internal Medicine* in 2009 found that neighborhoods with resources supporting physical activity and healthy eating had fewer cases of type 2 diabetes during the 5-year study period.

As a physician, it's apparent to me that awakening our country to the importance of exercise and movement must be addressed at the community level. We cannot rely on a clinical, individual approach. Too many people would miss out. It is clear that we have to create communities that invite walking and provide open spaces for other forms of exercise and sport. This means supporting urban planning that includes the development of parks, sports fields, recreation centers, playgrounds, walking trails, better sidewalks, and pedestrian-safe streets. Communities must find the funds for fitness because their hospital budgets won't be big enough to handle their sick populations if they don't.

We also need to encourage more exercise in the workplace, whether it's lunchtime walking groups, or a gym in the building, or treadmill desks. Many companies big and small are finally recognizing the benefits of keeping their workforce healthy. And healthier employees means happier employees, fewer sick days, and more productivity. We must also make sure that public school curriculums include mandatory physical education and recess for younger children. Advocating for healthy changes in school lunch programs is critical, but it's not enough. Our kids need to move.

And let's not forget that fitness begins at home. You don't need expensive equipment or a gym membership to get yourself going. A couple of balls, a pair of sneakers, a mat, and a good exercise DVD can go a long way toward improving your fitness level and overall well-being—and that of your family too.

Finally, remember that whether it's walking to work or taking the stairs or playing Frisbee with the kids (and dog!), exercise can easily be incorporated throughout your day—and it all adds up.

CHAPTER 9

WAKE UP AND
GET SOME SLEEP!

A colleague recently showed me a satellite photograph of Earth that, through the magic of digital photography, simulated what the planet would look like if each country hit the stroke of midnight simultaneously. I was struck by the fact that, as we panned the globe, we saw vast portions of darkness over most of the planet, but when we looked at the United States, it shimmered like a lit Christmas tree. Here in the United States, young and old alike were awake into the wee hours of the night doing everything but the one thing they were all supposed to be doing: sleeping! Today we know that many maladies associated with our unhealthy lifestyle can be initiated or aggravated by the failure to get enough sleep. On the flip side, these health problems could probably be significantly reduced, if not averted in the first place, if we just got more shut-eye.

Unfortunately, many people still think of sleep as a luxury, not a necessity. We need to change that view because sleep is an essential part of a healthy lifestyle. While we have known about sleep apnea for some time, thanks to the proliferation of sleep labs and sleep specialists around the country, in the past few years the volume of valuable information about the effects of sleep has increased exponentially. What we have learned is that lack of sleep does not just leave you groggy the next day; its health implications are much broader. We know how important nutrition and exercise are to our health, and now we also know that sleep affects our general health in ways that we did not suspect until relatively recently. All the new research has convinced me that we need to wake up and think more about our critical need for sleep. When adults chronically miss sleep, we are more vulnerable to a whole slew of physical and emotional problems, including obesity, diabetes, heart disease, stroke, and depression, not to mention a weakened immune system. When our kids don't get enough sleep, they too are more likely to become obese, suffer from depression (and thoughts of suicide), exhibit behavioral problems and poor performance at school, and ultimately be more prone to prematurely developing many of the health issues adults are subject to. This sounds a lot like what happens when we eat badly and don't get enough exercise, but it is absolutely true. Sleep is critical for good health, regardless of one's age. Furthermore, getting more of it might save your life. While lack of sleep can lead to myriad life-threatening diseases down the road, being bleary-eyed can kill you in more immediate ways. Statistics show that some 100,000 car accidents and 1,500 deaths each year in this country are due to someone nodding off at the wheel. Teenagers are especially prone to falling asleep while driving (as if texting and driving isn't bad enough!).

A SLEEP-DEPRIVED NATION

As a nation, we get 1.5 fewer hours of sleep a night than we did a century ago and way less than our hunter-gatherer ancestors were accustomed to—they are believed to have slept between 9 and 10 hours a night. Ideally, adults are supposed to get at least 8 hours nightly, and some (certainly those with health issues) may require even more. In contrast, adults today get 6.7 hours of sleep on average, and many of us get much less than that. According to a Stanford University study, 20 percent of American adults complain of excessive sleepiness during the day due to poor sleep at night.

Children are being cheated out of much-needed sleep as well. Toddlers are supposed to get between 12 and 14 hours of sleep at night; preschool-age kids need roughly 11 to 12 hours; school-age kids should get between 10 and 11 hours; and teenagers need up to 9.5 hours. In many homes, that's not close to happening. The American Psychological Association reports that 69 percent of children experience one or more sleep problems up to several times a week, which appears to impact their performance at school. According to a comprehensive poll from the National Sleep Foundation, about 40 percent of all schoolchildren show up in class at least once a week so tired from a lack of sleep that they can't function properly.

So what's preventing us from getting a good night's sleep? The major problem might be that many of us are simply not aware of the critical role a good night's sleep plays in our lives and just don't make time for it. Until recently, I included myself in that category. But experts tell us that most sleep problems are caused by poor sleep habits before bedtime, like e-mailing or texting or watching TV (computers and televisions actually stimulate the brain instead of calming it down, since the electronic screens emit light that interferes with the normal cycling of light-sensitive hormones at night). Other sleep problems come from being overstimulated by too much caffeine from one too many lattes or energy drinks during the day and evening, or from taking over-the-counter drugs like pain relievers and cold remedies that contain caffeine. Those who enjoy a little "nightcap" before bed to help them sleep may not realize that while alcohol can initially cause drowsiness, consuming even one drink up to a few hours before bedtime can disrupt deeper sleep later once that soporific effect wears off. And then there are the "night fretters"—those people (mainly women) who say that from the second they put their heads down on their pillows, they start worrying about everything from the bills that aren't paid to the kids' grades to the chores they need to do the next day.

Sometimes, sleeplessness is unavoidable: Having a new baby goes hand in hand with disrupted sleep. It can take some infants up to several months (and some even longer) to settle into a predictable sleep pattern, and until that happens, parents have to get their sleep catch-as-catch-can. Take it from someone who many moons ago spent plenty of nights pacing with a baby in his arms— it will pass. If a baby's sleep doesn't improve within the first 3 months, talk about the problem with your pediatrician. There are ways to help an infant sleep better, which often involve teaching parents better responses to the baby's awakenings.

People who work erratic schedules, especially those who work at night, often complain of sleep difficulties, which isn't surprising. As I will explain

(continued on page 148)

The Mystery of Sleep

Sleep is one of the most intriguing of all human activities: We spend up to one-third of our lives doing it, but nobody really quite knows why. Recent technology like the electroencephalograph (EEG), which allows us to measure brain waves during sleep, has shed some light on what actually happens when we doze off. But it still hasn't settled the debate over *why* we sleep.

One hypothesis, known as the evolutionary theory, contends that sleep evolved as a way of getting our hunter-gatherer ancestors out of harm's way in the dark of night, when they would be most vulnerable to predators. This theory suggests that sleep really doesn't serve any purpose beyond protection and that we still do it only because our genes are programmed that way. Given all the new research on sleep today, this explanation doesn't make much sense. Another widely held view, the so-called memory consolidation theory, suggests that sleep is a way of helping us process any new information we are exposed to during the course of a day so that our brains are fresh to absorb yet more new information the next day. This may be true, but it is only one of the ways that we benefit from sleep. And newer research reminds me of what my mom used to tell me as a child when she was encouraging me to cease my fun activities and get to bed: It's nature's way of giving the body time to rest and repair itself.

To further understand how sleep affects your body, you need to know about the process of sleep itself. There are two types of sleep: non-REM sleep and REM sleep (REM stands for rapid eye movement). Non-REM sleep is divided into four phases. Phase 1 is when you are hovering between sleep and wakefulness and can easily be awakened. Phase 2 is a period of light sleep when your body temperature drops, your muscles relax, and your heart rate and pulse are lowered. Phases 3 and 4 are the times during which you experience an increasingly deep stage of sleep called delta sleep. During this restorative stage, your body is repairing itself, building bone and muscle and releasing certain hormones. This is when your body performs the vital maintenance work that keeps you and your cells functioning at their best.

After you've gone through the four non-REM phases, you end the cycle with REM sleep, during which you have your dreams. As its name implies, during REM sleep, unlike the other sleep phases, your eyes move rapidly under your closed eyelids but your muscles are very still. This is called "sleep paralysis," but it's a good kind of paralysis. REM sleep is not only linked to learning (i.e., memory consolidation) but is also associated with mood. If you don't get enough REM sleep, you are likely to be cranky and more prone to depression. Why? No one knows for sure, but we do know that lack of sleep is associated with higher amounts of stress hormones, which can result in anxiety. Researchers are also investigating the relationship between the different stages of sleep and the normal cycling of neurotransmitters in the brain—these are the chemicals that regulate important functions such as mood and appetite. One hypothesis is that REM sleep helps preserve serotonin, a neurotransmitter that is critical for the management of mood, in much the same way that some antidepressants work.

Each sleep cycle consists of anywhere from 60 to 100 minutes of non-REM sleep followed by a short period of REM sleep. Typically, you cycle through each of the five phases of sleep about five times a night.

Think of your time in bed as a nightly maintenance visit to the body shop, a spa of sorts for your internal organs. If you severely cut back on your time "in the shop," all kinds of problems can arise.

later, the human body is designed to be alert when it is light outside and to wind down and fall asleep when it gets dark. We also sleep better when we go to sleep and wake up at a set time. If you do work the night shift, it is even more critical for you to try to stick to a consistent sleeping schedule.

All this, of course, is not intended to ignore those who are being kept awake by more serious sleep issues. It's estimated that 40 million Americans have a bona fide sleep disorder like sleep apnea (in which breathing stops and starts), chronic insomnia (regularly having difficulty falling asleep and staying asleep), or sleepwalking. Others can't sleep because of discomfort or chronic pain from a condition like arthritis or restless leg syndrome (the constant urge to move the legs). And still others suffer wakefulness due to indigestion or acid reflux or emotional problems such as anxiety or depression.

And then there's the occasional co-sleeplessness of those who share mattresses. I usually hear this complaint from tired wives but also from bleary-eyed husbands. Typically I hear about snoring from both sides, but often I learn about a more serious sleep issue, like sleep apnea, from the one who's kept awake.

Luckily, most of the lifestyle-related sleep problems I mention above are readily resolved with some simple improvements in so-called sleep hygiene, which we review in our Strategy 7: Sleep Longer, Live Longer (see page 241). Other sleep issues, like apnea, however, are not so simply resolved. Because sleep apnea in particular is related to so many other conditions, including obesity, high blood pressure, and heart disease, and because it so often goes undiagnosed in both adults and children, I want to explain more about this disorder.

SLEEP APNEA: DO YOU HAVE IT?

The Greek word *apnea* means "without breath," which pretty much tells the story of this ailment. It is a condition that is characterized by the frequent stoppage of breathing during sleep. In the most common form of sleep apnea, called obstructive sleep apnea, a person temporarily stops breathing for a few seconds or up to a minute because his or her airway is obstructed or blocked by the soft tissue in the rear of the throat, which collapses and closes during sleep.

When breathing stops, the brain knows it's being deprived of oxygen and responds by alerting you that something is wrong. That's when you briefly arouse and start breathing again. But as a result, sleep becomes very fragmented. In serious cases of obstructive sleep apnea, sleep can be interrupted 100 or more times a night! People with this condition not only snore loudly but often sound as if they are gasping for breath, which they are. While people's perception of how often they wake up varies (many don't realize that they were ever awake at all), it is often quite upsetting for the bed partner, who is also repeatedly jolted out of sleep. Needless to say, both parties are typically exhausted the next day.

As I mentioned earlier, sleep apnea can be serious, leading to even more serious health problems like high blood pressure and heart disease, as well as memory problems and sexual disorders. It can also increase the risk of heart attack, stroke, and sudden premature death. And as if this isn't scary enough, it's made all the more troubling by the fact that while about 24 percent of men and 9 percent of women have some form of sleep apnea, only 10 percent of these cases are actually diagnosed. Sleep apnea also often goes unnoticed for years in the roughly 2 percent of kids who have it, which puts them at greater risk for health problems as adults.

While obesity is the most common cause of obstructive sleep apnea in both adults and children, other risk factors include being over age 40, having a large offensive-lineman-type neck (due to genetics or the weight room), and having a family history of the disorder. It can also be caused by enlarged tonsils and adenoids (often true in children) or by an anatomical deformity like an elongated uvula (the fleshy tissue at the back of the palate), which can obstruct the airway. (In the case of an elongated uvula, the excess tissue can vibrate with every breath, which causes snoring.) In those who are overweight, excess fat around the neck and in the jowls, as well as inside the throat, can also promote sleep apnea.

If I suspect that a patient has sleep apnea, I will request a take-home sleep study, called a polysomnogram, to monitor breathing. Until recently, sleep studies were fairly complicated affairs that had to be conducted overnight in a sleep-laboratory setting. In a lab study, the patient gets tethered to a machine that monitors his or her heart rate and blood pressure and wears a mask over the nose to check breathing and oxygen levels. "Have a good night's sleep," the technician kindly says before leaving the room. Needless to say, this isn't always so easy to do under the circumstances, and I often had trouble convincing patients to go through with this overnight "nightmare." With the newer polysomnogram, however, I have no such difficulty, and it has really been helpful in diagnosing sleep apnea in many patients in which it previously would have gone undetected. When we do get an abnormal test, we refer patients to a sleep specialist, a subspecialty of pulmonology or neurology.

When a patient is diagnosed with sleep apnea, the most common treatment options include wearing a nighttime dental appliance to open up the obstructed airway or using a continuous positive airway pressure (CPAP) machine, which forces air through the nose and/or mouth to keep the air passages open. In rare cases, throat surgery may be necessary.

It is also well known that taking off just a few pounds can often decrease or completely resolve sleep apnea, and I have frequently observed good results with weight loss. In fact, my experiences with this weight-loss "treatment" were validated by a study of 61 obese men ages 33 to 61 with moderate to severe sleep apnea performed by the Karolinska Institute in Stockholm and published in 2009 in the online *British Medical Journal*. All of the men used a CPAP machine to help them sleep better, and 30 of them were also put on a very low-calorie liquid weight-loss diet for 7 weeks, followed by the reintroduction of normal food over a 2-week period. After the 9 weeks, those who were not on the diet had lost no weight and had not improved their apnea symptoms. Those who were on the diet had lost an average of almost 42 pounds (73 of the men were no longer obese) and had reduced the number of sleep apnea incidents at night by about two-thirds, which signifies a great improvement in sleep quality. Furthermore, 17 percent of the men who had lost weight were cured of their apnea! In addition, complaints of daytime sleepiness were dramatically reduced among the men who had lost weight, compared with those who had not.

I saw the same thing happen with a 45-year-old patient of mine named

Hector, who wasn't sure he had apnea when he came to me but who had all the signs and symptoms. Hector was overweight with daytime drowsiness. In fact, he told me he was pretty sure that he had nodded off twice during his daily commute on the interstate, only to be awakened when he ran over the raised reflectors between the lanes. Although he was concerned about those near accidents, it was his wife's complaints about his snoring that ultimately convinced him to try the take-home sleep test. The results indicated a severe case of apnea. Hector quickly committed to adopting the South Beach Diet along with a regular exercise regimen, and he shed 25 pounds in just a few months. The results: no more snoring, almost no sleep apnea episodes, a happier marriage, and best of all, no more near misses on his commute.

I have heard some really impressive life-transformation stories from patients who have been successfully treated for sleep apnea. They (and their partners) are no longer dragging themselves around during the day, and many have told me that, for the first time in years, they feel energized and wide awake. Some had thought that being sleepy most of the time was normal. Problems like erectile dysfunction, depression, and irritability, which are closely associated with sleep apnea, are often diminished or even disappear. And those who have lost weight as part of their treatment are also more likely to improve their blood pressure, blood lipids, and other cardiac risk factors.

If you suspect that you have sleep apnea, I urge you to check with your own doctor about further testing.

MORE REASONS TO GET MORE SLEEP

When I first started practicing cardiology more than 30 years ago, there was no data connecting sleep with heart attacks and strokes or documenting the connection between sleep and weight. In fact, back then, as a tired young doctor, I worried about just one thing when it came to sleep, and that was how to get more of it by working some quick naps into my day (I come from a family of nappers). At the time, I happened to take my first trip to the Mayo Clinic to participate in a medical course on heart imaging. While there, I picked up a book about the Mayo brothers, the two founders of the Mayo Clinic. I inhaled the story and instantly became a huge fan of the clinic (and still am). The atmosphere of innovation, along with the cooperation between the teaching doctors and the public, started by the Mayo brothers in the late 1800s continues to this day. But what really made me very happy back then was to learn that Dr. Charles Mayo took a daily "power nap" after lunch.

As it happens, another one of my heroes, Winston Churchill, was also a power napper. In fact, thanks to his power nap during the day, he could work quite effectively well into the wee hours. According to one story, whenever Churchill was a visitor to the White House during World War II, President Franklin Roosevelt (who did not take naps) became frustrated and exhausted by Churchill's late-night energy. It apparently took Roosevelt quite some time

The Littlest Sleep Apneacs

If you are a parent and think that one of your children has sleep apnea because of his or her snoring or excessive daytime drowsiness, it is important to tell your pediatrician. The proper diagnosis and treatment of sleep apnea can lead to a happier, healthier, better behaved, and more alert child.

In a presentation at the June 2010 meeting of the Associated Professional Sleep Societies in San Antonio, researchers from Cincinnati Children's Hospital Medical Center revealed the results of a study showing that kids with sleep apnea were more likely to get low grades in school than kids who did not have this problem. The reason: a poor attention span in class and poor study habits at home—no doubt due to exhaustion.

In young children ages 3 to 5, sleep apnea is often caused by enlarged tonsils or adenoids, which block the airways. This can be treated by the removal of the tonsils or adenoids. But often the disorder in children, as in adults, is caused by carrying extra pounds, which means excess fat in the neck and throat are reducing the size of the airways and making breathing difficult. Often the first indication of apnea in an obese or overweight child to recover from Churchill's visits and from what Franklin and Eleanor called the "Winston hours."

At any rate, I have happily adopted the habit of the power nap when time permits; I sit back in my comfortable desk chair with my back toward the door and doze off for a few minutes. It's a great pick-me-up, and I now know why. In my interview with sleep expert Alejandro Chediak, MD, beginning on page 157, he explains that our bodies are actually hardwired to nap.

Today thanks to the work of Dr. Chediak and others, I have learned just how detrimental sleep deprivation can be. In addition to many studies linking sleep apnea to heart disease and weight gain, there is new research showing other ways that lack of sleep can affect your heart and your waistline.

may be snoring. An Italian study published in the May 2010 journal *Chest* examined the relationship between weight and snoring in 809 elementary school and pre–elementary school children. Of the children surveyed, 44 were found to be habitual snorers, 138 occasional snorers, and 627 did not snore at all. The group consisted of 64 children who were obese, 121 who were overweight, and 624 who were normal weight. The researchers found that the obese kids were almost three times as likely to snore as the normal-weight kids, and were twice as likely to have obstructive sleep apnea as the overweight or normal-weight kids. David Ludwig, MD, who runs the Optimal Weight for Life (OWL) Program at Children's Hospital Boston, has found that sleep apnea can put an overweight child's body under great stress, producing changes in hormones and metabolism that can lead to even more weight gain. But once the apnea is diagnosed and adequately treated, weight loss often begins, sometimes effortlessly, and the sleep apnea generally improves or resolves.

The bottom line: If you think your child has sleep apnea, get it diagnosed and treated. The earlier treatment starts, the brighter your child's days—and future.

For example, in a 2008 study that's near and dear to my heart, University of Chicago researchers discovered a link between getting too little sleep (less than 5 hours at night) and an increased risk for coronary calcium, an indicator of the amount of atherosclerotic plaque that is building up (or not) in the arteries of your heart. As I discussed in Chapter 2, the higher your Calcium Score, the more plaque you have clogging your coronary arteries and the greater your risk for symptomatic heart disease, angina, heart attack, stroke, and even sudden death. You therefore want to keep your arteries as calcium free (and plaque free) as possible, which is in itself a great reason for getting enough sleep.

Recent studies have also shown a complex interaction between how much sleep you get and how much you weigh: *People who sleep less tend to weigh more.* Moreover, several studies have shown that not getting enough sleep can make it more difficult for you to lose weight and to maintain a healthy weight once you've reached it. All this new data has given me yet another reason to look carefully at sleep patterns when taking patient histories and when evaluating cardiac risk and lifestyle steps that can be made to improve a patient's risk profile.

In the relationship between sleep and weight, a number of factors are at play, some psychological, some physiological, and some a combination of the two. First, on the behavioral side, when you are extremely tired, you are more likely to "forget" to follow a healthy lifestyle because you are simply too worn out even to contemplate any exercise, much less think about shopping for healthy food and cooking a healthy meal. I certainly know that my own discipline for watching what I eat is diminished when I am exhausted at the end of a particularly long day. At times like this, it is tempting to seek the sanctuary of the couch, some mindless TV, and those comforting sugary and starchy carbs for a quick pick-me-up. Your blood sugar rises and falls and the hunger cycle begins, along with the weight gain.

This also happens when you're stressed (which can be both psychological and physical). Lack of sleep itself is a huge stressor on the body and can increase the production of adrenaline and cortisol, your body's "flight or fight" hormones. Many people experience feelings of agitation and jitteriness after missing a night's sleep, even if there is nothing going on in their lives that is particularly stressful, and that is because these hormones are revved up for action.

The problem for some is that cortisol also acts as an appetite stimulant. It actually turns up glucose production by the liver, which in turn stimulates an increase in insulin production. The increased levels of insulin decrease your blood sugar, causing hunger, which is most easily satisfied by eating sugary and starchy carbs. Sadly, just as lack of sleep can cause stress, being under chronic stress can also interfere with sleep, which contributes to a vicious cycle. You're already upset, so your body pumps out more stress hormones, and the lack of sleep makes a bad situation worse. Weight gain often follows.

Again on the physiological side, lack of sleep affects the production of two other important hormones that help regulate your hunger levels and your metabolism. The first, produced in fat cells, is called leptin. It suppresses hunger and lets your brain know when your stomach is full. The second, produced in stomach cells, is called ghrelin. It stimulates your appetite, slows your metabolism, and decreases your body's ability to burn fat. Levels of ghrelin normally increase before meals and decrease afterward. It turns out that not getting enough sleep means that your body produces lower levels of appetite suppressing leptin and higher levels of appetite-boosting ghrelin. So when you sleep too little, you are not only tired, but you're also hungry from too much ghrelin. And even after you eat, you don't feel satisfied because your leptin levels are not rising the way they should. This is yet another mechanism whereby insufficient sleep can set the stage for long-term overeating and weight gain.

In fact, a study conducted by Stanford University and the University of Wisconsin was the first to document the relationship of leptin and ghrelin to sleep and weight gain. Beginning in 1989, the researchers followed 1,024 people involved in the long-term Wisconsin Sleep Cohort Study, charting their hormone levels, the hours they slept, and their weight at regular intervals. They found that those who slept less than 8 hours a night not only had lower leptin and higher ghrelin levels, they also had higher levels of body fat. To summarize, those who slept the fewest hours per night weighed the most. In the study article, published in the December 2004 *PLoS Medicine,* the researchers concluded: "In Western societies, where chronic sleep deprivation is common and food is widely available, changes in appetite regulatory hormones with sleep curtailment may contribute to obesity."

But it gets worse. If you are on a diet, sleep deprivation could also result in the loss of muscle tone, which can undermine your efforts to keep the weight off. That's what researchers at the University of Chicago and the University of Wisconsin reported in the October 2010 *Annals of Internal Medicine*. In their small but important study of 3 women and 7 men on a weight-loss program, those who slept less than 5.5 hours per night were more likely to lose muscle mass and less likely to lose fat than those who got 8.5 hours of sleep per night. Remember, the goal of weight loss is to lose extra fat, not muscle. Muscle is what makes you strong, helps stabilize joints, and burns more calories than fat during rest. If you are trying to get to a healthy weight, muscle is the last thing that you want to lose.

Even lack of sleep during childhood can play a role in adult obesity. A 2008 study published in *Pediatrics* followed a group of 1,037 boys and girls who were born in New Zealand in 1972 or 1973. The parents were asked to keep track of the time that their children went to bed and the time they awoke at ages 5, 7, 9, and 11 years. In this fascinating study, the researchers found that less sleep during childhood meant more weight at age 32. This relationship is most likely explained by the childhood sleep deprivation, since other factors that could influence weight—including the weight of the participants' parents, their socioeconomic status, their childhood and adult TV viewing habits, and their adult sleep habits, smoking habits, and physical activity levels—were not factored into the results. So in addition to my appeal for all you Super Moms and Dads to work toward better nutrition and physical education programs in your children's schools, I also encourage you to lobby for a later start to the school day (which some schools have actually adopted) and, if necessary, nap time for the younger kids. It's thanks to studies like those mentioned above that we now know how and why sleep is important for every aspect of our health from childhood on up. Considering how many people fail to get 8 hours of sleep of night, it is certainly time to add sleep issues to nutrition and exercise considerations when charting a strategy to reverse our country's obesity epidemic.

A Conversation with Alejandro Chediak, MD

I have known Alejandro "Alex" Chediak for more than 20 years, going back to the early days when "sleep" first became a subspecialty of pulmonary medicine. Alex is the medical director of the Miami Sleep Disorders Center and past president of the American Academy of Sleep Medicine. In fact, his staff at Mount Sinai Medical Center in Miami Beach were pioneers in studying sleep apnea, which has become the single most important focus of sleep medicine. Alex has always been my "go to" doctor for patients with sleep problems, and he has taught me a great deal about sleep issues.

Over the past few years, there has been a growing body of scientific evidence linking the importance of a good night's sleep to many of the cardiac problems that I deal with daily, including metabolic syndrome, inflammation, and weight gain. In reviewing this research, I realized that our sleep patterns have been changing over the past decades just like our diets and exercise have been—and not for the better. Alex was kind enough to agree to share some of his expertise on the relationship between sleep and health.

Millions of Americans are walking around chronically sleep deprived, and many don't realize it. How can you tell if you need more sleep?

First, ask yourself, "Do I wake up feeling fully refreshed, or do I wake up feeling tired?" In other words, do you feel completely restored after a night's sleep? If the answer is no, then you are not getting enough sleep. The second way is to monitor how you behave throughout the day. At work, do you have to do things to resist falling asleep? For example, at a meeting, do you find that you are fidgeting a great deal in your chair, or do you have to get up frequently to go to the coffee machine and a few minutes later get up to get something to eat? These are the sorts of behaviors that we resort to when we need to keep ourselves awake.

There are other obvious symptoms of sleep deprivation, like finding it difficult to stay awake when you are driving or feeling tired or irritable during the day. If these are happening to you on a consistent basis, then you probably do need more sleep. It's also possible that the number of hours of sleep that you get is sufficient, but there's something about the quality of the sleep that is causing it to be fragmented and not allowing your body to fully restore itself. Sleep apnea or involuntary movements could do this.

What causes insomnia?

Insomnia can be defined as repeated difficulty with falling asleep, staying asleep, and/or poor sleep quality despite having adequate time for sleep, which can all result in some form of impairment. Speaking in very general terms, there are two types of insomnia: primary insomnia and secondary, or comorbid, insomnia. So the cause depends on which type you are experiencing. Primary insomnia cannot be linked to a physical or emotional problem. In fact, you may never know the root cause. Secondary insomnia is often related to another medical problem like arthritic pain, to a sleep disorder like sleep apnea, or to a psychiatric disorder like depression. In my experience, the most common cause of abrupt-onset insomnia is an acute stressor, like a death in the family or a financial crisis, that keeps you up at night worrying or feeling upset.

I'd like to clear up a point of confusion: I frequently encounter people who claim that they have insomnia because they only get 6 hours of sleep a night. When I start to question them about their sleep habits, however, I learn that they don't have a physical problem preventing them from sleeping; rather, they have a time-management problem. They don't allocate enough hours for sleep! They stay up late puttering around the house or doing other things when they should be in bed. Or they may be overbooked with work or social events that cut into the time that they should spend sleeping. This is self-imposed sleep curtailment, not insomnia.

True insomnia is when you actually have 8 hours for sleep—in other words, you're actually in bed that long—but are only getting 6 hours and are experiencing some of the symptoms mentioned above.

What controls our sleep-wake cycles?

Each of us has an internal biological clock that is controlled by cells in our brains and that runs on a predictable rhythm and tell us when it's time to be active and when it's time to shut down and sleep. Our clock's cycle is a little longer than 24 hours, which means that we are naturally wired to go to bed a little later and to wake up a little later every day. So, for example, if you could stick someone in a cave where he is isolated from all the social and light cues that inform us when the day begins and when the day ends, and you let him pick what's day and what's night, you'll see that he will go to bed later every night and will wake up progressively later every day. That's what would happen to us if we didn't "reset" our clocks to zero by waking up and going to sleep at a predictable time. Exposure to morning sunlight at a fixed time reinforces the notion of daytime versus nighttime and is the best natural method of keeping our internal sleep-wake clock on time.

Do our sleeping habits change as we age?

Yes, very much so. Our sleep-wake cycles do change as we get older. For example, many parents of teenagers are upset that their children are up late at night and are difficult to wake up in the morning, but that's how their biological clocks are wired. It's hard for them to fall asleep at the times that you and I would fall asleep, and it's hard for them to be awake at 6 or 7, when we would be pretty awake if we had slept well.

Some school districts have actually pushed their start time later by 1 hour to accommodate the sleep needs of the students. In Minnesota, for example, there was a purposeful change in the school start time for high school students, and there was a measurable improvement in school attendance and standardized testing outcomes.

Your biological clock cycle starts to advance in your middle to late twenties and thirties, meaning you fall asleep earlier and get up earlier. But it shifts again in your later decades, when you tend to fall asleep much earlier than you used to and wake up much earlier in the morning. This may be one reason why early-bird specials are popular in retirement areas.

How can you tell if your children are getting enough sleep?

It depends on their age. Before the age of about 10 or so, some children tend to get hyperactive when they're sleep deprived. In fact, some of the hyperactivity in children this young and in some young adolescents is really related to sleep loss, not to underlying neurological disease. Of course, if your child is hard to awaken, visibly sleepy, not performing well in school, and runs out of energy in the afternoon, it's also a sign that he or she is sleep deprived. Teenagers generally manifest lack of sleep more or less the same way adults do. They look tired and may be cranky and can unintentionally doze when not engaged.

Is it a good idea to take a nap every day?

We are biologically hardwired to nap. The neurons in one part of the brain that help to keep you awake fire actively until about 1 p.m., when there is a dip in activity for about 2 hours before they return to full activity. So it's not abnormal to feel a bit sleepy after lunch. As it turns out, a short nap of between 20 and 30 minutes is the optimal length required to restore the feeling of alertness. Studies also show that a daytime nap can help improve learning and memory and enhance feelings of well-being.

What do you recommend for people who have difficulty sleeping?

It depends on the kind of insomnia the person is experiencing. If someone has acute insomnia that is caused by a death in the family or the loss of a job, then sleeping pills are great because they work immediately and can help restore normal sleep patterns without interfering with daily activities. There are several different types of sleep medications, including some nonprescription ones like the hormone melatonin, which is sold over the counter and can help restore normal sleep cycles in some circumstances, such as insomnia due to jet lag. Before taking any sleep medication, prescription or otherwise, talk to your doctor or to a sleep medicine specialist.

If you have chronic insomnia and you've acquired a lot of bad habits to compensate for the sleep loss, like relying on caffeinated beverages all day to stay awake or staying up all night watching TV to pass the time, then cognitive behavioral therapy may help. Along with making some simple lifestyle changes, like setting your alarm to wake you up at the same time as often as possible, cognitive behavioral therapy has proven to be better than sleeping pills for treating chronic insomnia because it identifies the issues that allow insomnia to persist and gives you tools to permanently reverse those behaviors. Cognitive behavioral therapy for chronic insomnia is more than a simple set of rules that you follow to achieve good sleep. In order for it to be most effective, it is best delivered by a sleep medicine specialist or a sleep therapist.

Can you ever make up for lost sleep?

The answer is yes and no, depending on the circumstances. In the case of acute sleep loss, yes. If I take a normal individual and deprive him of sleep for a week   that is, I let him sleep for only 5 or 6 hours a night—there will be some predictable changes in behavior and in metabolism. If, however, I allow him to have recovery sleep for the next 4 or 5 nights— that is, I let him sleep as long as he needs to—within a few days he will be back to normal and feel fully refreshed.

The other scenario, and this is the more typical one, is the individual who gets only 6 hours of sleep during the workweek and then tries to make up for the sleep loss on the weekend. That won't work. Unless you change your sleeping habits so that you are consistently getting enough sleep, even during the workweek, you won't ever feel fully restored and your body will not get back to normal.

PART 2

The South Beach Diet Wake-Up Program

7 SIMPLE STRATEGIES FOR BETTER HEALTH

In the first part of this book, I described the destructive behaviors that are threatening your future and the future of your children. I explained how our unhealthy way of life is overwhelming the gains we have made in medicine over the past century and how, if we stay on this path, we will for the first time in modern history see a decline in average life span.

Now comes the good news. In the pages that follow, you will learn how to stop the downward spiral.

The South Beach Diet Wake-Up Program is a holistic lifestyle program that we have designed over the years to help individuals and families achieve optimal health and wellness. The goal of this program is twofold: to help you create a healthful environment in your home and daily life—protecting you from the potential fate of living out your years in sickness and pain—and to improve the health outlook for generations to come.

We show you how to shop, cook, and eat better and how to move from a sedentary to an active lifestyle. We also give you a plan for assessing your sleep habits and for making simple changes to achieve a restorative night's sleep. I have seen how these strategies can lead to sustainable changes that result in a healthier and happier life.

HOW DOES THE PLAN WORK?

The South Beach Diet Wake-Up Program consists of seven simple strategies that add up to a powerful and positive way of life:

1. **Control the Clutter, Free Your Mind**
2. **Make Every Meal Matter**
3. **Shop Right!**
4. **Cook As If Your Life Depends on It**
5. **Eat In More, Dine Out Smart**
6. **Get Moving, Get Fit**
7. **Sleep Better, Live Longer**

The sooner you embrace them, the sooner you will free yourself from the reckless behaviors that are killing you. I do, however, want you to tackle these strategies in a way that will make them stick.

So, before you dive in, I suggest that you take some time to review all seven strategies and decide how best to implement them in your own life. Some ideas may resonate with you more than others. If you are up all night tossing and turning, you may be eager to try my suggestions for getting better sleep sooner rather than later. The way you approach one strategy may be influenced by your approach to another. For example, in Strategy 7, Sleep Better, Live Longer, there are tips on how to create a restful environment in your bedroom, and these tips may also be useful for Strategy 1, Control the Clutter, Free Your Mind, as you prepare your living space for your new, healthier lifestyle. And while you are cleaning up your home, you may also want to be thinking about the main message of Strategy 6, Get Moving, Get Fit, and consider your cleaning time as an excellent opportunity to bring more functional exercise into your day. Although these strategies are presented separately, they are meant to work together and there is some overlap; feel free to take on more than one strategy at a time.

While I encourage people to work at their own pace, your goal should be to implement all seven strategies within 30 days. If you find yourself slacking off, I recommend that you reread Chapter 2 to remind yourself how a toxic lifestyle is slowly destroying every cell in your body. That should motivate you to get back on track. Regardless of how you approach making these changes, if you are committed to doing so, by the end of 30 days you should begin to see and feel a real difference in your health and well-being.

As part of each strategy, I offer special tips for parents created with the help of Andrea Vazzana, PhD, a clinical assistant professor in the Department of Child and Adolescent Psychiatry at New York University. Dr. Vazzana works directly with children and their parents, and her insights will help parents better incorporate each of these strategies into family life. Dr. Alejandro Chediak, a nationally recognized expert in sleep medicine, whose interview appears in Chapter 9, was instrumental in developing our sleep strategies.

BEFORE BEGINNING THE STRATEGIES: ASSESS YOUR LIFESTYLE

Before you even tackle Strategy 1 of the South Beach Diet Wake-Up Program, you need to ask yourself, "Just how toxic is my lifestyle?" and "What areas need the most improvement in my life?" For example, if you're 30 to 45 years old and grew up on fast food like so many of your peers (and maybe you're still eating too much of it), are you worried about the long-term impact of a poor diet on your health? Do you walk around feeling exhausted much of the time because you are stressed and not sleeping? Would you like to be exercising regularly but haven't managed to work it into your busy schedule? In sum, what is it about your life that you would like to change when it comes to improving your health? If you're not sure of the answer, I suggest you take our "Do You Need a Wake-Up Call?" online quiz at southbeachdiet.com/wakeupcall.

Of course, it's one thing to reflect on what you would like to do and quite another to actually take that first step and get started. Don't be discouraged if it takes you a little time to move from thought to action. Your persistence will pay off.

MAKE THE COMMITMENT

I've found that the people who do the best in transforming their lifestyle—those who sustain changes and don't revert back to their old bad habits—are the ones who are fully committed because they are aware of the benefits that will accrue. I hope the first part of this book has provided you with an understanding of why good nutrition, exercise, and sleep are so essential to your good health and well-being and that this will motivate you to take action.

When I work with my patients, I try to encourage them to lead a healthier life by explaining that some simple changes, like eating better and exercising regularly, can vastly improve their blood lipids and blood pressure, perhaps to the point where they no longer need medication. And of course I add that they will lose weight and generally look and feel better. For most people, these

If You Are a Parent

Once you've made the commitment to change your lifestyle for the better, you need to help your children feel a part of the process. Remember that your children take their cues from you. If you are positive and excited about what you are doing and explain in simple terms why you are doing it ("I want our family to be as healthy as we can be"), your kids will likely be cooperative—even enthusiastic. We have observed this in elementary schools where we have worked with the children of friends and patients.

It's very important for other adults in your home not to undermine your efforts; that is, if you have decided to stock the house with food that is compatible with the healthy eating principles of the South Beach lifestyle, you can't have your spouse, your children's grandparents, or caregivers paying lip service to your efforts and then bringing in junk food. By the same token, if you ask that everybody in the household turn off their electronic devices during a meal, everyone should comply.

Actions speak louder than words. Remember, kids pick up on the culture of a household, and what you do is more important than what you say. You can't exhort the benefits of living an active lifestyle as you

are very compelling—and convincing—arguments, and usually they are anxious to get started.

That said, I hear my fair share of excuses too. For every willing patient, there are those who claim to be too busy at work or at home to make even the slightest effort. So I tell them that while it may seem difficult in the beginning, once healthy lifestyle measures become a habit and they start to look and feel better, they'll wonder why they didn't make these changes sooner. I also tell them that they will find it easier to deal with stress and that more energy and less illness will lead to a healthier, happier, and more productive life.

channel surf from the couch. If you expect your kids to make fitness a habit, you need to exercise regularly yourself. If you believe that bedtime should be enforced, then you need to make sure that the household runs in a way that allows your children to go to sleep at a designated time every night. If you really want to reinforce the importance of sleep, you need to stick to a regular bedtime yourself as well.

All for one and one for all. If you have an overweight child, you must be careful that you are not singling him or her out—or appear as if you are—when it comes to adopting healthier eating habits or making other lifestyle changes. The South Beach Diet Wake-Up Program strategies are designed to benefit everyone in the household, including family members who are at a healthy weight and simply want to keep it that way. I want to stress that our program is not about putting children or teens on a diet. It is about helping young children learn how healthy food choices can give them energy, make them strong, and help them grow. It is about giving older kids the tools they need to transform their health and feel better about themselves. When children are provided with healthy food choices and opportunities for outdoor play and exercise, the weight takes care of itself. Kids do not have to "diet."

For some of you, the thought of saving your own life—or at least saving yourself from a debilitating old age—may be all the motivation you need to get started. If that still seems too abstract, then you'll need to find your own reasons for motivating yourself (and ideally, your entire family). Perhaps you need to reenter the job market and want to project health and confidence. Maybe you've just emerged from a divorce and want to look (and feel) your best so that you can resume dating. Perhaps your life's passion is to play a killer game of tennis or to go snorkeling on vacation and you can't muster the energy in your current physical condition. Or maybe, like the Super Moms whose stories appeared earlier in the book, you are determined to give your kids the best chance in life by creating a lifestyle for them that does not promote obesity and chronic disease.

Once you make the commitment and get started on the South Beach Diet Wake-Up Program, you will be taking a big step toward beginning the process of change. By implementing these strategies, you will be laying the foundation for a lifetime of healthy living for you and your family.

It's particularly important to keep in mind that successful change does not follow a continuously upward trajectory. There will be times when you may stumble or backtrack, and hate yourself for it in the morning. Don't allow setbacks to get you down. Simply pick up where you left off and keep looking forward. Remember, the goal is to learn how to make good choices in all aspects of your life *most of the time*. I don't expect perfection and neither should you. As my mom used to tell me, "Perfection is paralysis."

CONTROL THE CLUTTER, FREE YOUR MIND

You can't embark on a healthy new lifestyle if you are suffocating under the debris of the toxic old one. As you begin to make significant changes in your life, you need to feel emotionally strong and capable of performing the tasks that lie ahead. If you feel out of control, you will often end up doing what's most expedient at the time—skipping your workout or grabbing junk food instead of a healthy snack—and you will not be able to sustain these positive changes.

I have often been told that the process of housecleaning is exhilarating, not just because one's surroundings look better but also because people actually feel more focused and energized afterward. Outer clutter is often a sign of inner clutter, or emotional turmoil that is preventing you from moving forward. De-cluttering forces you to confront the contradictions in your life. For example, if you are trying to maintain a healthy weight, why is your refrigerator packed with so many take-out containers that you can't find your healthy snacks? If you are truly committed to using your home treadmill, why is it draped with clothes? Clearly, there is a disconnect between what your brain *thinks* you want and what you're actually *doing*. The process of de-cluttering will help close that gap and will help you put your thoughts into action.

This process is easier for some than for others. I admit to a particular problem keeping my desk clean at work and at home, and my wife refers to my nightstand drawer as "the pit." It's definitely better now than it used to be. If you are basically tidy but have not been careful about the food that you have been bringing into your home, de-cluttering may be as simple as cleaning out the fridge and pantry. If you look around your home and can't see a clear surface, you may need to spend a bit more time on de-cluttering; it will be well worth the effort.

ASSESS THE MESS

Walk through your home, room by room, with a pad, a pen, and a critical eye. Look around each room carefully and assess your living space. Make notes! When you see a problem area, write down what needs to be done on your to-do list. The big question: Is the room being utilized in the best possible way, or is it so overloaded with junk that you are not getting the full benefit of the space? Let's go room by room, then outdoors:

Is your kitchen functional and well stocked? Can you find counter space to prepare a meal, or is your kitchen the repository for everyone's backpacks, toys, work papers, and everything else no one knows what to do with? Is there a place to set up a cutting board and chop? Check the drawers: Are your cooking utensils accessible, even visible? Now look in the refrigerator and freezer. Has the fridge become a burial ground for last week's dinner leftovers and half-used condiments that should be tossed? Are the vegetable drawers filled with rotting produce? Do prehistoric meat packages fall from the freezer when you open it? Can you even find the lean ground turkey you bought on sale and froze last week? Check the pantry and cupboards. Do you see cans of sugary soda, packages of chips and cookies, bags and boxes of white flour, white pasta, and white rice, and nothing remotely healthy?

Are your dining surfaces clear? Or is your dining table covered with books, newspapers, magazines, and unpaid bills? Is your kitchen table overrun by craft projects or piles of junk mail? When was the last time you could actually see the table to set it?

Is your bedroom conducive to sleep? Or is it a home for distracting electronic equipment: a TV, computer, and/or DVR? Is the bed unmade and covered with clothing, paperwork, dog hair?

Is there a space to exercise indoors? If you have a family room or finished basement, is there room for you to do jumping jacks or dance moves or yoga there?

Is the outdoor sports equipment handy? Or do your kids have to climb through a packed closet or garage to find their bikes, basketballs, baseball bats and gloves, roller skates, ice skates, jump ropes, and the like?

Is the backyard well tended? Or has it become a dumping ground for the things you couldn't fit indoors or in the garage? Is it overgrown with weeds? Could you be using the space to grow a vegetable garden? Could you exercise out there? If you have younger kids, is there play equipment that is safe and inviting to use?

Now that you've taken the tour, I'm sure that you may be dismayed by the clutter you've ignored for so long. It's time to start fresh.

TAKE ACTION!

The next step is turning the preliminary to-do list you've made into action. Go through the list, room by room, checking off each task as you complete it. Expect that this job could take a few days, but try to get all your rooms in order before you move on to the rest of the strategies. It will make improving your lifestyle so much easier.

Get out the garbage can and recycling bin. Gather up all the papers and other clutter on the kitchen counters, on the dining and kitchen table, and in your bedroom. Separate out anything important and recycle what you don't need. Be ruthless. Then dust!

Use organizers. Buy some file boxes for your important papers and attractive holders for your kitchen utensils. Place empty baskets in every room for members of your household to stash newspapers and other reading material (and remind everyone to recycle the junk mail and newspapers daily).

Set some new ground rules. Make sure that everybody in the family understands that, from now on, no one is to park his or her stuff on the counters or dining tables. Be sure to follow your own rules and set a good example for the others.

(continued on page 174)

Foods to Remove from Your Pantry, Cupboards, and Fridge

Here's a quick checklist of foods that should be removed from your kitchen to help you stick to a healthy, South Beach–friendly way of eating. Exceptions can be made for special occasions, of course, and for children, since kids are not meant to be on a "diet" or a restricted eating plan. Our goal for children, as for adults, is to get them to make better food choices most of the time. Use your good judgment and buy empty-calorie foods only as a special treat. In fact, put "special treat" foods in opaque containers at the back of the fridge or on a high shelf. Out of sight, out of mind.

Baked goods All baked goods made with refined flour, including breads, bagels, rolls, cakes, cookies, crackers, cupcakes, muffins, waffles, and so on (see page 184 for a primer on replacing these with 100% whole wheat and whole-grain products)

Beverages All concentrated no-pulp fruit juices, sodas, alcohol, and any other drinks containing added sugars (see page 202 for a list of added sugars)

Candy All candy, except sugar-free and some dark chocolate

Cereals All varieties of sugary cereal, as well as cornflakes, cream of wheat, and instant oatmeal

Condiments, dressings, and seasonings Barbecue sauce, honey mustard, ketchup (recognizing that if you have children, you may want to keep some ketchup around for their burgers and healthy chicken tenders now and then), and any other condiment, sauce, or salad dressing made with corn syrup, molasses, or sugar

Dairy and cheese Whole milk; cheeses made with anything but 1%, part-skim, or fat-free milk; creamy cheeses, except for fat-free or low-fat cottage cheese; full-fat yogurt; ice cream

Flour All white flour and packaged products made with white flour, including pancake and waffle mixes (white whole-wheat flour is OK for baking)

Fruit Canned fruit in syrup; sugared fruit jams and jellies

Meat and poultry Anything processed using sugars (honey-baked or maple-cured ham, for instance); fatty fowl such as goose and duck legs; pâté; dark-meat chicken and turkey (legs and wings); processed fowl such as packaged chicken nuggets or patties; beef brisket, liver, rib steaks, skirt steak, bacon, bologna, pepperoni, salami, and other fatty meats

Oils and fats All solid vegetable shortening or lard, butter, and hydrogenated oils

Pasta All pasta made from refined grains (replace with those made from brown rice, soy, spelt, whole wheat, or quinoa)

Potatoes White and instant

Rice White rice (except white basmati), jasmine rice, sticky rice

Soy Full-fat soy milk

Snacks All unhealthy snacks are off-limits (such as chips and cookies)

Soup All powdered soup mixes (many are full of trans fats and lots of sodium)

Sweeteners All sweeteners, except sugar substitutes. You can keep some natural sugar or stevia around for the kids and yourself, for those times when you may want a little sprinkled on steel-cut oatmeal or other high-fiber whole-grain cereals.

Transform the Kitchen

The biggest part of turning a kitchen into a healthy place to cook and eat is to get rid of the bad food to make room for the good. (Then you can go shopping using our Master Shopping List, on page 307–13, which you can adapt week by week.)

Start with your pantry, cupboards, and fridge. Use the list on pages 172–73 as a guide for what to toss. Or, if you have unopened packages that you think might be right for a local food bank, by all means give the food away. Once you've done so, look at what's left and dump any perishables that have exceeded their expiration date or that look less than savory. Also open up containers of herbs and spices and put them to the "smell test." If any smell musty or have no smell at all, they are too old and should be thrown out and replaced next time you go shopping. Smell or taste all your salad and cooking oils to make sure that they haven't become rancid. If they smell or taste acrid, throw them out.

Clear out the freezer. Toss out anything undated or that has passed its expiration date (including food you froze yourself) and anything with freezer burn. Toss the half-finished cartons of ice cream and any frozen entrées or desserts that contain sugar, saturated fat, or a lot of sodium. You will need an organized freezer to store the meals you'll now (ideally) be cooking ahead for quick dinners during the week, and you'll want to have room to freeze plenty of lean meats, seafood, vegetables, and fruits, as well as homemade broth.

Create a Peaceful Bedroom

Keep in mind that your bedroom is supposed to be used for just two purposes at night: sleep and sex. You should strive to make this room a sanctuary of tranquility, which may take some doing, especially if yours doubles as a home office.

Remove the electronics (or at least make them disappear at night). The blue light emitted from computers and TVs can suppress melatonin production and disrupt sleep. And tuning in to the often-disturbing late-night news isn't conducive to a good night's rest either. If possible, move home computers,

TVs, and any other equipment not related to sleep to another room or behind a room divider. If you can't do that, turn them off and keep them off.

Keep the desktop clear. If you do need to use part of the bedroom for a home office, keep your desk tidy and, if possible, use a laptop, which you can stash away when you're finished working for the day.

Make a Space to Exercise

If you choose to work out at home, you need to make sure that you have a clear space to do your exercises. Find a corner of the living room, den, bedroom, or basement that you can convert into your exercise space. Keep it clear of clutter so that you don't have to clean it up every time you want to work out. It's a good idea to keep your exercise mat or towel, and whatever other small equipment you may use, in a basket or small chest near the exercise area so it is close at hand when you need it. (See pages 228–37 for an interval walking plan that you can adapt to a treadmill, exercise bike, or elliptical trainer indoors along with some strength-training exercises.)

Improve Your Outdoor Space

If you are lucky enough to have a yard or a terrace, take full advantage of it.

Create an outdoor play area. If you have small children, consider getting some basic playground equipment like swings or a slide, which will encourage them to be physically active. Remember, it doesn't take a lot of space to put up a basketball hoop.

Plant an edible garden. Is there a corner of the yard that can be used to plant a vegetable or herb garden? Can you devote part of a terrace to growing herbs, tomatoes, and other edible plants? Kids love to eat what they grow, and they will be willing to taste many more vegetables when they see how the plants bloom in "their" garden.

Make a space for alfresco dining. If you have the space, consider buying an outdoor dining table and chairs. Eating outdoors in good weather is a real treat and a great incentive for families to eat together. If you have an outdoor barbecue, the kids can run around and play while you grill dinner (lean protein and wholesome veggies, of course).

If You Are a Parent

Keep your family informed about why you are cleaning up and why it is so important. In other words, tell them that it is essential to make space for your new, healthier lifestyle. Let them know that the junk food you are throwing out will be replaced with good-tasting healthy food you're sure they'll like. Get them excited about the prospect of an active lifestyle.

Get the little kids involved. Younger children enjoy being called upon to do "adult tasks," and they will probably jump at the chance to work with you. Declare a "Clean-Up Day" and have them help you clear a space for their outdoor play or indoor exercise. If you plan to install some play equipment in your yard, get them involved in helping you chose the equipment so they have a stake in using it. Reward them when their work is done by enjoying a picnic or bike ride together.

Encourage older kids to support the plan. Adolescents and teenagers may be more recalcitrant about change, especially if it is being instigated by their parents. Expect to be greeted with the usual eye-rolling. Your job is to help them understand what's in it for them. Keep in mind that teenagers often do not respond to long-term goals like "If we get healthier food in the house, you won't have a heart attack in 20 years" or to being badgered about their weight. They *are* receptive to more immediate rewards, however. For example, an overweight or unfit teenager may be motivated to start a walking program to develop more stamina so he can shoot some hoops with the kids next door. Overweight teens who gorge on junk food may be encouraged to participate in a healthier lifestyle by being reminded that eating healthy—not necessarily eating less—could help them shed some pounds so that they can wear more fashionable clothes, or eventually join a sports team, or feel confident enough to ask someone on a date. And you can confidently tell them that better nutrition and exercise will improve their complexion. It's the best and most natural way to fight acne.

MAKE EVERY MEAL MATTER

Many of my patients ask me how much of what foods to eat at meals. They have seen the latest federal dietary guidelines and they want to know how these new recommendations dovetail with our South Beach eating principles. What I like to say is that, finally, the dietary guidelines have come around to our way of thinking, by recommending, in a nutshell, that Americans consume more nutrient-dense foods. In summary, the USDA says to fill at least half of your plate with fruits and vegetables and the other half with grains (ideally whole grains) and protein (lean, please). It recommends that you drink low-fat dairy and cut down on processed foods high in sodium, saturated fat, and sugars.

When you eat a satisfying, healthy diet like this, you don't have to worry about counting grams of fat, carbs, or protein or resort to weighing or measuring your food. That's because when you create meals focusing on nutrient- and fiber-rich carbohydrates (vegetables, fruits, whole grains), lean sources of protein, good unsaturated fats, and low-fat dairy, you will feel satisfied and have little desire to overeat. In other words, if you eat nutrient-dense foods, portion control takes care of itself. Furthermore, counting, weighing, and measuring simply aren't conducive to a pleasant and sustainable lifestyle.

Another essential in a healthy diet (and I use "diet" here to mean a healthy way of eating, not simply a means of losing weight) is to eat three meals and at least two snacks each day. This helps prevent the drop in blood sugar that typically results when you don't eat often enough, leading to fatigue and then cravings. It also reduces the need to reach for a sugary or starchy infusion to feel better. I realize how hard eating regularly may seem in this hectic world, but if you or members of your family start skipping meals and healthy snacks, or start grabbing chips, pretzels, or candy from a vending machine when you have the 11 a.m. or 4 p.m. munchies, these bad decisions will become a habit that will take a toll on your health.

I covered our basic South Beach eating principles in the first part of this book, but when it comes to eating for good health, there are some things I can't seem to explain enough. In general, many people don't believe they need to eat breakfast every day (in fact, only 46 percent of Americans do so 7 days a week), especially when they're racing to get out the door in the morning. Many also don't understand why snacking is so important to their health and why these mini-meals won't make them fat. And of course many don't want to start a diet because they think they'll have to permanently give up chocolate cake.

Here's what I tell them.

START THE DAY RIGHT

There's no question that my mom (and probably yours too) was right. Breakfast is the most important meal of the day. Why? As numerous studies now confirm, people who skip a morning meal tend to eat more poorly throughout the day than those who eat breakfast. They also exercise less. Furthermore, adults who regularly miss breakfast tend to have higher cholesterol, elevated insulin levels, and larger waist circumferences (all risk factors for heart disease). Children who miss breakfast (and some 34 percent of youngsters regularly do) tend to have weight issues and more instances of type 2 diabetes. They also have trouble concentrating, have higher absenteeism rates at school, and, not surprisingly, do worse academically. And breakfast skippers open themselves up to hunger, cravings, and the tendency to grab whatever unhealthy foods are available.

Choose lean protein and fiber. The best breakfast consists of some lean protein and fiber. Both help stabilize your blood sugar and keep you feeling satisfied until at least midmorning, when you should enjoy your first snack of the day. I usually start my day off with a couple of scrambled eggs or an omelet made with chopped vegetables, reduced-fat cheese, or salmon. Chopped frozen spinach and tofu are also good choices for a healthy breakfast omelet. The reality is, it doesn't take very much time to whip up a couple of eggs, and while eggs do have a fair amount of dietary cholesterol (185 milligrams in one yolk), studies have found that dietary cholesterol doesn't raise levels of blood cholesterol in most people, even when eggs are eaten most days of the week.

If you are not an egg fan, there are plenty of other choices that will start you off on the right track. Spread some nut butter on whole-grain bread or have some reduced-fat cottage cheese or nonfat Greek yogurt. Add some seasonal berries, an apple, a banana, or another fresh fruit and you're good to go. (See our Sample Meal Plan for a Healthy Week, on page 194, for more breakfast ideas.)

Be ready to grab and go when necessary. Many patients tell me that they would love to eat breakfast but that they're so busy in the morning, trying to get the kids fed and to school and/or themselves to work, that the idea of eating anything seems overwhelming. My answer is, you don't have to cook breakfast from scratch every morning, and you can often make the whole meal, or at least do some of the prep work, ahead of time.

When you are in the kitchen preparing dinner, hard boil some eggs or start some steel-cut oatmeal cooking in a slow cooker to be ready in the morning. When you're ready to head out, just put them in a container (microwavable for the oatmeal) and go. Or make our Sweet and Savory Breakfast Burritos with Sautéed Apples (page 262), Pumpkin-Cranberry Breakfast Bread (page 264), or Blueberry Buttermilk Muffins with Almonds (page 266) in advance and wrap and store them for easy portability when you're in a rush.

Another quick breakfast option is a healthy smoothie, which can be whipped up in a blender in minutes. Just toss in your favorite fresh or frozen fruit, some reduced-fat milk or plain nonfat yogurt or silken tofu, and maybe some flaxmeal, and you have a quick protein- and fiber-rich breakfast drink that can be enjoyed either at home or on the road. You can also buy single-serving containers of cottage cheese or yogurt to grab and go.

Not hungry in the morning? Some patients tell me that they just don't feel hungry first thing in the morning. If you're like these people, do what I tell them to do: Eat something anyway. Start off with a light breakfast, like one hard-boiled egg and half a banana, or a half cup of fat-free Greek yogurt and a handful of nuts, or a small serving of oatmeal. Once you see how much better you feel and how much more energy you have, you can increase the amount of food you're eating, or not. I've found that patients who used to avoid breakfast altogether soon become breakfast fanatics—and they tell me they'll never go without this important meal again.

SNACK STRATEGICALLY

When I tell patients that they *really should* eat at least two snacks daily in addition to three meals, some are very skeptical, especially those who are struggling with their weight. They have trouble believing that eating more can actually help them weigh less and maintain a healthy weight once they get there. The point of snacking an hour or two before lunch and dinner is to keep your blood sugar stable throughout the morning and afternoon, which prevents hunger and cravings between meals and keeps you from overdoing it when you do sit down to eat.

The most satisfying and energizing snacks contain some fiber-rich good carbohydrates and protein. The trick is to make sure you always have snacks at the ready—in your refrigerator at home and at work, in your desk drawer, and/or in your backpack and car for the times when you're out and about. You'll also want to be able to snack within 15 minutes after a workout to keep your energy up. Make sure your kids are provided with healthy snacks as well.

Here are some suggestions for nutritious and satisfying snacks that you can put in individual to-go bags or containers:

◆ A handful of almonds, cashews, pumpkin seeds, soy nuts, or dry-roasted edamame

◆ Apple slices with 1 or 2 tablespoons of natural no-sugar-added peanut butter or almond butter

◆ Carrot or celery sticks with a 2-ounce container of hummus

- ½ of a whole-wheat mini bagel topped with 1 or 2 tablespoons of fat-free or reduced-fat cream cheese
- ½ can of olive-oil or water-packed packed sardines with 8 whole-wheat crackers (look for crackers with the most fiber)
- 3 slices of turkey breast and 2 tablespoons of salsa in a small whole-wheat tortilla or half of a large tortilla
- 1 hard-boiled egg and 1 small sliced pear
- 1 cup of microwavable homemade bean or lentil soup
- 1 small peach and a reduced-fat spreadable cheese wedge
- Cottage cheese (1%, 2%, or fat-free) with salsa or chopped cucumber

ENJOY DESSERT IN MODERATION

I am quick to admit that I am a chocoholic who does enjoy a decadent dessert from time to time. In our South Beach eating plan, we have always made sure that a healthier dessert (ideally one that contains some filling protein) is a part of all phases, and I always tell my patients who ask that they can certainly enjoy a few bites of an empty-calorie dessert now and then. The fact is, once you have learned to make smart, healthy food choices most of the time, you can occasionally enjoy a decadent dessert in moderation. The problem in this country is that people have forgotten what the word "moderation" means, particularly when it comes to sugary confections.

If you are trying to lose weight, then having what we like to call a dessert "snack" after dinner—consisting of some nonfat yogurt or a piece of reduced-fat cheese and some almonds, or some melon or berries and a handful of nuts—can go a long way toward keeping you satisfied and preventing you from succumbing to the late-night munchies.

On pages 304–6, we've included two of my favorite special-occasion desserts, Chocolate Bark with Cranberries, Almonds, and Pecans and Multigrain Blueberry Cobbler, both of which include some of the best health-giving ingredients around. (Yes, bittersweet chocolate chips do have antioxidants!)

Here are some dessert pointers:

Take three bites. When you are confronted with a dessert that looks too good to pass up, just follow the South Beach Diet "Three-Bite Rule." Take three bites of the dessert, eating it as slowly as possible so you can savor each wonderful mouthful. And then pass your plate to a fellow diner, or to the busboy if you're in a restaurant. You'll soon see that enjoying just three bites of a decadent dessert can be as pleasurable as eating the whole thing and that your sweet tooth will be very satisfied with just a small portion.

Don't let the occasional splurge derail you. There will be occasions when you will inevitably eat the whole piece of cake. But don't let this become a pattern. If you continue to make healthy food choices most of the time, the occasional splurge is fine. It becomes a problem when you adopt an "I guess I blew it" attitude and allow yourself to get permanently off track, particularly if you are trying to lose weight. If you do detour, simply count it as that, and not as a derailment, and resume your healthful eating at the next opportunity.

Keep temptations out of sight. As noted in our Control the Clutter, Free Your Mind strategy, we recommend that if you do have indulgent desserts in the house (and we all do from time to time, particularly around birthdays and holidays), make sure that they aren't staring you in the face, especially if you or someone you live with is trying to make healthy eating changes. Keep cookies and cakes in the freezer until serving time, and when there are leftovers, send extras home with guests or cut them into bite-size pieces and store them in individual freezer bags.

CONSIDER YOUR EATING TRIGGERS

If you are eating three meals a day and snacks and yet still find yourself foraging through the refrigerator at odd times or buying chips and candy bars on the fly, you need to question what's triggering that behavior:

Are you really hungry? Hunger is the feeling you get when you experience a normal and gradual drop in blood sugar about 4 or 5 hours after a meal. It's your body's way of telling you that eating is overdue. Hunger signals can come from your stomach (in the form of growls, pangs, or a hollow feeling), as well as from your brain (which may include headachy sensations or fatigue).

Cravings, on the other hand, usually happen within a couple of hours of your last meal and are caused by exaggerated spikes and dips in blood sugar that can occur after you've eaten highly processed carbohydrates (like white bread, white pasta, or white rice), sugary baked goods, or candy bars. They're what drive you to want more of the same.

If you are eating three wholesome meals and snacks each day, then you probably won't be hungry. But if these meals and snacks still contain refined carbs and sugars, they could be what's driving you back to the fridge. You need to take a hard look at everything you eat and keep a food diary for a week or two. Also take a look at our "Quick Guide to Choosing the Right Carbs," on page 184, to remind yourself again of what's good and what you need to avoid.

If you are more than 10 pounds overweight and find that you are craving sugary and starchy carbs, you may want to try Phase 1 of the South Beach Diet, which is specifically designed to stabilize your blood sugar. See page 68 for a summary of the phases of our diet.

Are you eating because you're tired? If you are not getting enough sleep, your body will crave fuel, in the form of carbohydrates, to keep you going. Don't resort to sugars and refined starches, which will ultimately make you feel more tired and put you on the fast track to poorer health. Check out Strategy 7: Sleep Better, Live Longer, beginning on page 241, for tips on how to get enough rest at night so that you are not droopy during the day. And don't forget to eat your healthy snacks!

Are you eating for comfort? Moods and emotions play a huge role in how vulnerable we are to food and in our ability to stay in control of what we eat. There's no question that many people are "emotional" eaters; they eat when they are lonely, bored, upset, and sometimes even when they are happy. Stress is also a major trigger that can lead to cravings for "comfort foods" high in fat and refined sugary and starchy carbs. They don't call them "comfort foods" for nothing.

In fact, there are solid biological reasons why we are drawn to such foods. When stress strikes, the body releases hormones (specifically adrenaline and cortisol) to initiate a "fight or flight" response. This reaction is a holdover from

(continued on page 186)

A Quick Guide to Choosing the Right Carbs

If you have trouble remembering the difference between a good carbohydrate and a bad one, use this crib sheet for quick reference. But remember, a list of good carbs and bad carbs should not be seen as an absolute. While you should get most of your carbs each day from the "good" list, you certainly don't have to skip your birthday cake or that celebratory cocktail on occasion. Just don't make foods from the "bad" list an everyday thing, particularly if you have weight to lose.

For a Master Shopping List that specifically covers what good-carb foods to buy in each of these categories, and many other healthy foods as well, see pages 307–13 or download it from southbeachdiet.com/wakeupcall.

Good Carbohydrates

Also referred to as complex carbohydrates, good carbohydrates are digested slowly and release their sugar steadily, so they don't cause the fluctuations in blood sugar (the way refined carbs can) that can lead to hunger and cravings. Also, because of their high fiber content, good carbs help you feel fuller longer.

Enjoy these good carbs:

Whole fruits

Whole vegetables

Beans and other legumes (such as lentils and chickpeas)

Whole grains (such as 100% whole wheat, brown rice, quinoa, and
buckwheat)

100% whole-wheat and whole-grain breads

100% whole-wheat and whole-grain cereals

Whole-grain pastas

Bad Carbohydrates

Also referred to as simple carbohydrates, bad carbs are refined, highly processed sugary and starchy foods that have had all or most of their natural nutrients and fiber removed. Because the fiber has been stripped away, simple carbohydrates are rapidly digested and release their energy almost immediately, resulting in exaggerated swings in blood sugar that can cause hunger and cravings.

Avoid these bad carbs:

Processed refined grains (such as white flour and white rice)

Bread, bagels, crackers, and pasta made with any refined flour

White potatoes (which are technically a complex carb but act more like simple carbs in the body, especially when eaten without the skin)

Cakes, cookies, muffins, doughnuts, and other baked goods

Biscuit, pancake, and waffle mixes made with refined flour

Unhealthy snack foods (like chips and pretzels)

Sugary cereals

All candy (except sugar-free and dark chocolate in moderation)

Jellies and jams with sugar added

Non-diet soft drinks

Fruit juices and fruit drinks with sugar added and fiber removed

Puddings and custards

Sugary alcoholic drinks and mixers

our hunter-gatherer days, when we had to be able to outrun or outwit lurking prey—or we would perish. While adrenaline levels normalize pretty quickly, cortisol levels take longer. And even though today we generally don't have to beat the bushes for our next meal, the underlying physiological process still kicks in when we feel pressured, leaving chronically stressed people with constantly elevated levels of cortisol. And cortisol, unfortunately, acts as an appetite stimulant, one best satisfied by quick-energy-producing fats and carbohydrates.

The worst part about comforting yourself this way is that you feel terrible about yourself after you've done it, which turns up the stress hormones even further and starts the cycle all over again. The solution is to find a more positive way to respond to these feelings. Exercise is one of the best ways to counteract stress hormones, as well as to improve your overall health. It is also a natural mood booster. So instead of reaching for food when you are feeling emotional, reach for your sneakers instead. (For more on walking, see page 228).

MAKE THE MOST OF YOUR DINING TABLE

Once you've made the commitment to eat more meals at home, and have cleared the clutter off your dining room table, kitchen table, or breakfast counter, I urge you to actually sit at that table, alone or with family or friends, and enjoy your food. As I described in Chapter 7, if you are a parent, eating five or more meals a week with the family—whether it's breakfast, lunch, or dinner—has been shown to have numerous health and social benefits for children.

Don't let everyone's crazy schedules be a deterrent. If, as I suggest, you've planned a week's worth of meals, you will have already figured out (more or less) who's going to be home when and can set the table accordingly.

Here are some other suggestions for maximizing mealtime:

Actually set the table. An attractive table, set before the food is served, automatically draws people to it and creates a pleasant tone for the entire meal. It doesn't take more than a minute or two to put out some placemats, dishes, flatware, and maybe even some flowers. This is a great job for kids—as long as they are old enough to handle dishware and cutlery safely. Also, keeping the table semi-set most of the time will keep people from using it as a junk repository.

Turn off the TV. Eating while the TV is blaring in the same room or nearby is a bad combination. Not only does it distract from conversation; it also distracts everyone from paying attention to what they are eating. Numerous studies have confirmed that when a TV is on during meals, people mindlessly devour more food more quickly than they would if they were totally focused on their plates or one another.

Ban all other electronics. Today we live in a world in which it's nearly impossible to have a dinner or breakfast table conversation without the intrusion of an electronic device. Someone is always distracted by an e-mail, a text, or a call. Make sure that you, and all family members, switch off any electronic devices that can interfere with your meal; or better yet, leave the devices in another room and on silent. And don't answer the house phone during meals either (let the answering machine do it). If you like, you can enjoy quiet relaxing music (without headphones and with everyone listening) while you eat.

Encourage conversation. If silence reigns at your dining table, come prepared with some conversation starters for the kids, but avoid asking questions like "What did you do today?" that can result in a one word answer like "Nothing." Instead, ask "What was the funniest/most surprising/worst thing that happened to you today?" Or ask each child to describe the day's events in 1 minute. If you're a twosome who's gotten into the habit of reading at meals rather than making conversation, relegate the books and newspapers to another time and place.

Eat slowly and savor each bite. Eating should be a pleasurable, relaxing, *fulfilling* experience. If everyone actually enjoys their food, and gets the most out of each morsel, there will be more satisfaction and contentment at the end of each meal. Encourage everyone to put down their forks in between bites and to chew slowly. Remember, it takes the stomach about 20 minutes to signal the brain that it's full. Today there is plenty of research showing that

(continued on page 190)

If You Are a Parent

As I discussed in Chapter 7, children and teenagers who sit down for meals with their parents eat healthier food, do better at school, and are at less risk for drug abuse and other problematic behaviors. It is well worth the effort to make family meals a regular part of your life. If you can't carve out time to sit down together for at least five meals a week, it could be a sign that it's time to reassess priorities and make some changes. A family meal doesn't have to be dinner—any meal that you can share is fine—just don't expect teenagers to be too talkative in the morning.

Here are a few parental ground rules:

Set a mealtime schedule and stick to it. If everyone in the family knows what time dinner (or breakfast) will be served and that you're not cooking for anyone before or after that time, it makes it more likely they'll show up and eat it and less likely they'll be asking for meals to order. (You can obviously make exceptions for small children who go to bed early and need to eat sooner.) Of course, some flexibility for prior commitments can be factored in.

Set the tone. Mealtime should be harmonious: No arguing or teasing should be allowed at the table. Parents should set an example by keeping adult controversies out of the dining room. Furthermore, any discussion of a family member's weight should be off limits. Siblings can be very cruel to an overweight brother or sister, and if the subject of weight arises at mealtime, it's important for parents to nip it in the bud immediately. Parents must also be models for trying new foods, for eating slowly, and for encouraging conversation.

Encourage a taste. Although it is a terrible idea to force children to eat something they despise (or at least *think* that they do), I do believe it's important to urge kids to at least have a small bite of a food before rejecting it, even if they have tasted it before. In some cases, it may take up to 20 exposures to a new food (presented in different ways, of course) before a child decides that he or she likes it, and tastes certainly change as children get older. The point is, don't give up trying and don't use a bribe like dessert as a reward. Bribes only fuel suspicion that there's something wrong with what you're serving.

Never force children to eat everything on their plate. Parents have the responsibility of providing healthy food and a wholesome atmosphere in which to eat it. It's up to each child to determine how much to eat, and that decision should be based on the child's own perception of feeling full. Parents should put a reasonable serving of food on their children's plates—not pile it sky-high—and let them eat until they say they've had enough. Never push a child to eat more and never use the line "If you don't finish dinner, you won't get dessert." The "Clean Plate Club" threat has encouraged too many kids to ignore their own appetite cues and eat more than they would have or probably should have. It is a tradition that should end. If a child refuses to eat, simply put his plate in the fridge and bring it out later to reheat when he says he's hungry. This way, you don't become a short-order cook and your consistency will help prevent random demands.

Say yes to seconds. If a child wants a second helping of something, let him have it, even if you are worried about his weight. If he is provided with healthy choices and is engaging in regular physical activity, in most cases eating a second serving won't contribute to weight gain or impede weight loss. My only caveat is that it's very important for children to learn how to recognize real hunger as opposed to eating seconds out of habit. Therefore, after finishing a meal, all family members (not just the ones who need to shed some pounds) should be sure they are still truly hungry before taking another helping. (As I noted earlier, it takes about 20 minutes for the stomach to signal to the brain that it is full.) Of course, parents must set a good example by following this advice themselves.

routinely galloping through meals often leads to chronic overeating and obe-sity. This is because putting too much food in your stomach too quickly can interfere with your body's feedback mechanisms, prompting you to continue to take in calories even though you're full.

Recently, I came across a small study published in the *Journal of Clinical Endocrinology and Metabolism* that provides more evidence for why this hap-pens. Greek researchers found that speed eating limits the release of appetite-regulating hormones called peptides in the digestive system (or gut) and promotes overeating. In the study, the scientists compared blood samples from volunteers who had eaten about 675 calories' worth (about 10 ounces) of ice cream very rapidly (in 5 minutes) with those who had eaten more slowly (over 30 minutes). Those who had eaten more slowly, savoring the ice cream over half an hour, had the highest levels of two peptides that signal fullness, or satiety, and actually felt more full than the group who had eaten quickly. While I don't recommend that you start eating ice cream, the point is, if you slow down and focus on every mouthful of food, you will not only enjoy it more, but it will also permit your body's natural satiety-signaling systems to work more effectively.

SHOP RIGHT!

You've cleared the clutter and set up your kitchen for healthy cooking. Now it's time to start preparing more meals at home, if you aren't doing so already. Of course, you should use the healthiest ingredients, and this may mean changing your shopping habits. Whether you're eating at home on your own, dining with your family, filling a child's lunch box, or nibbling food from a brown bag at your desk, it helps to plan your menus and shop ahead so you always have the makings for healthy breakfasts, lunches, dinners, and snacks. By buying your own food and preparing it yourself, you can ensure you're getting the maximum nutrients in each meal. Or to put it another way, if you don't know what you're having for dinner on any given night, it increases the odds that (1) you will likely be searching out convenience food when the hunger pangs finally do strike and (2) you won't be having dinner as a family (or at all).

Whether you're trying to lose weight or simply to stay healthy, the importance of eating three meals a day and strategic snacks cannot be underestimated. It's also important to be aware that a key remedy for preventing obesity, prediabetes, type 2 diabetes, and a host of other ailments plaguing our nation today can be found right in your own kitchen—in your refrigerator, pantry, and cupboards. But that's only if they're filled with the right foods.

On the following pages you'll find ways to shop that will save you money without sacrificing the nutritional quality of the foods you buy. While there will always be new studies touting the health benefits of one food over another, there is no question that when it comes to healthy eating, a diet that contains plenty of nutrient-dense, high-fiber vegetables (including legumes);

fruits; whole grains; lean protein; good fats; and low-fat dairy (if you eat dairy) is the right way to eat. Additionally, if you serve a wide variety of these foods at most meals most of the time, you will make great strides in improving your own health and the health of your family.

MAKE A WEEKLY MEAL PLAN

No busy home cook wants to be running in and out of the supermarket every day for lack of planning. That's why creating menus for the week (building in a night out for fun), and a shopping list to match, saves time (and money).

To plan menus, however, you need to think about who's home when and also to consider changing up your same-old, same-old repertoire with some tasty new mealtime ideas. Making some meals using leftovers should be factored in, as should preparing on-the-go breakfasts and office and school lunches. For inspiration, take a look at our Sample Meal Plan for a Healthy Week, on page 194, which utilizes a number of the recipes in this book. (For those of you on the South Beach Diet, be aware that these menu ideas are consistent with Phase 2 of the diet.)

Remember, nothing can derail a week's menu planning quicker than becoming a "short-order cook," acquiescing to everyone's personal tastes at mealtime. I recently saw a sign in a friend's kitchen that said, "You have two choices for dinner. Take it or leave it." This may be a little harsh, but the point is that catering to picky eaters creates picky eaters and destroys the best-laid plans for serving the healthiest meals. When planning menus for the week, try to think of meals that have at least one key element that everyone will enjoy and also consider dishes that can be easily customized. For example, provide various veggie toppings for whole-wheat pizzas and let each person design his or her own pizza. Do the same for taco fillings and toppings. And consider a make-your-own salad night. Even if you get complaints that "there's nothing to eat," I assure you that your family won't starve.

Consider everyone's schedule. Plan your meals around your own and your family's weekly schedule as much as possible. Do you or your spouse (or other family members) come home later on some nights than others (or not at all if someone is traveling or working nights)? If that's the case, prepare a big meal and package the leftovers for those who can't make the original dinnertime. Or cook ahead and refrigerate or freeze individual portions.

Consider a "meatless weekday" or two. The idea of Meatless Mondays has been around for a while to encourage plant-based eating and reduce the amount of saturated fat in our diet, but eating meatless meals any day of the week is fine. Whether you choose one based on beans, eggs, or tofu or another soy protein, there are plenty of dishes that you and your family will enjoy. For example, try a wholesome dish like Black Bean Chili with Tangerine-Avocado Salsa (page 286), which you can make on the weekend, or Mighty Mac and "Cheese" (page 290), which requires less than 15 minutes of hands-on time. Both are great sources of protein and contain plenty of fiber and antioxidants as well. Meatless meals are often more economical too.

Consider ethnic nights. Plan dinners around ethnic themes; it's a great way to make mealtime fun, and if you have kids, they'll look forward to Italian Wednesdays or Chinese Fridays. (It's also a conversation-starter about what's most nutritious in these cuisines and what to stay away from.) Use the recipes on pages 259–306 for ideas. For example, on Italian night serve Mega-Meatballs and Sauce (page 276) with whole-wheat pasta preceded by a vegetable antipasto. (You can make the meatballs ahead of time and freeze them.) For Middle Eastern night, start the meal with Lemony Tomato Hummus with Carrot Chips (page 269) followed by Lentil-Bulgur Salad with Summer Squash and Walnuts (page 292). For Asian night, try Stir-Fried Garlic Shrimp with Bok Choy (page 289) served with brown rice rather than white.

Plan for leftovers. Recycling leftovers into next-day meals and snacks not only saves you cooking time, it also helps keep your food budget in check. Leftover flank steak (page 279), for example, can be sliced and tossed with veggies for a lunchtime salad; extra chicken (pages 275 and 278) can be turned into a chicken salad sandwich on whole-grain bread or be sliced, reheated, and served with vegetables over brown rice for dinner; leftover grilled salmon (page 288) makes a great salad paired with greens and a mustardy yogurt dressing; leftover broccoli (page 297) or sweet potatoes (page 303) can be used the next day for a vegetable omelet or frittata for breakfast or dinner.

SAMPLE MEAL PLAN FOR A HEALTHY WEEK

	BREAKFAST	LUNCH	DINNER	SNACKS
MEATLESS MONDAY	• Vegetable juice blend • Toasted Pecan Muesli with Dried Fruit (page 268) • ½ cup nonfat Greek yogurt • Coffee or tea	• Lentil-Bulgur Salad with Summer Squash and Walnuts (page 292) • Tomato slices with fresh basil	• Black Bean Chili with Tangerine-Avocado Salsa (page 286) • Slice of whole-wheat baguette • Chocolate Bark with Cranberries, Almonds, and Pecans (page 306)	• Lemony Tomato Hummus with Carrot Chips (page 269) • Feta cheese cubes (marinated in 2 tablespoons low-sugar vinaigrette) with bell pepper slices
TUESDAY	• Cantaloupe wedge • Poached egg and Canadian bacon atop ½ whole-wheat English muffin • Coffee or tea	• Cobb salad (top chopped romaine with diced reduced-sodium deli chicken, crumbled turkey bacon, and chopped avocado, tomato, and red onion) with balsamic vinaigrette	• Stir-Fried Garlic Shrimp with Bok Choy (page 289) • Brown rice • Sliced cucumber and radish salad drizzled with extra-virgin olive oil and vinegar • Sliced kiwi with a squeeze of lemon	• Red bell peppers with a spreadable reduced-fat cheese wedge • Asparagus spears with ham (wrap baby asparagus with lean ham and sprinkle with extra-virgin olive oil, lemon juice, and black pepper)
WEDNESDAY	• Blueberry Buttermilk Muffin with Almonds (page 266) • Scrambled eggs with chopped chives • Coffee or tea	• Tuscan Kale and Mushroom Soup (page 274) • ½ lean roast beef sandwich on whole wheat bread with horseradish	• Chicken Cutlets with Apricot Sauce and Pistachios (page 278) • Sweet Potato Salad with Fresh Basil (page 303) • Sugar-free vanilla pudding cup	• Tuna "boats" (fill celery stalks with tuna salad) • Granny Smith apple slices with 1 slice reduced-fat Cheddar cheese
THURSDAY	• Sweet and Savory Breakfast Burrito with Sautéed Apples (page 262) • Coffee or tea	• Greek salad (top chopped romaine with diced cucumbers and tomatoes, kalamata olives, and reduced-fat feta cheese) with 2 tablespoons red wine vinaigrette	• MegaMeatballs and Sauce (page 276) • Whole-wheat couscous • Mixed green salad with 2 tablespoons low-sugar prepared dressing • ½ cup fat-free Greek yogurt with berries	• 2 deviled egg halves with cherry tomatoes • "Cheesesteak" bundles (wrap cubes of string cheese in lean deli-sliced roast beef; microwave for 15 seconds)

	BREAKFAST	LUNCH	DINNER	SNACKS
FRIDAY	• Cheddar cheese toast (melt reduced-fat Cheddar on 1 slice 100% whole-grain bread) • Fresh berries • Coffee or tea	• Super Veggie Minestrone (page 272) • Hearts of romaine with 2 tablespoons low-sugar Greek Goddess dressing	• Grilled Salmon with Cucumbers and Ginger Dressing (page 288) • Greens Gratin with Turkey Bacon (page 299) • Quinoa • Raspberries with mint	• Fresh pear slices with ½ cup fat-free Greek yogurt and 6 walnut halves • Turkey roll-up (spread deli-sliced turkey with Dijon mustard, top with a slice of reduced-fat provolone cheese, and roll up)
SATURDAY	• ½ grapefruit • Scrambled eggs • Turkey bacon • Coffee or tea	• Mighty Mac and "Cheese" (page 290) • Assorted vegetable crudités	• Chicken in Mexican Mole Sauce (page 275) • Chunky Guacamole Salad (page 301) • Sugar-free gelatin with sliced banana	• Individual 3-ounce can water-packed light tuna with 8 whole-wheat crackers • Snow peas with red pepper dip (purée jarred roasted red peppers with fat-free or reduced-fat cottage cheese)
SUNDAY	• Fresh orange segments • Chickpea and Carrot Frittata (page 263) • Coffee or tea	• Layered Salad with Creamy Cilantro Dressing (page 294) • Small whole-wheat pita	• Better Beef Burgundy (page 280) • Watercress and endive salad with fresh lemon juice and extra-virgin olive oil • Baked apple with chopped walnuts	• Salmon Mousse with Vegetable Dippers (page 270) • Caprese snack (toss mini mozzarella balls and grape tomatoes with extra-virgin olive oil and red pepper flakes)

MAKE A HEALTHY GROCERY LIST

Before heading out to the supermarket, farmers' market, or co-op, review your meal plan for the week and make a grocery list that includes all the ingredients for each meal. A list is essential for efficient shopping, for figuring out expenses ahead of time, and for keeping unhealthy impulse items out of your shopping cart. Divide the list by food/product type. Your basic categories should include Vegetables; Fruits; Lean Protein (Meat, Seafood, and Poultry); Soy-Based Meat Substitutes; Whole Grains; Beans and Other Legumes; Dairy,

The Lowdown on Buying Whole-Grain Products

If you don't read the ingredient list on a food package, you can't be truly sure that a product that purports to be whole grain actually is. But how do you separate the true whole-grain products from the huge number of imposters on the supermarket shelves? Before buying any grain product—bread, crackers, cereal, or pasta—check the ingredient list to make sure it says "100% whole wheat," "100% whole oats," or "100% whole rye," for example. Skip products that simply say "whole wheat"; they may be predominantly whole wheat, but it's not a guarantee. Also pass up any products that just use terms like "wheat flour," "enriched wheat," or "enriched white flour." Other commonly used words like "multigrain," "3-grain," or even "10-grain," which may make a product sound more wholesome, mean only that the product contains several different types of grains and are no assurance that any of them are whole grains. Even the word "organic," which describes how a product may be grown and processed, does not mean it's made with whole grains.

Cheese, and Eggs; Healthy Oils and Other Fats; Nuts and Seeds; Seasonings and Condiments; Beverages; and my favorite Special Treat, dark chocolate.

Then list the specific items you need under the appropriate headings. On pages 307–13 we have provided suggestions for healthy foods in each of these categories to help you get started. You can either photocopy this list or download it from southbeachdiet.com/wakeupcall. Once you've come up with your weekly meal plan and made your shopping list based on the recipes you want to prepare, go through your pantry, refrigerator, and freezer and cross off any items you already have. Although it's more efficient and economical to shop

So why is it so important to eat only whole grains? The term "whole grain" means that all parts of the grain kernel—the bran, germ, and endosperm—are kept intact, which is beneficial because the complete grain kernel contains the vitamins, minerals, and phytonutrients, as well as fiber, which appear to be protective against so many different types of diseases. The latest federal dietary guidelines recommend that everyone (except those who are already gluten-free) significantly reduce the amount of refined grains in their diet and replace them with whole grains.

Once you begin looking at grain packages, you will notice that some display a very visible black and yellow stamp from the Whole Grains Council, a nonprofit consumer advocacy group. There are two types of stamps: "100% whole grain," meaning that a product is made entirely from whole grains and "whole grain," meaning it may contain some refined grains. It's best to look for the 100 percent stamp. Just because a product does not have a Whole Grains Council stamp, however, does not mean that it is not whole grain. Once again, you need to read the label carefully. And please, try to get your kids used to doing so too.

once a week, there will, of course, be times that you'll want to purchase fresh ingredients more often. Consider how many times you can actually get to the market as you write up your shopping list.

Some In-Store Reminders

It's not that hard to shop, right? When it comes to making the healthiest meals, however, there are a few things people often forget:

Timing is everything. In considering when to shop for the week, keep in mind that most grocery store chains get deliveries on Mondays and Tuesdays and the freshest food is usually available on Wednesdays. Also, the best store sales tend to run Wednesdays to Sundays in many chains. Look at the weekend newspapers and supermarket circulars for sale items and coupons, or go to your favorite supermarket's Web site to see what will be on sale in the coming week. You may find "buy one, get one free" offers. Shopping close to closing time may also provide additional discounts, since perishable items sometimes must be sold by the end of the day.

Often the biggest bargains aren't at the grocery store. Consider shopping for some items at big box stores and also getting fresh produce from a local food co-op (see also "Shop Healthy on a Budget," on page 202).

Eat before you shop. You've heard this advice before, but it bears repeating. Never go shopping when you are hungry. You will be more vulnerable to the sights and smells of food and end up with a shopping cart full of items you wouldn't succumb to if your hunger were in check. Have a healthy snack at home or in your car before setting foot in the store.

Stick to your shopping list but be flexible. Having an easily readable list in hand will keep you from wandering aimlessly down the aisles, randomly tossing things into your cart that you may or may not ever use or that you'll regret later (like that box of cookies!). Be flexible, however, and don't pass up any super-sale items that you know you can use for present or future meals. You should be especially flexible when it comes to buying produce, purchasing what looks the freshest rather than just sticking to what's on your list.

Don't just shop the perimeter. It used to be standard advice to tell people trying to eat healthy to shop only the perimeter of the store—where you typically find fresh dairy, meat, poultry, produce, and fish—and to avoid shopping the center aisles, where the processed foods and sugary drinks are stocked. While the perimeter continues to be your main source for healthy items, these days shopping the center aisles is also essential for a well-rounded, healthy diet. It's here that you'll likely find whole-grain breads, cereals, and pastas; monounsaturated olive and canola oils; great vinegars; flavorful herbs and spices; and, of course, all manner of canned goods, including beans, fish (light tuna, salmon, and sardines), and vegetables (tomatoes being an important one), no-sugar-added jams and jellies, natural peanut butter, and lower-sodium soups.

Read the food labels. While about half of grocery shoppers say they read food labels to help them figure out what to buy, less than half of these people say they even bother to read the ingredient list after scanning the Nutrition Facts panel. There's no question that both can help you make better in-store decisions. And by the time this book comes out, there may finally be a front-of-package nutrition panel that is clearer and more helpful.

Since so many people are in a rush when grocery shopping (the average shopper purchases 61 items in 26 minutes), we suggest that you *look for a few key things on the Nutrition Facts panel:*

- **Serving size.** What you assume is a serving for one may actually be a serving for four, so read carefully.

- **Grams of dietary fiber.** The American diet is sorely lacking in this essential nutrient; see "Facts about Fiber," page 78.

- **Grams of sugar.** We're getting way too much of this empty-calorie nutrient; see the information on added sugars, page 202.

- **Protein.** Like fiber, it's very important for maintaining stable blood sugar levels, suppressing hunger, and controlling weight.

And when it comes to reading the ingredient list, we recommend that you look particularly for whole grains (see "The Lowdown on Buying Whole-Grain Products," on pages 196–97) and watch out for added sugars. Added sugars

(continued on page 202)

A Sugar Experiment

If you are following the typical toxic American diet, you are consuming 35 teaspoons of added sugar in your food *every day.* According to a 2011 USDA report, that adds up to an average of 132 pounds of sugar a year for every man, woman, and child in the United States.

I want you to conduct an experiment. If you have kids, invite them to join you.

Equipment needed: One box of granulated sugar, a teaspoon, a bowl, and a glass of water (which you'll need later)

Step 1: Carefully measure 35 teaspoons of sugar into the bowl.

Step 2: Eat all 35 teaspoons of sugar, one teaspoon at a time.

I bet most of you are horrified at the thought of eating all that sugar, and frankly, so am I. *Of course I don't want you to eat it!* I suggested this experiment to help you visualize your daily sugar intake.

If you eat processed foods regularly, chances are you're getting added sugar under a variety of guises—corn syrup, high-fructose corn syrup, glucose, honey, dextrose, fructose, crystalline fructose, maltose, malt syrup, and molasses, just to name a few (for others, see page 202). We all know that products like cookies, snack cakes, and candy bars are high in added sugar, but you may be surprised to learn how many other so-called "wholesome" foods are swimming in it, including breakfast cereals, commercial salad dressings, spaghetti sauces, canned fruit in syrup, and many granola bars. Read labels!

When you eat (or drink) something sugary, it produces a spike in blood glucose that turns on the production of insulin, which is the hormone that ushers sugar and fat into your cells and tissues. If you ingest sugar in the absence of fiber or protein, it breaks down very rapidly, producing a sudden drop in blood glucose that leaves you feeling ravenous—this is the source of most food cravings. Although added sugar has not been directly linked to heart disease, it is clearly associated with risk factors such as obesity, high blood pressure, increased levels of triglycerides, and high levels of C-reactive protein, a marker for arterial inflammation. An overly sweet diet also increases the potential for diabetes, another major risk factor for heart disease.

The 35 teaspoons of added sugar that many Americans are averaging daily is in addition to other sugar that is naturally occurring in foods like fruits, vegetables, milk, and whole grains. While these foods do have fiber and other healthful nutrients, the natural sugar they contain is still sugar, though it is digested more slowly than sugar coming from processed food.

Now to Step 3: Stir 8 teaspoons of sugar into a glass of water. This time, really do take a little taste. This is the amount of sugar in a typical 12-ounce non-diet soda, or 130 empty calories.

Sugar-sweetened beverages, including many sports drinks, fruit drinks, flavored teas, and punches, are little more than liquid candy. But many parents don't seem to realize this. A position paper in *Pediatrics* on sugar-sweetened beverage consumption and its role in adolescent obesity showed that soft drink consumption among kids has increased by *300 percent* since the mid-1980s, with 56 to 85 percent of schoolchildren consuming at least one soft drink daily. Dr. David Ludwig of Children's Hospital Boston, whom I interviewed in Chapter 2, notes that if a child were to drink just one 12-ounce sugary soft drink every day, it would add up to the equivalent of a 40-pound bag of sugar by the end of the year.

Given all the hidden added sugar in foods, saying no to sweetened beverages is one of the easiest ways to cut out excess sugar from your diet. The latest American Heart Association dietary guidelines suggest that most women should eat or drink no more than 100 calories per day from added sugars (1 gram of sugar has 4.5 calories, so look at the Nutrition Facts panel carefully) and that most men should eat or drink no more than 150 calories per day from added sugars—that's 6 and 10 teaspoons, respectively, not 35! For children, the American Heart Association recommends no more than 3 teaspoons (48 calories) of added sugars a day, which is why I hope you invite your kids to participate in this experiment.

are those that don't naturally occur in foods—not to be confused with the fructose in fruit or the lactose in milk, for example, which do. While the Nutrition Facts panel does provide the total amount of sugar in grams per serving for a food or beverage, what it doesn't provide is how much of that sugar is "added" to make a food taste sweeter. That's because the FDA requires that these added sugars appear only in the ingredient list. Since all ingredients are listed in descending order by weight, manufacturers can "disguise" the amount of added sugar in a product by using more than one type of sweetener, which means each added sugar weighs less and can be buried far down in the ingredient list. That's why it's important to read the ingredient list all the way through to look for added sugars under a variety of names.

Here's a list of added sugars to look for:

Agave nectar	Honey
Barley malt syrup	Invert sugar
Brown sugar	Lactose
Cane crystals	Malt syrup
Cane sugar	Maltodextrin
Corn sweetener	Maltose
Corn syrup	Molasses
Crystalline fructose	Raw sugar
Dextrin	Rice syrup
Dextrose	Saccharose
Evaporated cane juice	Sorghum or sorghum sugar
Fructose	Sucrose
Fruit juice concentrates	Syrup
Glucose	Turbinado sugar
High-fructose corn syrup	Xylose

SHOP HEALTHY ON A BUDGET

I understand that in this era of tight budgets, it may be tempting (and certainly easier) to buy cheap fast food instead of fresh whole foods. My response?

Don't even think about it! If you are feeding your kids fast food on a regular basis, you are likely sentencing them to acute illness in the present and chronic illness in the future. If you are feeding yourself a diet of fast food, you are committing slow suicide. The truth is, given the importance that nutrition plays in our health and well-being, we can't afford *not* to eat the healthiest food available.

I've never bought into the "healthy food is too expensive" argument. I think that in many cases we've been given a false choice between health and saving money. The reality is, when you stop buying junk and start buying only high-quality food, you will be surprised by how far your dollar can go. There's no question that as a nation we are throwing vast amounts of money away on empty calories—on food and drink with little nutritive value—and that those dollars could be better spent on healthier options like low-fat milk instead of sugary drinks, or whole grains or fresh produce instead of highly processed sugary and starchy snacks. Furthermore, savvy shoppers, like the Super Moms I interviewed for this book, know how to get the best value for their dollars, and that means finding high-quality food at reasonable prices. It also means going to the store armed with a shopping list so you don't buy items you don't really need; reading food labels to be sure that you are getting the biggest bang for your buck in terms of nutrient content; and clipping circular coupons or printing online coupons to take advantage of supermarket sales.

Here are some ways to manage your healthy-food budget:

Leave your credit cards at home. Studies show that people are much more likely to make impulse buys when they use credit cards than when they fork over cold, hard cash. In particular, they are more likely to buy junk food when using a credit or debit card. If you typically pay by credit card and find that you are winding up with a lot of stuff in your cart that isn't healthy or necessary, switch to cash and see if it transforms you into a more disciplined shopper.

Use customer loyalty cards. Most major supermarket chains and even some local groceries sponsor customer loyalty programs that offer substantial savings. In return for discounts on many products, the supermarket tracks your purchases, which provides it with information on what products appeal to specific customers so it can monitor trends and better target its advertising and promotional campaigns. Very often, after you've shopped at the store a few times, you will be offered extra discounts on the products that you regularly buy when you swipe your card at the cash register, or be sent notices about trying new products. Joining such a program is great way to remind yourself of just how healthy a shopper you are and to encourage the supermarket to carry more healthy products.

Join a buying club or warehouse club. For a nominal fee, you can get a membership in a buying club or warehouse club that offers brand-name products at a substantial discount. These products are often sold in huge packages containing multiple boxes or individually in larger sizes than you would find in a supermarket. This is a boon for big families who can polish off five boxes of whole-grain cereal or a five-pound bag of almonds in a matter of weeks, but it can prove to be wasteful for single people and smaller families. If you don't have a lot of mouths to feed, but still want the benefits of bulk buying, check to see whether you can get a fractional share in the membership.

Look for Best Buys on Produce

The first rule for buying produce at a good price is to buy it fresh and in season. For example, berries can be dirt cheap in the summer and priced through the roof in the winter, and vice versa for citrus fruit. Here are some other tips on how to cut the cost of fruits and vegetables:

Join a food co-op. Several Super Moms have told me that they save a good deal of money on produce by joining local food cooperatives, or co-ops, which are essentially grocery stores that are owned and operated by their members. The local co-ops buy their goods directly from co-op food distributors or farmers, and they can usually offer better prices than a commercial store because they don't have to turn a profit. They're not in business to make money; they're in business to save money for their members. The co-op members get to partake in the savings in exchange for helping to run the business and a small initiation fee. Plus, members have access to a wide variety of fruits and vegetables.

Many co-ops support local agriculture and buy organic and other responsibly produced goods. Some co-ops, like the famous Park Slope food cooperative in Brooklyn, New York, have thousands of members; others scattered across the Unites States may have just a few dozen. Some offer a selection of goods that rivals any supermarket; others may specialize in particular types of products, like organic produce, that may not be available in local stores. Food co-ops can be found in virtually every state in the United States and in many countries worldwide. If you are interested in joining one or learning more about the food co-op movement, check out coopdirectory.org.

Patronize farmers' markets. A favorite late-afternoon snack at our house is freshly picked heirloom tomatoes with thin slices of part-skim mozzarella cheese. We find the best and most reasonably priced tomatoes at various farmers' markets around Miami, where South Florida farmers display their vegetables, fruits, herbs, whole-wheat bread and pastas, and many other items. More than 7,000 farmers' markets are already established all over the country, and they are especially popular in urban areas. Farmers' markets give local farmers an opportunity to sell their goods directly to consumers, and by patronizing them, you are helping to sustain local agriculture.

Farmers' markets are a terrific resource for the freshest produce. If you're a first-time visitor, walk around the various stands to familiarize yourself with all the options before making a purchase. If you typically shop in supermarkets, you may see more unusual types of greens or different varieties of produce than what you're used to. Farmers' markets can sometimes be cheaper than traditional produce stands and supermarkets, especially for products like organic fruits and vegetables (as well as organic eggs and grass-fed beef). Many farmers' markets also now accept cards from the Supplemental Nutrition Assistance Program (SNAP; formerly the Federal Food Stamp Program), which can be exchanged for tokens for purchasing items; and more and more farmers' markets nationwide are doubling the value of these cards, thanks to the Double Value Coupon Program from the nonprofit Wholesome Wave (see wholesomewave.org). For additional bargains, browse through the market as the farmers pack up to leave at the end of the day. They'll often drop their prices to avoid having to haul the food back to the farm. To find a farmers' market near you, check out apps.ams.usda.gov/farmersmarkets.

Join a community-supported agriculture (CSA) group. Another way to ensure that you're getting the freshest food possible, especially if you live in a city, is to join a CSA group. The way it works is that you purchase a share (a membership or subscription) in a farmer's harvest, and then every week or every other week throughout the farming season you pick up or receive a box, bag, or basket of seasonal produce (and sometimes eggs or meat as well, if desired) from that farm. Today there are thousands of CSA farms all across the United States (see the database at localharvest.org/csa to find one near you). While a CSA may seem expensive to join (many memberships range from $400 to $600 per season, paid up front), if you share the expense with a neighbor or two, it can be a great way to have direct access to the highest-quality produce while also supporting local agriculture. Many CSAs offer flexible payment plans, including paying in installments, and some accept SNAP cards, offer sliding scale fees, and provide scholarship shares. Many CSA farmers allow visits to the farm once a season, and parents often find that their kids are far more willing to try new foods when they know they're from "their farm."

Buy frozen veggies and fruits. Frozen vegetables and fruits are a terrific, convenient, price-conscious alternative when fresh local produce isn't in season. Frozen products can be considerably cheaper than fresh and, of course, can be stored for a long time. Most frozen food companies now use a technique called flash freezing, which means that the produce is frozen immediately after it is picked to preserve flavor and nutrients. It can be argued (and frozen food companies make this assertion) that flash-frozen vegetables and fruits are more nutritious than fresh produce that has been shipped thousands of miles after it has been picked. To me, that long-distance shipping is instantly a good reason to buy fresh *local* produce when possible. But in the off-season, frozen is fine (and way cheaper than the many items that need to be shipped cross-country or internationally).

There are scores of different brands of frozen products to choose from, including some inexpensive store brands that are excellent. There are also organic lines of frozen foods sold in both supermarkets and natural foods markets. Browse through the frozen food section of your local store to familiarize yourself with the wide variety of frozen vegetable and fruit choices. And be sure to purchase those without high-fat sauces or added sugar.

Don't overlook canned fruits and vegetables. Canned produce typically costs considerably less than fresh or frozen and can be comparable to or better than fresh in terms of nutrient content (especially when the fresh produce is imported and has been sitting around the supermarket for days). Some of you may have childhood memories of mushy, overcooked canned peas or that ubiquitous casserole made with canned string beans and condensed mushroom soup (and canned french-fried onions!). If that's the case, you should give canned vegetables (as well as canned beans and other legumes) another try. Today, many brands offer products that taste almost as good as fresh. And you can even find organic canned fruits and vegetables in many supermarkets.

The downside is that canned goods often have very high amounts of sodium added as a preservative. Look for reduced-sodium or no-salt-added canned products, or remove some of the sodium yourself by draining the liquid from the can and lightly rinsing the contents with cold water before using. Avoid canned vegetables in high-fat sauces and any canned fruits that have added sugar or syrup.

Remember, when it comes to getting dinner on the table quickly, canned beans, tomatoes, and broth (look for fat-free, lower-sodium brands in cans or boxes) are three staples you'll always want to have on hand in your pantry. We use all three in the recipes on pages 259–306.

Look for the Best Buys on Protein

Consuming lean protein is an essential part of a healthy diet, but lean cuts can be among the most expensive items on your shopping list. Fortunately, most grocery stores and big box stores run regular sales on lean ground beef, chicken and turkey breast cutlets, and ground chicken and turkey (and to really save money you can always buy a whole bird and cut it up yourself). Buy more than you need when the price is good and freeze what you don't need. Most frozen meat will stay fresh for at least 6 months. If you're interested

(continued on page 210)

If You Are a Parent

There is no better way to teach children about healthy eating than to allow them to help you with the meal planning and shopping. If a child is invested in the process, he or she will be more likely to eat the food that's put on the table. Here's how to get them involved:

Let the kids help with the menus. If you're planning a week's worth of meals at one time, as we suggest above, let the kids who are old enough have a say in some of them, beginning with "ethnic nights." There are plenty of books on cooking healthy with kids that you can pore over with your child for easy recipe ideas, and many farmers' markets now give out recipes utilizing the foods that they sell. Let your child search the Internet for recipes. Reading the recipes together also strengthens that skill and lets you share in a project. We have found in our public school nutrition experiences that when kids are involved in tastings and meal planning, they become enthusiastic about healthy food.

Take the kids shopping. Some of you may be tempted to leave your children at home when you shop because you fear that they will distract you from buying wisely and clamor for every type of junk food that they see. Personally, I think *not* involving kids in shopping is a big mistake, although I do recommend taking one at a time so the experience is worthwhile. And it's not just the grocery store they should visit with you. Make sure they see the farmers' market and the food co-op too. Kids need to be taught early on about where food comes from (a chat with a real farmer can help with that), need to see how the markets are organized, and need to learn how to differentiate between wholesome food and the junk food.

Do some homework before you go. Before you bring a child into the store or market, you need to prepare them for the experience. Let them know that you are counting on them to help you pick out *healthy* food. At home, show them what the Nutrition Facts panel and ingredient list look like on different products. Explain to them what can be learned from looking at packages. Teach older kids about serving sizes and show them how sugar is often disguised in many different forms in the ingredient list (see the list of added sugars on page 202). Even young nonreaders can learn to identify the whole-grains stamp (see page 197), which is a great way to teach them how to home in on healthy breads and cereals, or they can be taught to recognize the organic symbol on fruits and vegetables.

When children grow up learning about the best-tasting, healthiest foods, they will be less likely to accept inferior options. This early learning will go a long way in making them more demanding consumers.

Find teachable moments. One good place to start is the produce section at the supermarket. Stroll down the aisle to see which fruits and vegetables your child can already identify. Then introduce a few new ones and ask if there are some that he or she would like to try. You can also use produce to teach younger children about colors and older children about how each of these colors offers unique health benefits (see our MegaFoods list on pages 254–58 for a quick tutorial). If the good cereals and bad cereals are stocked together, make a game out of who can find the cereal with the lowest amount of sugar first. If your child is old enough to read and do math, have him or her figure out the cost per ounce times the number of ounces per serving of a particular brand of whole-wheat pasta, cereal, or bread. This will help a child better understand the cost of feeding a family and why it's so important to spend money wisely on food that provides good nutrition.

Allow a healthy treat. To avoid an endless wail of "I want that," let your child know in advance that one treat can be picked out on the shopping trip, but be sure to limit the options. For example, give her a choice among three healthy things: a piece of fresh fruit, a fruit ice made from real fruit with no added sugar, or a low-sugar frozen yogurt bar. If something else is clamored for, just say it's not part of the deal.

in the best buys on grass-fed beef and pastured chicken, for example, shop the big box stores or visit a local farmer.

Don't forget about dried legumes. Beans and other legumes, like lentils and chickpeas, not only provide high-quality protein but are also a good buy, especially when purchased in bulk. Food co-ops and natural foods stores often offer the best bargains. Check out our recipes for Chickpea and Carrot Frittata (page 263) and Super Veggie Minestrone (page 272), both of which can easily be made with dried beans. Simply do a quick soak (bring the beans to a boil in a large pot with about 3 inches of water, cover them, remove them from the heat, and let them sit for an hour), then simmer the beans until they're tender before adding them to your recipe. One-third of a 1-pound package is equal to a 15-ounce can of beans. Buy no more beans than you will use in a year, and store them in resealable glass or plastic containers at room temperature.

Don't overlook frozen and canned fish. Unless you are a vegetarian, eating fish at least twice a week is recommended on a healthy diet. If you are fortunate enough to live near a reputable fish market with good prices, or a supermarket that carries good fresh fish, by all means become a "regular" and shop the bargains. If not, canned and frozen fish are a fine alternative. Frozen seafood is often as good as fresh, and in some cases could actually be "fresher." New flash-freezing techniques enable fishermen to freeze seafood within minutes of catching it, which means it retains its flavor and nutrients. Typically, frozen fish costs less than fresh, and it can stay in your freezer for weeks if it's not allowed to thaw before you get it home.

Canned fish is usually much more economical than fresh fish and is definitely more convenient. Stock a few cans of salmon, light tuna, or sardines (packed in water or olive oil) in your pantry for a quick lunch or dinner.

Avoid fish high in mercury, such as such as marlin, swordfish, shark, tilefish, orange roughy, king mackerel, big-eye and ahi tuna, and canned albacore tuna (use light tuna instead).

COOK AS IF YOUR LIFE DEPENDS ON IT

As I so strongly suggested in Chapter 7, it is time to finally break the fast-food take-out habit that has resulted because we're too busy to cook at home. If we are to become a healthier society and reverse the trends toward obesity, diabetes, and heart disease, we need to take back the responsibility for cooking our own meals, and ideally involve our children in the process. When you eat many of your meals out, you lose that control and are literally putting your health—and the health of your family—in somebody else's hands.

As it happens, I don't cook (except eggs for breakfast), so I am deeply appreciative of those, like my wife and the Super Moms whose stories are told in the book, who do manage to put healthy meals on the table on a regular and timely basis. Not long ago, I came across an observation in the *Economist* from chef and author Jamie Oliver, whom I was fortunate enough to spend time with when he came to Miami for a symposium the Agatston Research Foundation sponsored on childhood obesity. Jamie said: "The beauty of knowing how to cook is that it makes you resilient, adaptable and resourceful, no matter what ingredients you have in front of you." I would of course insert the word "healthy" in front of "ingredients," and I have no doubt that Jamie would agree with my edit, since he is one of those at the forefront of trying to change our abysmal eating habits.

DON'T LET LACK OF TIME OR SKILLS STOP YOU

There's no question that most of us are time-challenged these days and that home cooking often takes a back seat to the drive-thru. But I urge you not to let lack of time be the dictator when it comes to your own health and that of your family. Plenty of delicious and nourishing recipes can easily be made from start to finish in 30 minutes or less. You can find some of them, like our Chicken Cutlets with Apricot Sauce and Pistachios (page 278) and our Chunky Guacamole Salad (page 301), in this book and others in *The South Beach Diet Quick & Easy Cookbook* and *The South Beach Diet Super Quick Cookbook*.

Nor should you let lack of cooking skills be a deterrent. The good news is that once you have organized your kitchen, planned your menus, and shopped for a week's worth of food, the actual cooking itself can be surprisingly easy— and many meals require little or no stove or oven time at all. Cooking can truly be enjoyable when you feel in control and aren't panicking because you haven't figured out what's for dinner or are missing a vital ingredient. If your pantry, fridge, and freezer are well stocked, putting a meal together doesn't have to be a nerve-racking experience.

Here are a few additional recommendations to make home cooking easier:

Cook in advance. Knowing there's a meal already prepared in the fridge or freezer to simply reheat is certainly a busy person's stress-reliever. On weekends, when possible, cook a few meals ahead of time to serve midweek or later. Enjoy weekend cooking as a family activity, or make a date with just your spouse to cook together while sipping a glass of red wine and listening to music. Soups, casseroles, stews, brown rice, oven "fried" sweet potatoes, and lightly steamed vegetables are just a few examples of dishes that can be made ahead and frozen.

If weekend cooking is impossible, try to do some advance prepping in the evenings when you can. Cut up veggies, chop herbs, make pasta and rice, and precook ground beef, turkey, and chicken, for example, and then refrigerate them so you can put a meal together faster when you get home from work or your day's activities.

A slow cooker can be a big boon when you know you're going to get home late. If you have some extra time in the morning, get a nice meat or legume and vegetable stew going and look forward to being greeted by the aroma of a fully cooked meal when you return home at night.

Rely on the pantry. Dinners don't have to be elaborate affairs. On days when you are especially pressed for time, look to your well-stocked pantry. You can do a lot with canned beans (black, red, pinto, garbanzo), dried lentils, canned tomatoes (diced, crushed, whole, paste), whole-wheat pasta (thin spaghetti, rotini, elbows), quinoa, broth (chicken, vegetable, beef), nuts and dried fruits, extra-virgin olive oil, vinegar (balsamic, white wine, red wine, cider), dried herbs and spices (all kinds), and some onions and garlic, of course.

For example, a meal of whole-grain pasta with a low-sodium canned tomato sauce or some store bought jarred pesto simply requires boiling water and heating up the sauce. If you have some meatballs in the freezer, reheat them in the microwave and throw them on top. Add to that a simple salad of romaine or another lettuce with some canned garbanzo beans, and you have the perfect quick dinner. Or make a pilaf in 15 minutes with whole-wheat couscous, nuts, and dried fruit. Or toss together a three-bean salad dressed with a prepared sugar-free dressing of your choice.

Take advantage of prepared foods. Healthy home cooking doesn't mean that everything at every meal has to be made from scratch. Many supermarkets offer a wide variety of prepared foods that work well as main dishes, like rotisserie chicken or turkey breast, baked salmon, steamed shrimp, and turkey chili; check how they are prepared to avoid those with a lot of added sodium, sugar, and fat. All you need to do is add your own salad or sides. You can also use a store-bought roast chicken breast as the basis for chicken salad or as a quick addition to a vegetable stir-fry. Take off the skin.

If you're really pressed for time and budget isn't a major factor, most large supermarkets also offer a wide variety of prechopped and shredded vegetables, bagged lettuce mixes, sliced and chopped fruits, shredded reduced-fat cheeses, chopped garlic and onions, and all manner of sauces and salsas. Be creative: Figure out ways to supplement your own home-cooked fare with these convenience foods—just be sure to check the ingredient list.

Make healthy "fast food" at home. There are healthy ways to make the fast-food favorites that your kids clamor for or that perhaps you occasionally crave yourself. Cheeseburgers and fries and chicken nuggets not only can be nutritious; they also can take less time to prepare than you would spend driving to the fast-food establishment to pick them up.

A cheeseburger, for example, doesn't have to be off the charts in terms of saturated fat if it's made from lean ground beef (or ground turkey or chicken) and topped with reduced-fat Cheddar cheese. When served on a 100 percent whole-wheat bun with lettuce and tomato and a little low-sugar ketchup, it's a far healthier option than the typical cheeseburger made with full-fat beef and cheese and served with loads of mayo and ketchup on a white roll, which can quickly tally up 700 calories and 45 grams of fat, 17 grams of that saturated.

Also remember that french fries made from white potatoes aren't the only option to have with burgers. Sweet potatoes can be cut up and oven "fried" with just a little olive oil and a pinch of coarse sea salt. The end result is an absolutely delicious "fast food" that is loaded with vitamins, minerals, and beneficial antioxidants. If your kids *must* have standard french fries, you can also oven-fry white potatoes the same way; you just won't get the added nutrition found in sweet potatoes. (Leave the skins on for added fiber and other nutrients.)

And remember, chicken nuggets don't have to come from the deep-fat fryer. You can dip chicken pieces in a small amount of olive oil, fat-free or reduced-fat milk or egg whites, coat them in whole-wheat breadcrumbs mixed with some Parmesan cheese, and "fry" them in the oven.

Make every recipe count. Once you are committed to cooking at home, you'll want to maximize every recipe in terms of nutrients. That's why on pages 259–306 we offer MegaRecipes that utilize as many healthy ingredients as possible. Take a look at the list of my favorite MegaFoods on pages 254–58, then come up with some recipes of your own using as many of these nutrient-rich foods as possible. I bet your older kids will give you some great ideas if you ask.

If You Are a Parent

Most kids love to spend time with a parent, especially if it's one-on-one time when they have you all to themselves. And cooking is a great way to get that time together. Invite one child at a time into the kitchen to assist you, but be sure that you don't get so wrapped up in your part of the process that you forget this is a bonding opportunity. There's no question that by joining you in the kitchen, your child will learn a lot more than just how to cook. (Always bear in mind that safety comes first and that children need supervision.)

Here are some age-related considerations:

Preschoolers. Give them pots and pans and safe utensils and let them "pretend cook" with you, or simply let them bang away on the pans. Fine motor skills can be honed with pouring and stirring, even if it's just water. Spread a plastic mat on the kitchen floor and let them assist you in their own way.

Grade schoolers. Kids ages 6 and older can learn how to measure and do other physical tasks like scrambling eggs, pouring in liquids, or making sandwiches. You can also teach them why you chose the ingredients you're using and why they're healthy. Math, science, and reading skills can be improved. Try to be patient and keep your sense of humor. Messes are part of the fun.

Middle schoolers. Older children can help make salads and dressings, cut up vegetables and fruits, and eventually do some of the real cooking themselves. In addition to basic nutrition principles, some world history and geography can be taught by preparing ethnic foods.

Teens. Many parents don't think teens can cook, but you'll be pleasantly surprised at what happens when they're given a little guidance and the chance to be alone in the kitchen. Offer them some cookbooks and the opportunity to shop for and produce an entire meal, if possible. You'll be amazed at the amount of self-esteem it can generate.

EAT IN MORE,
DINE OUT SMART

Not surprisingly, dining out is one of the biggest challenges faced by anyone who wants to maintain a healthy lifestyle. Studies show that those who eat in restaurants generally consume 500 more calories per meal than they would if they had eaten a similar meal at home, in large part because of the number of courses and unknown ingredients. Just do the math: If you actually do eat out three times a week and consume 500 extra calories each time, that's 78,000 extra calories a year! Not only will this potentially show up on the scale, but it will also set the stage for prediabetes, diabetes, high blood pressure, heart disease, and many other obesity-related ailments.

CHOOSE THE RIGHT RESTAURANTS

I am not suggesting that people stop dining out or start skipping the salad course. By all means, eat the salad course—just ask for oil and vinegar or dressing on the side. Try to make the best food choices you can. And, as with any meal, eat slowly to a point of satisfaction and remember that you don't have to finish everything on your plate.

The real problem today is that many restaurants do not routinely use healthy ingredients or prepare food using healthy cooking methods. This is especially true of fast-food restaurants, where so much of the menu is fried, overly salted, and high in sugar to appeal to our primal urges for fatty, salty, and sweet foods. And even though many fast-food chains are making an effort to include healthier options on their menus (and are legally required to list calorie counts in some states), it's still better to skip these venues when possible and enjoy a meal out at a restaurant where you can discuss how the food is prepared with your server and actually influence what ends up on your plate.

A trick that I use when dining out is to ask for something light as soon as I sit down—such as gazpacho, a clear soup, or a green salad. You can turn away the bread basket, or ask whether whole-grain bread is available.

Here are some other tips for getting the best from restaurant meals:

Use the menu as a resource. Be sure to read over the descriptions of the dishes that you are considering and don't be afraid to ask the server questions about how a dish is prepared, even in a fancy restaurant. Is the fish, for example, sautéed, baked, or fried? Does a sauce contain a lot of butter or cream? What are the sides? Can vegetables be steamed or sautéed in a little olive oil?

Some menus are more detailed than others and will include calorie counts as well as a breakdown of fat grams and carbs, which can be very useful in seeing how one appetizer or entrée compares with others. If you are on the South Beach Diet, I don't recommend counting calories, though we all know that calories do count and the better the quality of those calories the better. In a restaurant, where you have no control over ingredients, plenty of calories (along with fat and sodium) can creep into sauces, marinades, salad dressings, and so on, depending on how a dish is prepared.

Order it your way. Many restaurants will accommodate dietary preferences, which means you can adapt virtually any meal to be in line with our South Beach eating principles. For an appetizer, enjoy a soup or a salad, as I suggested earlier, then scan the menu for the lean protein entrées, like chicken or turkey breast, sirloin steak or filet mignon, any type of seafood, or a meatless dish made with tofu, beans, and/or vegetables. Request that your entrée be baked, grilled, or sautéed (using olive oil, not butter). Ask for dressings and sauces on the side.

See if you can replace the white potato with a sweet potato or with a salad or extra green vegetables like broccoli or spinach (and order those vegetables without sauces or butter). If you do choose to eat bread with your meal, make sure that you specifically request only the whole-grain options (also ask for

If You Must Eat Fast Food

As a rule, I think it's a good idea to limit your visits to popular fast-food franchises, and this includes family/casual restaurants where the food can be just as "deadly." If you do find yourself in one, look for the healthy options. Although fried chicken, cheeseburgers, and other fast-food fare may be tempting, it's better to scan the menu for grilled chicken or turkey dishes—and always skip the fries and onion rings. Other good choices are green salads with lean meat or seafood toppings, vegetarian chili, and broth-based soups.

Better Fast-Food Options

Lean "bunless" burgers

Caesar salad, without croutons and with the dressing on the side (use half the packet where available or ask for oil and vinegar)

Green salad topped with grilled chicken or shrimp, with the dressing on the side (choose ranch, Caesar, or a vinaigrette; use half the packet where available)

Roasted or grilled poultry, seafood, or meat

Vegetarian chili

Broth-based soups

olive oil to dip your bread in instead of slathering on butter). See if you can replace the white rice with brown rice, wild rice, barley, or whole-wheat couscous and the white pasta with whole-wheat pasta. And request a tomato-based sauce made with olive oil and vegetables over a vodka sauce or carbonara sauce.

If you are concerned about gluten, tell your server that you have a food "allergy" and that you need to know how the food is prepared. If your server

Fresh fruit with reduced-fat yogurt (if available)

Diet soda, coffee, tea, fat-free or low-fat milk, club soda, water

Fast Foods to Avoid

Bacon cheeseburgers

Panini sandwiches

White bread or white rolls

Breaded and deep-fried foods

Potato and pasta salads, coleslaw

Creamy soups, such as cream of tomato, cream of mushroom, or New England clam chowder

Buffalo wings

Nachos, potato skins, and other fried appetizers

Cookies, pies, cheesecake, and other pastries

Full-fat ice cream and milkshakes

Sugary drinks

appears not to understand, which many won't, ask to speak with the restaurant manager or the chef.

Watch the cocktails. If you're following a healthy eating plan, what you drink in a restaurant is just as important as what you eat. If you start drinking before you order, it may sabotage your willpower, so it's better to wait and have a drink with your meal. It's recommended that women limit their intake to one alcoholic beverage a day, and men to one or two a day. Choose red or

(continued on page 222)

If You Are a Parent

Studies show that the more meals a child eats outside of the home, the more likely that child is to gain weight and develop high blood pressure, high cholesterol, and other risk factors for heart disease, diabetes, and other diseases. Clearly, the problem is that kids are not eating as healthy on the go as they would at home and are consuming more calories and fat, drinking more sugary soda, and eating fewer fruits and vegetables. And while you may have committed to eating more meals at home, there will be times when this isn't possible. Therefore, when eating on the run is the only option, you need to make sure that you prepare ahead and make the best choices for your kids.

Keep the following in mind when you're on the go with children:

Pack healthy snacks. Whether you're taking your children with you to run errands or you're on a long-distance trip, be sure that you bring a stock of healthy snacks. That way, when the kids get hungry, you won't have to patronize the nearest vending machine or fast-food restaurant, and they won't be starving when mealtime does arrive. For some healthy snack ideas, see pages 180–81.

Stay out of fast-food restaurants. Don't get your kids into the fast-food habit just because you're in a rush. Even if you order some of the healthier options for them, they will likely be exposed to other kids' french fries and sodas and will inevitably want some too. Instead, find a family-friendly restaurant, like a diner, that has more good choices.

Never order from the kids' menu. Even good family restaurants tend to offer the worst possible choices on their kids' menus: Macaroni and cheese, hot dogs, cheeseburgers, fried chicken fingers, and buttered pasta are just a few of the typical offerings. Not surprisingly, a 2008 Center for Science in the Public Interest analysis of 1,474 kids' meals from national chain restaurants found that 93 percent were excessively high in calories for a single meal and that 45 percent were high in bad saturated fat and trans fats.

If your child has a small appetite, order a full adult portion and take half home for another meal to avoid wasting food. Or simply ask for a separate plate and serve her a little bit of your meal, or suggest things from the appetizer or soups section of the menu. Breakfast at any time of day can also be a healthy option: An egg, some Canadian bacon, a slice of whole-wheat toast, and a fruit cup can make a kid's meal.

Use dining out as an educational opportunity. Just as you teach your kids about healthy eating at your own dining table, you can do the same in a restaurant. Use the opportunity to read the menu together and let them select from the healthiest options you've steered them toward. Discuss how the dishes are prepared and why some are good and some are not so good. If you're eating ethnic cuisine, talk about the new ingredients, foods, flavors, and tastes. Let the older kids check the bill.

Use the power of the purse strings. There comes a time when adolescents and teens begin to spend most of their time with friends outside of your home and start to make their own decisions about what to eat. If you have given them the best guidance you can by teaching them the principles of good nutrition, you hope that they will make good decisions most of the time, but that may not always be the case. If you suspect that your teen is loading up on junk food in the afternoons, think about how he is paying for it. If you are providing the money, you need to exercise control, but not necessarily in a heavy-handed way. Rather than cutting his allowance or lunch money, use a different tactic. For example, if your child has been talking about saving up for something special, like a new pair of expensive jeans, computer speakers, or even a car, you can offer to contribute to the fund if he puts the money he is spending on junk food toward his special purchase. Of course, there will be times when your teenager will be gathering with friends after school at such places, and you want to encourage him to socialize. Just talk with him casually about choosing the better-for-you menu options.

white wine, extra brut champagne, or light beer. Or if you want a cocktail, opt for one made with a sugar-free mixer like diet soda, club soda, or seltzer.

Enjoy dessert, in moderation. Dessert is often hard to pass up at a restaurant, especially when it's a special occasion or when you're out with friends who insist on having it. If you do order dessert, simply use common sense and choose fruit or a little cheese. If you can't resist a decadent dessert, follow the "Three-Bite Rule," described on pages 181–82. Or order a dessert "for the table" with forks for everyone.

MANAGE MEALS WHEN TRAVELING

I know firsthand how tough it can be to maintain a healthy diet when you are looking for food in the middle of an airport or a train station or facing endless miles of fast-food joints along the highway. Traveling generally means you're off your usual schedule, and often tired and stressed, so you end up grabbing whatever is easiest, including a candy bar from the minibar in your hotel room.

Sometimes even I have to remind myself that the rules of the road when it comes to food are no different from those at home: Eat three meals and at least two snacks a day, and try to make good choices most of the time. That means you may need to do some pre-trip planning, but it's worth a small investment of your time to maintain your healthy lifestyle.

Here are some tips to abide by when it comes to travel and food:

Eat a healthy meal before you leave. If you fuel up with a good meal at home before you start your trip, you'll be less likely to overindulge on unhealthy snacks in the traveler's lounge or feel compelled to stop at a drive-thru because you're suddenly starving.

Always bring snacks. Keep a healthy assortment of snacks with you at all times. Invest in an inexpensive, lightweight reusable lunch bag that you can fill with small bags of mixed nuts, part-skim mozzarella sticks, cut-up raw vegetables, lean deli meats like turkey slices, some air-popped popcorn, or mini "sandwiches" of whole-grain crackers with nut butter. When you are hungry, reach for one of these healthy choices instead of succumbing to the sugary, salty, high-fat packaged snacks available at concession stands. It's also important to stay well hydrated when traveling, particularly if it's by air. Once you've gone through the security screening, buy yourself a big bottle of water for the trip. In fact, carry water no matter what the mode of transport.

Do some research ahead of time. We live in an age when, with the click of a mouse or the downloading of an app, you can learn virtually everything about your destination before you leave. Let technology work for you: Use it to check out the menus in restaurants near your motel or hotel so you can choose the ones that offer the healthiest options.

Find a local supermarket or deli. Whether you're on the road or have already arrived at your destination, a supermarket or good deli can be a terrific source of healthy "road food." Look for lean chicken and turkey breast, reduced-fat cheeses, 100 percent whole-grain bread or crackers, fresh veggies and fruits, nuts, and so on, which you can eat in the car or store in the minifridge in your hotel.

GET MOVING, GET FIT

In Chapter 8, I detailed the health hazards of spending most of the day sitting, or the "chair sentence," as one doctor so aptly put it. There is only one antidote to the sedentary lifestyle that is slowly killing us: You have to get up out of your chair or off that couch and MOVE!

I like to think of fitness as a three-legged stool.

The first two legs are cardiovascular conditioning and core strengthening. Doing both types of exercise, as I describe in this chapter, can take less than half an hour a day of your time, and you will reap enormous health benefits in return. The third leg of the stool is *moving*—that is, making the effort to incorporate more physical activity into your daily life even when you are not exercising. I'm talking about walking a few blocks instead of driving everywhere, or taking the stairs instead of the elevator, or getting up and walking over to a colleague's office instead of sending an e-mail. These are the kinds of simple, everyday activities that kept human beings healthy before technology rendered getting out of our chairs obsolete. (I provide more suggestions on how to get moving on pages 237–40.)

The Wake Up and Move 2-Week Quick-Start Plan on pages 228–37 combines both cardio and core-strengthening exercises, which you can do on alternate days. When it comes to aerobics, I've found that interval walking—whether done outdoors or indoors on a treadmill or elliptical machine—is the form of exercise my patients are most willing to try and stick with, though intervals can also be done while riding a stationary or regular bike, or while doing laps in a pool. When you do intervals (which means alternating short bursts of intensive effort—15 to 60 seconds—with easier recovery periods to catch your breath), you can burn more calories and fat in 20 minutes than you would doing about 40 minutes of steady-state exercise, which is why it's so appealing to busy (and overweight) people.

When you do interval walking, you are working harder than you normally would in a conventional steady-state walking program, though it is only for brief spurts and they are over before you even realize it. This is a much more effective workout in every way, and as you get fitter and increase your level of intensity, you will not only be conditioning your heart and lungs but also improving your muscle metabolism, boosting your "good" HDL cholesterol, and helping your body to handle insulin and sugar more efficiently. All this and you don't get bored!

On the days when you're not doing intervals, you'll want to do some core-strengthening exercises to target the vital muscles in your back, abdomen, pelvis, and hips, which are critical for posture, flexibility, balance, and stability. Since they involve working against your own body weight, which provides resistance, core exercises are also good for strengthening and toning the peripheral muscles in your arms and legs. When you have a strong core, you'll find that day-to-day tasks like lifting grocery bags and luggage become much easier and that you are less likely to succumb to the myriad injuries related to poor muscle tone.

GETTING STARTED

I know that there are plenty of reasons why people don't exercise, because I hear them every day from my patients. The excuses run the gamut from "I hate exercise" to "I would exercise but I don't know what to do" to "I feel ridiculous working out next to those body builders at the gym" to "I have young kids and a full-time job and I just can't find the time."

What's not surprising to me, but often surprising to them, is that many of these so-called exercise haters find that once they experience a workout program that is both fun and effective, they actually enjoy it and find the time to fit it into their schedules. They quickly discover that the benefits of vigorous exercise extend far beyond taut muscles and a svelte physique. They find that exercise reduces the level of stress hormones, revs up the production of the feel-good hormones called endorphins, and gets their blood pumping, which produces a feeling of exhilaration as their cells take in more oxygen.

Those who have been struggling to get off a weight-loss plateau are delighted to see that regular aerobic and core functional (resistance) exercise makes it easier to keep the scale heading downward and ultimately keep unwanted pounds at bay (assuming they stick to a healthy eating plan too). Patients with arthritis, who are often reluctant to begin an exercise program out of fear of injury, find that working their joints in a safe fashion feels much better than doing nothing at all. And my patients with children, who frequently say that they have no time to exercise, are surprised to discover that once they find 20 minutes to add regular physical activity to their routine, they have more stamina, which translates to being better able to cope with the demands of work and home. As an added benefit, many have told me that once they start exercising, their children develop an interest in exercising with them.

If you need a little impetus to get back on the exercise track or to start exercising for the first time, here are some tips on getting started:

Make sure that you are healthy enough to exercise. Most people will be fine starting an exercise program, even after not exercising for a while, and will certainly benefit from it. But do talk with your doctor before making any change in activity level, especially if you are 50 years of age or older, have been inactive, have difficulty keeping your balance, have periods of dizziness, or have heart problems.

Make a date with yourself. Take out your iPad, datebook, BlackBerry, or whatever device you use to keep track of your appointments, and carve out about 20 minutes or so every day for exercise (plus whatever time it takes you to change into and out of your exercise clothes). Study your schedule and figure out which part of the day will work best for you. For stay-at-home moms, the best time may be right after dropping the kids off at school and before getting caught up in chores. For parents who work outside the home, you may find that early morning is best for exercising because if you don't do it first thing, it's likely you won't do it at all. I fall into this category. I like to roll out of bed and do my intervals and core-strengthening exercises before I go to the office. I find that it energizes me for the day, and if I decide to put exercising off until evening, I just don't do it. If you are not a morning person, consider doing your workout during your lunch break, or go to the gym after work or exercise as soon as you get home. Unless there is a true emergency, the time that you set aside for exercise should be nonnegotiable. And if the kids are clamoring for attention, let them exercise with you.

There's no reason not to fit in a workout when you're traveling for business. Most hotels have fitness rooms where you can do intervals on a machine, and the core exercises we recommend can be done anywhere, as long as you have a few feet of floor space to lie on. Of course, you can always do interval walking outside if you're in an area safe for walking.

As an aside, I am often asked whether there are better times than others to do cardiovascular or core workouts in terms of fat burning. Current research suggests that slightly more fat is utilized following the overnight fast. That said, exercise can usually be performed at a higher intensity in the late afternoon, when the body's temperature and hormone levels peak. If you try to do both your interval workout and your core workout on the same day, the exercise that's done later in the day may very well suffer because of muscle fatigue. That's why I suggest alternating days for cardio and core.

Find a buddy. I have found that people who make a commitment to exercise with a friend are more likely to do it consistently, primarily because they know that someone else is counting on them. This even works long distance. On days when you want to beg off, call a friend. It's good to have someone on the other end of the phone urging you to get moving.

Don't give up if you mess up. There may be times that you need to skip a day. Don't beat yourself up about it; we know that no one is perfect. Don't fall into the "I missed my workout yesterday, so I quit" syndrome. A lifestyle is a marathon not a sprint. Just pick up where you left off, and try not to let too many days elapse between your workouts.

THE WAKE UP AND MOVE 2-WEEK QUICK-START PLAN

On pages 230–31, you'll find a 2-week day-by-day guide to getting started with interval walking and core exercises, which you should do on alternate days. (For more on the core exercises, see pages 233–37.)

Interval Walking

As you look at the chart, you'll see that the intervals have four levels of intensity:

Easy Pace. This feels like you're taking a stroll through town or the mall (but no stopping to window shop!). Your breathing is normal and you can carry on a conversation. You will be working at Easy Pace when you do your warmup before beginning the actual intervals and when you cool down afterward.

Moderate Pace. You're walking faster and breathing harder than when you are walking at Easy Pace. You can still carry on a conversation, but it will be a little harder to do so.

Revved Up. When you're revved up, you're really moving. You're short of breath and it's difficult to carrying on a conversation at this level of intensity.

Supercharged. You are working at your maximum level. You are walking as fast as you can, and it is impossible to sustain this pace for very long. As you get fitter, however, you will find that even this exhausting pace can be sustained longer.

On some days the walking will be more difficult than others. This is intentional. Don't be tempted to work at your highest level of intensity all the time; it's a good way to expose your body to overuse injuries. Also, don't leave out the recovery periods between intervals. They are important for recharging your muscles. Depending on your level of fitness, you may find that the intervals suggested here are too easy. If that's the case, simply increase the number of reps, your speed, and the length of time you do them.

Keep in mind that when you are doing your interval walking, you will be switching between slow and fast walking speeds for specific time periods. While it's important that you keep track of time to a point, you don't have to be accurate to the nanosecond. You could use a stopwatch, but why bother?

Try the tried and true "one Mississippi, two Mississippi" method of counting seconds, or purchase one of the new sports apps for your smart phone that keeps track of your interval-training program. Or watch a second hand if you'd like to.

Whether you do your intervals outdoors or in, poor foot support will put you on the fast track to injury. Throw away the worn-out sneakers and invest in a comfortable pair that gives adequate support. A good walking shoe will provide stability and keep you correctly aligned so that you don't experience aches and pains in your feet or anyplace else the next day. Make sure that your shoes fit snugly around the heel so that your foot doesn't slide around, but make sure you also have ample room in the toe box. Socks made from a synthetic material are best for wicking moisture away from the foot.

Finally, don't forget about your posture: Keep your belly drawn in as you move, your chest lifted, and your chin parallel to the ground. With each step, strike the ground from heel to toe, which will help tone your buttocks and the back of your legs as you walk.

Tips for an Outdoor Interval Workout

I'm lucky enough to live near the beach, which is ideal for walking because it's flat, it has great scenery, and there's no traffic to worry about. And walking on sand, especially soft sand, takes some extra work. But most often I walk in my neighborhood. If you don't live near a beach, a park, or a dedicated walking trail, you can still do intervals on the sidewalks or roads of your city or town; you just have to be careful. Here are a few things to think about when walking outdoors:

Avoid heavily trafficked areas. Whether you exercise during the day or evening, you need to choose a venue that ideally isn't too crowded with people or vehicles and that is well lit. If you must walk on the road, stay off to one side, and walk against traffic so that you can see oncoming cars, buses, trucks, and bikes. I don't recommend walking during rush hour if your roads get crowded; the risk of an accident is too great. If you must walk at night, do so in a familiar place and wear a white reflective top (or even a headband) and shoes with reflective material so that you are visible.

(continued on page 232)

WAKE UP AND MOVE 2-WEEK QUICK-START PLAN

	Day 1	Day 2	Day 3	
WEEK 1	**Interval Walking** Warm up with a 5-minute walk at Easy Pace.* • Walk 15 seconds at Moderate Pace. • Walk 60 seconds at Easy Pace. • Repeat 6 times. Cool down with a 2-minute walk at Easy Pace.	**Core Exercises** Do core exercises: See pages 233–37. Take a recreational walk at Easy Pace for 15–20 minutes (optional).	**Interval Walking** Warm up with a 5-minute walk at Easy Pace. • Walk 15 seconds at Moderate Pace. • Walk 45 seconds at Easy Pace. • Repeat 8 times. Cool down with a 2-minute walk at Easy Pace.	
	Day 1	**Day 2**	**Day 3**	
WEEK 2	**Core Exercises** Do core exercises: See pages 233–37. Take a recreational walk at Easy Pace for 15–20 minutes (optional).	**Interval Walking** Warm up with a 5-minute walk at Easy Pace. • Walk 15 seconds at Revved Up. • Walk 45 seconds at Easy Pace. • Repeat 10 times. Cool down with a 2-minute walk at Easy Pace.	**Core Exercises** Do core exercises: See pages 233–37. Take a recreational walk at Easy Pace for 15–20 minutes (optional).	

See page 228 for information on intensity levels.

Day 4	Day 5	Day 6	Day 7
Core Exercises	**Interval Walking**	**Core Exercises**	**Interval Walking**
Do core exercises: See pages 233–37.	Warm up with a 5-minute walk at Easy Pace.	Do core exercises: See pages 233–37.	Warm up with a 5-minute walk at Easy Pace.
Take a recreational walk at Easy Pace for 15–20 minutes (optional).	• Walk 15 seconds at Moderate Pace.	Take a recreational walk at Easy Pace for 15–20 minutes (optional).	• Walk 15 seconds at Revved Up.
	• Walk 60 seconds at Easy Pace.		• Walk 60 seconds at Easy Pace.
	• Repeat 11 times.		• Repeat 8 times.
	Cool down with a 2-minute walk at Easy Pace.		Cool down with a 2-minute walk at Easy Pace.

Day 4	Day 5	Day 6	Day 7
Interval Walking	**Core Exercises**	**Interval Walking**	**Core Exercises**
Warm up with a 5-minute walk at Easy Pace.	Do core exercises: See pages 233–37.	Warm up with a 5-minute walk at Easy Pace.	Do core exercises: See pages 233–37.
• Walk 15 seconds at Revved Up.	Take a recreational walk at Easy Pace for 15–20 minutes (optional).	• Walk 15 seconds at Supercharged!	Take a recreational walk at Easy Pace for 15–20 minutes (optional).
• Walk 30 seconds at Easy Pace.		• Walk 60 seconds at Easy Pace.	
• Repeat 12 times.		• Repeat 8 times.	
Cool down with a 2-minute walk at Easy Pace.		Cool down with a 2-minute walk at Easy Pace.	

Keep the music low. Listening to music on a headset is a great way to get yourself revved up and supercharged, but make sure that you aren't playing it so loudly that you can't hear the traffic noise over the Beatles or Lady Gaga.

Bring a water bottle. Having water with you, even on a short 20-minute walk, is a good idea. Be sure to take sips even if you don't think you are thirsty; it's easy to dehydrate when you are exercising, especially if it is hot and sunny out. And you'll be surprised by how much you sweat when you actually get to the Supercharged intervals.

Protect against the sun. Even if it's not that sunny out, wear UV-protective sunglasses and a hat, and always wear sunscreen on your exposed areas, even in the cooler months. Remember, in the summer, the rays can penetrate your clothing, so either slather on the sunscreen under your clothes or wear clothes made with sun-protective fabric.

Wear light colors in warm weather. On warm days, light colors will keep you cooler by reflecting sunlight. If there is a chill in the air, wear a light jacket that you can remove and tie around your waist once you are warmed up.

Wear several layers of clothing in cooler weather. On cold days, wearing several layers provides better insulation. But be prepared to remove your outer layer if you get too warm, which could happen if you are exercising at a high intensity. Wear a lightweight winter jacket, a sweater, and a moisture-wicking synthetic-fabric top to help keep the sweat away from your skin; if your sweat is not wicked away, it could make you colder. Always wear a hat and gloves to retain body heat. And if it's icy, snowing, or raining, take your interval walking indoors. (I don't recommend doing intervals in these slippery conditions.)

Tips for an Indoor Interval Workout

If you own a treadmill, elliptical machine, or stationary bike, you are in luck. You can do your interval program on any of these machines. Or, if you belong to a gym, you can obviously use the cardio equipment there. Knowing that you can get better conditioning and fat burning with just 20 minutes of interval exercises should be the motivation to finally take advantage of that unused gym membership. As with walking outdoors, always start off slowly, at Easy Pace, and gradually work up to Supercharged on whatever machine you choose.

Treadmill tips. Walking on a treadmill feels different from walking outdoors, and you need to have fairly good balance to stay stable. If you have back problems, increase your intensity by picking up speed, but keep your incline level at the lowest setting or it could further aggravate your back.

Elliptical machine tips. As with the treadmill, you use your muscles somewhat differently on this machine than you do when you are walking outside. Do a few sessions on the elliptical to get familiar with it before you begin a serious interval program. Most brands allow you to adjust the grade and resistance to increase intensity, but again, it is preferable to increase your speed as opposed to just boosting the resistance. Only turn up the resistance when you have achieved all you can with the maximal speed. As with the treadmill, I recommend keeping the grade at the lowest setting to prevent back problems, and be sure to keep your heels down (which makes it a lot harder).

Stationary bike tips. Make sure that you adjust the seat so that each leg is only slightly bent at the bottom of the pedal stroke. You can change your intensity by either cycling faster or increasing resistance. Try not to apply so much resistance that you can't turn the pedals at least 60 times per minute. As with the elliptical machine, speed is the goal. Only increase resistance when you have achieved all you can at maximal speed.

Work out without a machine. You can also do a great indoor interval workout without a machine. Try jumping rope (if your knees can take it), jogging in place, or doing jumping jacks. Just speed up and slow down as you would if you were walking.

Core-Building Exercises

As noted above, at the same time that you are improving your vascular system, you should also begin a regimen of stretching and strengthening exercises to utilize all the different muscle groups in your body and promote functional fitness. Try to incorporate the exercises on the following pages into your fitness routine about three times a week, alternating them with interval exercise. All are low-impact and suitable for almost any age and fitness level.

Here are a few things to consider:

Use a mat. You don't want to lie on a hard floor. If you have a yoga mat, you can use it; if you don't, a thick towel will do.

Dress right. Wear comfortable clothing that allows for maximum movement. Do all your exercises barefoot, which will allow you to flex and point your toes more easily. Don't wear socks—you could slip.

Focus on your movements. You can listen to music, but turn off the TV. To get the most out of this workout, you need to concentrate on what you are doing. Work slowly and think about each movement. Breathe through each exercise. Make sure that you are following proper form (reviewing the photographs will help) and are doing the exercises carefully. If the instructions tell you to contract your abs, even though you may be working a different part of your body, it's for a good reason. These core muscles provide stability, and if you're not engaging them, you're not getting the most out of your workout.

As with interval walking, it's important to start with the minimum number of reps and add more as you get fitter.

TOE DIP

A Lie on your back with your hands at your sides, palms down, and your legs up and bent at a 90-degree angle. Keep your abs contracted and press your lower back toward the floor.

B Inhale and lower your left leg for a count of two ("down, down"), moving only from the hip and dipping your toes toward the floor. Exhale and raise your leg back to the starting position for a count of two ("up, up"). Repeat with your right leg and continue alternating until you've done 12 reps with each leg.

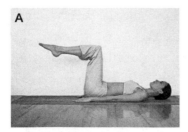
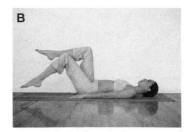

LEG CIRCLE

A Lie on your back with your legs straight and your hands at your sides, palms down. Raise your left leg toward the ceiling, with your toe pointed, and hold for 10 to 60 seconds. (To make it easier, you can bend your right leg and place your right foot flat on the floor.)

B Draw a small circle with your left toes, rotating your leg from the hip. Inhale as you begin the circle and exhale as you finish. Keep your body still—no rocking—by tightening your abs. Do 6 circles, then reverse the direction and do 6 more. Repeat with your right leg.

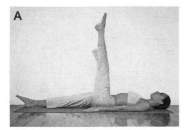
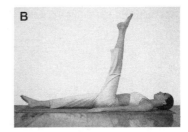

CRISSCROSS

A Start as in the Toe Dip but with your hands behind your head and your elbows out to the side. Curl up to raise your head, neck, and shoulders off the floor.

B As you inhale, rotate your torso to the right, bringing your right knee and left shoulder toward each other and extending your left leg toward the ceiling in a diagonal line from your hip. As you exhale, rotate to the left, bringing your left knee toward your right shoulder and extending your right leg. That's 1 rep. Do 6 reps.

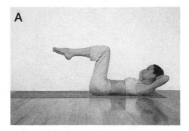
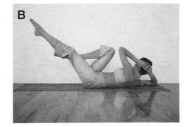

LEG KICK

A Lie on your left side with your legs straight and together so your body forms one long line. Prop yourself up on your left elbow and forearm, lifting your ribs off the floor and your head toward the ceiling. Place your right hand lightly in front of you for balance. (If this position is uncomfortable, extend your left arm on the floor and rest your head on your arm.) Raise your right leg to hip level and flex your foot so your toes are pointing forward.

B Exhale as you kick, swinging your right leg forward as far as comfortably possible and pulsing for two counts ("kick, kick"). Inhale, point your toes, and swing your leg back past your left leg for two counts. That's 1 rep. Do 6 reps without lowering your leg. Then switch sides and repeat.

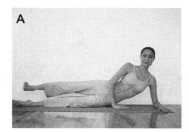
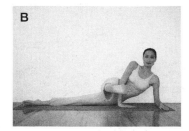

BACK EXTENSION WITH ROTATION

A Lie on your stomach with your forehead on your hands, palms on the floor. Separate your feet to a hip-width apart. Pull your abs in.

B Raise your head, shoulders, and chest off the floor. Rotate your upper body to the right and back to the center, then lower. Repeat to the left side and continue alternating until you've done 6 rotations to each side.

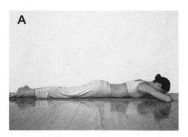
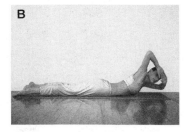

SIDE BEND

A Sit on your left hip with your left leg bent in front of you and your left hand beneath your shoulder. Place your right foot flat on the floor just in front of your left foot, so your right knee points toward the ceiling. Rest your right arm on your right knee.

B Pull your abs in, press into your left hand, and lift your hips off the floor. As you come up onto your left knee, straighten your right leg and raise your right arm over your head so you form a line from your right fingers to your right toes. Hold for 10 to 30 seconds. Lower and repeat on the other side. Gradually work up to more than one rep.

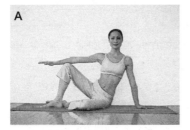
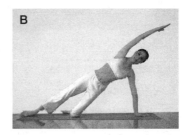

FIND CREATIVE WAYS TO MOVE

As I noted earlier, the third leg of the fitness stool is to simply move more, and it's not that hard to do. It's actually easy to work different forms of movement into your daily routines, whether you're at home, at the office, or outdoors. While none of the ideas suggested below will replace a really good interval-training session or a core workout, over time these small actions will definitely help you burn calories, build muscle, and get out of the sitting habit. And when incorporated throughout your day, they will certainly make you feel better.

Timed superclean. Once you've cleaned up your living space (Strategy 1), you'll want to keep it uncluttered. Why not combine your subsequent clean-up efforts with some exercise? Set the timer on the oven or your cell phone for 10 minutes, and then see how much of your house you can tidy up before the buzzer goes off. This will probably mean running from room to room, upstairs and down. Under pressure from the timer, you're sure to zip around faster and faster. And there's a double benefit: You'll get moving and the house will get picked up too.

If You Are a Parent

As more and more schools cut out recess and physical education, it is imperative for parents to pick up the slack and make sure that their children get enough physical activity. Although you can't force children to exercise, you can encourage them by exposing them to different ways to get moving. Some kids may gravitate to competitive sports; others may prefer dance, karate, yoga, bike riding, or, if they're old enough, even walking fast on a treadmill. The key is to find something that your child enjoys and provide opportunities to do it.

Make an exercise date with your child. If your child is beginning to develop sedentary habits, try to bring more movement into his or her life. Make a date on the weekend when the two of you can go for a walk or go ice-skating. Shoot some hoops in the backyard or at the schoolyard. Go swimming together at a local pool. Make it your special time together and your child will look forward to it. Encourage elementary age children to have friends over, then provide them with equipment for outdoor play.

Limit screen time. Kids should not be *sitting* playing video games, socializing online, or watching TV for hours on end. If your children are enamored of video games, get them hooked on Wii sports games and/or Wii Fit, the Nintendo play system that contains more than 40 activities designed to engage the player in physical exercise, such as yoga, strength

Kitchen workout. If you've heeded the "wake-up call" in Strategy 3, you'll be spending more time cooking, which means more kitchen clean-up. It's a boring job, so relieve the tedium with some mini-sets. While you're doing the dishes, for instance, try for 10 leg raises to each side and 10 to the rear. As you're cleaning the counters, work in some countertop pushups. Stand back, put your hands on the edge of the counter, and do some half pushups. Start with 5 and work up from there.

Office mini-moves. Don't slouch in your chair. Sit with your feet on the training, aerobics, balance games, and dance. Wii Fit combines fitness with fun and is designed for everyone, young and old. Wii Fit players work toward personal fitness goals, and they block soccer balls, swivel hips to power hula hoops, and ski big jumps to get themselves there. There are also numerous other video exercise games to choose from, and kids who may feel uncomfortable at the thought of beginning a competitive sport at school may gain body confidence by mastering these virtual games in the privacy of their own home.

Motivate, but don't demand. Children who lack body confidence may be slow to adopt exercise. You may need to expose them to many different forms of fitness before they find one that they feel comfortable doing. Be encouraging, but don't make them feel worse about themselves than they already do. The motivation to change has to come from within, but gentle coaxing can be useful. Help children to understand that watching less television and walking a few blocks every day, or dancing along to a video, could go a long way toward helping them fit into clothes that they thought they could never wear and give them more energy to keep up with school and a social life. Don't give up. If a child is reluctant to listen at first, bring up the subject a few days later. Be patient. Keep trying.

floor, and your knees over your toes. Maintain a tight core, keep your back straight, and keep your neck relaxed. No need to stay glued to your chair all day, though. You'll burn more calories if you make it a habit to stand up when you're talking on the phone and move around. Periodically (or even permanently), switch out your chair for a stability ball; you'll improve your balance and strengthen your core while at your desk. Instead of e-mailing or instant-messaging, walk to your colleagues' desks and talk to them in person. Take the stairs, not the elevator.

Stand Tall

Get up out of your chair, stand up tall, suck in your abdominals, relax your shoulders, and keep your chin parallel to the floor. Now go look at yourself in the mirror. This is what good posture looks like. When you are standing correctly, your shoulders aren't hunched over and your stomach isn't protruding. You look taller, slimmer, and more attractive. But posture is not just a matter of aesthetics. When your muscles and bones are properly aligned, you are able to move better and stay injury free.

Working your core doesn't end when you finish your 20-minute workout: You will begin to incorporate core-strengthening movements into your daily activities. By that I mean you will develop a much greater consciousness about how to hold your body even when you are not officially "exercising." When you are sitting at your desk, or washing the dishes, or making a bed, you will not let your stomach sag and your shoulders cave in, but you will maintain healthy posture. As you get stronger and more limber, standing tall will become second nature. Being core strong will become a lifestyle.

Desk strengthening. Keep some fitness equipment in your desk drawer or next to your desk, where you can see it and be reminded to use it. Use resistance bands or light hand weights at least twice a day. Think how easy it is to do some arm curls while you're reading through a long report or listening in on a conference call.

Group gallop. Recruit some co-workers to go for early-morning or lunchtime walks. Not only will this help build camaraderie and be a good break from the office, it will also help keep your muscles toned and get your blood circulating too. The fittest office groups try to walk three times a week or so.

While none of these activities is particularly taxing on its own, taken together they can make a real difference in how you feel. So, get moving! Pretty soon you'll be coming up with mini-exercises of your own.

SLEEP BETTER, LIVE LONGER

No matter how well you eat, how often you exercise, and how much time you spend planning and cooking your meals, you can never be truly healthy if you don't get enough quality sleep. Lack of sleep can alter your metabolism, making you prone to weight gain, diabetes, and heart disease. It can interfere with your ability to learn and perform at your peak. It can rev up your stress hormones and make you depressed. It can dampen your immune response, leaving you susceptible to colds and flu. Not getting enough sleep can make you feel so overwhelmed and exhausted that you stop making good choices and end up doing what is easiest at the time.

If you are one of the fortunate few who can put your head down on your pillow at night and wake up 8 hours later feeling revived, count your blessings and keep doing what you're doing. If, however, you are one of the 70 million or so Americans who struggle with sleep, who have difficulty either falling asleep or staying asleep, and who often wake up feeling exhausted, then you need to reevaluate your "sleep style."

SOLVE YOUR OWN SLEEP PROBLEMS

So what's keeping you up? If you've had a longstanding problem with sleep, this may be a difficult question for you to answer. For you, not sleeping has become a way of life. You are so accustomed to being a fitful sleeper that you no longer even expect to have a good night's sleep. One of my missions is to raise your expectations: There is no reason why most people can't get a good night's sleep, but it may take a bit of effort on your part to get there.

Some people are kept awake by bona fide sleep disorders, like sleep apnea, which I discussed in Chapter 9. If you snore loudly and suspect you have apnea, consult with your doctor or see a sleep specialist. There are many effective treatments for sleep apnea, and you don't have to live with it. Nor should you suffer in silence if you are up at night in pain. If you have arthritis, restless leg syndrome, or any other medical condition that could be interfering with your sleep, see your doctor.

There are times in all of our lives when we experience emotional turmoil that interferes with our ability to sleep. The loss of a loved one or an illness in the family can be very upsetting. Don't suffer alone. Walking around exhausted will only make matters worse. There are some excellent sleep medications that can be used on a temporary basis to restore sleep. This is a time to seek help from your doctor.

In the vast majority of cases, however, people are sabotaging their own sleep because they don't know any better. For most of us, sleep medication is not necessary. Very often, making some simple changes in lifestyle and environment can help resolve typical sleep problems over time.

KEEP A SLEEP LOG

So how do you know what's standing between you and a good night's sleep? Is it something that you're doing or eating or drinking during the day? We provide a Sleep Quiz at southbeachdiet.com/wakeupcall to help you analyze your sleep habits, as well as a Sleep Log to help you keep track of how long and how well you sleep at night and what aspects of your lifestyle may be disrupting your sleep.

MAKE YOUR BEDROOM A GOOD PLACE FOR SLEEPING

You spend (or should be spending) a third of your life in your bedroom. So it's important to make it a pleasant, relaxing environment that is conducive to good sleep. If you've followed our suggestions in Strategy 1 for de-cluttering the room and removing electronic equipment at night, you've already made a good start.

A comfortable bed is essential. After a long day, you should look forward to crawling into your bed for 8 hours of restorative sleep. If that's not the case, is it because your bed isn't comfortable? Do you wake up with aches and pains? Is your mattress sagging or too hard or lumpy? Can you feel the coils when you lie down? Are there uncomfortable patches of mattress that you avoid? If any of these problems exist, maybe it's time to buy a new mattress and box spring. The rule of thumb is that a mattress should be replaced every 7 to 10 years; however, if you're not getting the sleep you need and think your mattress may be contributing to the problem, you should consider doing it sooner. If you can afford to purchase a new one, go to a department store or bedding store and try out a few mattresses to see which ones you find comfortable. Ideally, bring your sleep partner with you. A bed can feel different when there is someone lying next to you. If your partner's tossing and turning is keeping you awake, consider purchasing a mattress made from memory foam, a type of material that doesn't shift when you change position.

If you can't afford to buy a new mattress, try a foam or down mattress topper, which, as its name suggests, you place on top of your mattress to make it more comfortable. A mattress topper is a lot cheaper than a whole new mattress; however, it does need to be replaced every few years.

Keep your room cool but not cold. The ideal temperature for sleeping is somewhere between 65°F and 72°F; some people prefer a cooler room, and others like it warmer. If you are constantly throwing the covers off at night, consider turning the thermostat down a few degrees. If you are freezing, turn the heat up a few degrees. A room that is either too warm or too cool (below 60°F) will disrupt sleep, so it is important to find the right temperature for you.

Make sure your room is quiet. If outside noise is keeping you awake, consider moving your bedroom to another, quieter room if you have one, or invest in double-glazed windows, which can shut out street noise, and/or heavy drapes. If you are hearing noisy neighbors, move your bed to a quieter part of the bedroom. If you are extremely noise sensitive, try using a white noise machine, which muffles ambient sound.

AVOID FOOD AND BEVERAGES THAT CAN KEEP YOU AWAKE

The food and drink that you consume during the day and evening can have a significant impact on how well you sleep at night.

Snack but don't gorge before bedtime. A big meal at night can rev up your metabolism and make it hard for your body to wind down. So eat light at night, but don't go to bed hungry. Hunger pangs will make it difficult to get to sleep and to stay asleep. Some foods have a slightly soporific effect, like turkey, hummus, dairy, pumpkin seeds, whole grains, hazelnuts, and bananas, which contain the amino acid tryptophan, known to induce mild sleepiness. Other foods, especially those that are spicy, can induce wakefulness. Eating highly spiced meals at night can cause heartburn or aggravate gastric reflux, both major causes of sleep problems.

Limit caffeine in the afternoon. We live in a caffeinated world, where up to 90 percent of the population ingests this stimulant in one form or another. Caffeine perks up your central nervous system, making you feel more focused and alert. Found naturally in coffee, tea, chocolate, and the cola nut, caffeine is added to many brands of soda and energy drinks. In fact, caffeine is so ubiquitous in our food supply that it's hard to keep track of how much you are ingesting unless you make a conscious effort to do so.

Even then, it's difficult to really know how much caffeine is in a particular product because manufacturers are not required to list it on the label. For example, some brands of brewed coffee have 75 grams of caffeine per serving, but others can have 120 or more grams; instant coffee typically has about a third less than most brewed coffees. Even decaf coffee has a few milligrams per cup, which could affect caffeine-sensitive people. Tea contains between 20 and 90 milligrams of caffeine, depending on the type. If you drink a lot of diet cola with caffeine, be aware that many brands have a whopping 45 grams of caffeine per serving (diet orange soda has 40 grams). I usually advise patients to avoid caffeinated foods and beverages at least 6 hours before bedtime, and even longer if they find that an early-afternoon cup of coffee or iced tea makes it difficult for them to sleep. If you are having sleep problems, be vigilant about limiting your caffeine intake after noon and see if it helps. Maintaining a sleep diary can help you keep track of your caffeine intake to see whether there is any correlation between caffeine consumption and disordered sleep.

But don't cut out caffeinated beverages cold turkey; it could cause caffeine withdrawal, which includes some uncomfortable symptoms like headache, nausea, anxiety, and even panic attacks in some people. If you are a habitual user—that is, you have a cup or two of coffee or consume other caffeinated products on a daily basis—gradually taper off by cutting back by half a cup of coffee or diet soda daily until your body gets accustomed to less caffeine.

Say no to nightcaps. For most people, a glass of wine at dinner is fine, but it's best not to drink alcohol right before you go to bed. Although a drink may make you drowsy at first, in some people it can disrupt normal sleep cycles and leave them wide awake a few hours later. In highly sensitive people, drinking alcohol up to 6 hours before bedtime could cause wakefulness. On the South Beach Diet, we suggest no more than one drink daily for women and two for men (beginning on Phase 2). If you are having trouble sleeping, try cutting out the alcohol altogether for a while and see if it helps.

WIND DOWN BEFORE BEDTIME

Your body and mind need time to transition from alert to drowsy. If you are upset or revved up over things that have occurred during the day, sleep will not come easy. An hour or two before bedtime, begin winding down in preparation for sleep.

Put out that cigarette. First of all, don't smoke. Smoking is the worst thing that you can do for your health, and if you are still smoking, you should make every effort to stop. Having said that, I know that there are people who say that they "must" have a cigarette at night to calm down. Although the act of smoking a cigarette may initially relax you, in reality the nicotine is a stimulant that can interfere with sleep. Another reason to quit.

Get enough physical activity, but at the right time. Several studies have shown inactivity to be a major cause of insomnia. Among my patients, I have found that people who complain of insomnia are often "cured" when they take up exercise. My only caveat is that you shouldn't exercise too close to bedtime because it can be overly stimulating.

Sex before bedtime can be relaxing . . . or not. Some people find that having sex at bedtime helps them to sleep better, but others tell me that it excites them so much that they have difficulty sleeping. There are no rules here; do what works best for you. If you find that you need to unwind after having sex, suggest to your partner that you enjoy sex earlier in the evening. If both of you find that you are wide awake afterward, consider having sex in the morning.

Follow a bedtime ritual. Doing the same thing every night before sleep will signal to your brain that you are prepping for bedtime. Turn on soothing music, take a lavender-scented bath, read an entertaining but not-too-exciting book or magazine article, do some mild stretching or deep breathing. Now is not the time to have family arguments or engage in stressful activities like paying bills or preparing your tax returns. Obviously, if you live with other people, you need to get their cooperation; teens have to agree not to blare loud music after a certain time of night, and a spouse must commit to not bringing his or her laptop into bed.

Turn down the lights. You know that you sleep better in a dark room, but you may not know why. Darkness—or rather, the absence of light—triggers the production of melatonin, a hormone that regulates sleep-wake cycles in addition to lowering blood pressure and body temperature in preparation for sleep. Under ideal circumstances, your body produces ample amounts of melatonin at night to allow you to sleep and then curtails production by morning so that you can wake up. Exposure to artificial light late in the evening, however, can suppress and shorten the duration of melatonin production, which could contribute to difficulty falling asleep and staying asleep.

As I discussed in Chapter 9, lack of sleep not only makes you feel lousy, but can also disrupt normal metabolism and increase the risk for weight gain and diabetes. Interestingly, contact with light at night might play a role. In a recent study, mice exposed to a dim light (like from a clock radio) while they slept gained 50 percent more weight over an 8-week period than mice sleeping in total darkness, even though they got the same amount of food and

Is Your Bed Partner a Snorer?

If your bed partner's snoring is keeping you awake, it's a real problem for both of you. First, he or she should be examined by a physician to see if it's due to a medical problem. It could be sleep apnea (see pages 148–51), which can be treated. If it is simply loud snoring, which is not life threatening to the person doing the snoring, there are some simple things that can be done that may improve matters:

✓ Alcohol can aggravate snoring by relaxing the muscles in the airways, which makes breathing harder. Eliminating alcohol at night may help silence the snorer.

✓ A stuffed nose or clogged nasal passages can make snoring worse by causing the snorer to breathe through his or her mouth. A nasal strip worn on the bridge of the nose can open nasal passages, which could reduce the need for mouth breathing.

✓ Dry heat can trigger snoring. A humidifier can help keep the room moist, and therefore prevent the mouth and nose from drying out.

✓ Losing even a few pounds can help reduce snoring.

✓ An anti-snoring mouthpiece may help reposition the mouth and jaw so that the snorer has an easier time breathing and thus makes less noise. There are many different types of over-the-counter mouthpieces to choose from. If the problem is severe, a mouthpiece made specifically for the individual by a dentist or sleep specialist is best.

✓ If all else fails, the nonsnoring partner can try wearing earplugs to shut out the noise or invest in a white noise machine to muffle the sound.

exercise. It's possible that even the dim light disrupted the cycling of melatonin, which could be at the root of the metabolic problem that caused the weight gain. Remember, this is a mouse study, but it is food for thought.

(continued on page 250)

If You Are a Parent

If you have children, it is absolutely critical for their mental and physical development that you make sure they are getting ample sleep. It is also essential for your own sanity. You can't be a good parent if you are exhausted and resentful from not getting enough rest because the kids are going to bed late or getting up throughout the night.

Of course, new parents will lose sleep because it can take infants several months to get into a sleep routine. By the toddler years, however, children should know how to go to sleep and how to get themselves back to sleep if they awaken at night, at least most of the time.

Sleep "rules" are the same for young and old. Almost all the sleep tips that I provide in this chapter apply to children. It is especially important for parents to maintain an orderly, predictable bedtime ritual that helps children know when it's time to wind down and prepare for bed. Kids should also understand that lights out means lights out, or else bedtime can drag on for hours into the night. Don't get your child into the habit of needing you to fall asleep. Teach her how to comfort herself by playing or singing quietly until she falls asleep on her own.

Don't ignore snoring. Sleep apnea often goes undiagnosed in children. If you have a child who snores loudly, alert your pediatrician. While it may not be apnea, snoring and breathing difficulties could be a sign of allergies or even asthma.

Watch the caffeine. Some adolescents and teens inadvertently consume large amounts of caffeine in soft drinks, coffee drinks, and in so-called energy drinks, which may contain as much caffeine as a cup or two of coffee. All these beverages can contribute not only to insomnia but also to anxiety and heart palpitations. Make sure that your children are aware of the potential dangers of these beverages and encourage them to stop drinking them.

Suggest a sleep log. If older children are having difficulty going to sleep or staying asleep, suggest that they keep a sleep log to see if there are things they're doing that could be sabotaging their sleep. Keeping track of the foods and beverages they consume and the amount of exercise they get and when could provide some clues to sleep problems. By giving children a chance to track their behavior, you will give them a sense of control and more motivation to be part of the solution.

No bed sharing (including the dog). Kids should understand that they sleep in their own beds, and that a parent is available to them if need be. For example, if a child has a nightmare or feels ill, by all means he should be allowed to wake up a parent. But in general, it is not good for anyone in the family to be popping in and out of bed at all hours. Kids should be able to get back into their own beds after a reassuring hug.

By the way, don't get into the habit of allowing a pet to share your child's (or your own) bed. Many people who sleep with their pets find that they lose sleep because, believe it or not, dogs can snore as loudly as people, not to mention take up space. So do yourself and your pet a favor—get Buddy his own mattress.

Get the computer and smart phone out of the bedroom. Allowing a computer or smart phone in the bedroom all evening will make it too tempting for an adolescent to talk, text, tweet, or e-mail until late into the night. If your child has a desktop computer, establish a shutdown time. A better option for kids may be a laptop, which can be removed from the room at bedtime. And don't forget to remove that smart phone. Older kids can hopefully be trusted.

You can try to keep your own melatonin production robust by dimming the lights an hour or two before bedtime and sleeping in a dark room. As noted earlier, avoid using a computer, watching TV, or even looking at your smart phone screen. After you go to sleep, avoid exposure to ambient light. Don't sleep near a lit screen (like an alarm clock); get drapes or blinds to block out light from the street; and if you get up at night to use the bathroom, use a night light instead of turning on a bright light.

Stick to a schedule. Each of us has a biological clock that regulates our bodily processes. This internal clock works best when we stick to a predictable schedule. Try to go to bed around the same time every night and awaken at roughly the same time every morning. There are days, however, when this may not be possible; often when work interferes or social engagements keep you up way past your bedtime. When this does happen, strive to get up around your usual time anyway. You may be a bit sleepier than normal when you awaken, so as quickly as possible, go outside and let your brain register that it's daylight. This will help reduce the drowsiness. Sleeping in will only further disrupt your schedule, and could interfere with your ability to fall asleep that night, which could trigger a cycle of disrupted sleep.

If you want to party late into the night on the weekend, it's better to do it on Friday than on Saturday. If you stay in bed a bit longer on Saturday morning but go to sleep Saturday night within an hour or so of your normal bedtime, you can awaken at your regular time on Sunday. This will enable you to go to sleep at your normal time Sunday night, so that you can wake up at your regular time on Monday and not feel exhausted at the beginning of the work or school week.

Make your bedroom a worry-free zone. You need to create a barrier between the "real world" and the world of sleep. We all have worries that can keep us up at night, but in our saner moments it's important to recognize that sleep deprivation is not conducive to problem solving or performing well. So leave anxiety outside the bedroom door. I mean this quite literally. If there is something nagging at you, write your thoughts down in a journal to be addressed the next day, and then stash it away somewhere outside your bedroom. When your head hits the pillow and you close your eyes, create a relaxing mental image that becomes your internal "screen saver." Think of walking on a beach, or hiking, or sleeping in a hammock, or whatever your ideal de-stressing scenario might be. Focus on it, don't allow your mind to wander, and allow yourself to drift off to sleep.

MAKE GOOD HEALTH A HABIT

Once you've completed the seven strategies of the South Beach Diet Wake-Up Program, your new healthy habits should be so seamlessly embedded into your life that that you can no longer imagine living any other way, nor should you want to. By now you should be reaping some of the many benefits of your new lifestyle: If you had some weight to lose, you should be well on your way to reaching your goal, thanks to shopping and eating better and avoiding fast-food venues. If you were tired and listless, you should be feeling more ener-gized and alert from your improved diet, exercise, and sleep habits. If you were sitting all day, simply moving more has no doubt helped improve a litany of ailments. If you hardly saw your family before, hopefully you're now grow-ing closer and enjoying one another's company, thanks to more frequent fam-ily dinners. Ideally, you and your children have cooked a few meals together, gone for walks after school, or planted a home garden that is beginning to bloom.

When it comes to making good health a permanent way of life, perhaps the most important piece of advice that I can give you is this: Don't be dis-couraged if you and your family are not perfect. We all have setbacks. Perhaps you will overindulge at a party or skip exercise for a few days. Maybe during an especially hectic week you'll eat out more than you should. Maybe you let the dog sleep in your bed. Things happen, but you shouldn't give up and slip back into your old ways. Always pause when setbacks occur, take a deep breath, and get back on track at the earliest opportunity.

Please keep this book handy so that you can refer to it from time to time when you need a "wake-up call." And do visit South Beach Diet Wake-Up Call online at southbeachdiet.com/wakeupcall for guidance and support and to become part of the larger community pledging to lead a healthier life.

PART 3

MegaFoods and MegaRecipes for Healthy Eating

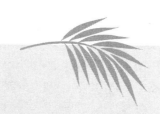

Over the years I have been asked many times about the best foods to eat for improving heart health and health in general. Coming up with a short list wasn't so easy, since every day researchers are discovering new health-giving phytonutrients in the foods we eat, to add to the thousands of phytonutrients already documented. It is these remarkable plant substances that we now know are responsible for helping the body neutralize cell-damaging free radicals, the unstable oxygen molecules that play a role in so many degenerative diseases. They also stimulate the body's immune cells and infection-fighting enzymes. Needless to say, I keep updating and adding to my MegaFoods list as new discoveries come up. And while the foods I list on the following pages are certainly some of the most nutritious, the real secret to staying well is to eat as wide a variety of health-giving foods as possible and to include some of these MegaFoods at as many meals as possible.

That's why, as I thought about the importance of re-establishing healthy home cooking as part of our program strategies, I wanted to bring something new to the table: Interesting and delicious recipes that provide a big health bang for the buck. With that in mind, I gave our South Beach test kitchen my MegaFoods list along with descriptions of the foods' health benefits, and asked them to create MegaRecipes for everything from breakfast to dessert that incorporate as many of these superfoods as possible. The recipes follow on pages 259–306.

MEGAFOODS
FOR HEALTHY EATING

The following 15 foods or groups of foods provide outstanding health benefits for people of all ages. Work as many of them into your daily meals as possible.

Avocados, Extra-Virgin Olive Oil, and Other Sources of Healthy Fats Among the healthiest fats are the monounsaturated fats found in avocados (and avocado oil), olive oil, peanut oil, and canola oil. They are essential for building cell membranes; for nerve, heart, and brain health; and for nearly all the body's basic functions. Avocados have been found to reduce the risk of heart disease because they contain beta-sitosterol, a plant sterol that can lower levels of bad (LDL) cholesterol and raise good (HDL) cholesterol. Avocados are also a good source of the B vitamin folate, as well as potassium and magnesium. Olive oil, in particular extra-virgin olive oil, contains powerful disease-fighting antioxidant compounds called polyphenols. Because all fats (even healthy ones) are calorie dense, they should be consumed in moderation.

Beans, Lentils, and Other Legumes All legumes—from black beans and kidney beans to chickpeas and lentils—are loaded with filling protein and plenty of fiber, as well as disease-fighting phytonutrients. The fiber in legumes can help lower total and LDL cholesterol and it also helps to slow the digestion process, preventing glucose and insulin levels from rising steeply. All this makes legumes a good choice for people with diabetes. While all legumes provide fiber, chickpeas and kidney beans have a whopping 7 grams per half-cup serving.

Blueberries, Cranberries, Raspberries, Blackberries, and Other High-Antioxidant Berries In general, berries are powerful sources of antioxidants, including vitamin C, but blueberries and cranberries in particular are stars. The flavonoids in blueberries are probably responsible for the fruit's antioxidant power, and recent studies show that the anthocyanins in blueberries may help prevent the development of hypertension. Blueberries (like cranberries and most berries) also contain ellagic acid, which has been shown to have anti-cancer properties, and the fruit is also packed with pectin (a type of soluble fiber that has been found to help reduce total and LDL cholesterol). In addition, blueberries may help prevent cataracts and the short-term memory loss associated with aging. Studies have found cranberries to be protective against a variety of cancers, and the flavonoids they contain (in particular quercetin) may play a role in preventing coronary artery disease thanks to their anti-inflammatory properties.

Broccoli and Other Cruciferous Vegetables Broccoli, cabbage, brussels sprouts, cauliflower, kale, bok choy, horseradish, and other cruciferous vegetables are antioxidant powerhouses that can help lower blood pressure and cholesterol, protect against macular degeneration, and reduce age-related memory loss. In addition, the sulfur compound called sulforaphane found in these vegetables may increase the activity of cancer-fighting enzymes in the body. Superstar broccoli is also packed with folate, riboflavin, and potassium, and contains considerable amounts of beta-carotene as well. Moreover, ounce for ounce, broccoli has more vitamin C than an orange and as much calcium as a glass of milk.

Coffee and Tea New studies show that drinking caffeinated coffee (in moderation) can reduce the risk of type 2 diabetes. This may be due to both the antioxidants in the coffee (the polyphenols in particular) and the caffeine (decaf has not shown the same results). Typical servings of caffeinated coffee contain more antioxidants than typical servings of other antioxidant-rich beverages, such as grape juice and orange juice. As for tea, the polyphenols in white, green, oolong, and black tea have been found to help lower LDL cholesterol. In addition, a recent study showed that regularly drinking green tea, which is rich in a type of polyphenol called catechins, may help promote exercise-induced abdominal fat loss. Catechins have also been shown to improve triglyceride levels and help protect against Alzheimer's disease and certain forms of cancer.

Dark Chocolate and Cocoa Powder Several studies have shown that eating dark chocolate in moderation can lower blood pressure (probably due to the beneficial effects of its polyphenols on blood vessel elasticity and blood flow) and reduce levels of C-reactive protein (CRP) in the body, a powerful predictor of heart disease and type 2 diabetes. The flavonoids in dark chocolate and cocoa powder may also help protect against certain forms of cancer and diabetes. Choose dark chocolate that contains at least 70 percent cacao (and thus the least sugar) and brands of cocoa powder labeled 100 percent cacao.

Flaxseeds and Other Edible Seeds Whether you choose pumpkin seeds, sunflower seeds, sesame seeds, or flaxseeds, all edible seeds are good sources of protein, fiber, and unsaturated fats. Pumpkin seeds are also rich in zinc, a potential immune-system booster; sunflower seeds are a good source of vitamin E and folate, possible cancer fighters; and sesame seeds are an excellent source of zinc, which vegans are often lacking in their diet. Flaxseeds (which can be used whole or ground) are rich in alpha-linolenic acid (ALA), a heart-healthy omega-3 fat that's highly unsaturated. Omega-3s have been found to help lower significantly elevated triglycerides and total cholesterol and to reduce the formation of blood clots (important for preventing a heart attack or stroke). They can also help to control high blood pressure. Because all seeds are calorie dense, be sure to enjoy them in moderation.

Low-Fat Dairy There is mounting evidence that something in dairy foods (milk, yogurt, and cheese), perhaps the vitamin D that's in the cheese or added to fortified milk and yogurt, not only strengthens bones but also protects the heart, reduces high blood pressure, and fights breast cancer. The jury is still out about whether dairy can aid weight loss. Choose fat-free or reduced-fat products to avoid excess saturated fat.

Mushrooms The only fruit or vegetable source of vitamin D, mushrooms contain ergosterol, a plant sterol that converts to vitamin D when exposed to real or artificial sunlight. In addition to vitamin D, mushrooms contain eight essential amino acids as well as niacin, riboflavin, thiamin, and dietary fiber. They are also an excellent source of potassium, a mineral that helps lower blood pressure. Shiitake mushrooms in particular have been found to help boost the immune system and may help protect against certain forms of cancer, as well as atherosclerosis and bacterial and viral conditions.

Oats, Barley, Wheat, and Other Whole Grains Recent studies have shown that eating high-fiber whole grains (oats, barley, wheat, wild rice, quinoa, millet, barley, spelt, and rye, for example) can actually lower the risk of diabetes by stabilizing blood sugar and controlling insulin production. The fiber in whole grains also helps prevent artery-clogging atherosclerosis by interfering with cholesterol absorption.

Red Wine A phytonutrient found in red grapes known as resveratrol may help suppress plaque development and protect against artery-damaging LDL cholesterol, thanks to its antioxidant and anti-inflammatory properties. Increasing evidence also indicates that resveratrol may help protect against cancer and type 2 diabetes and may activate a so-called survival gene that has been shown to extend the lives of mice. Enjoy a glass or two of red wine with a meal, but stop at one or two; more than one drink a day for women and two drinks daily for men can increase the risk of heart disease (and possibly breast cancer in women), and have other harmful effects on the body.

Salmon and Other Omega-3-Rich Fish Fatty cold-water fish such as salmon (buy wild if you can), herring, mackerel, anchovies, and sardines are all rich in heart-healthy omega-3 fatty acids. Studies have also found that including this type of seafood in your diet can help reduce blood pressure; play a positive role in mood, memory loss, and other brain functions; and reduce inflammation. Try to eat omega-3-rich seafood two or three times a week, avoiding any high in mercury (see page 210).

Sweet Potatoes and Other Bright Orange Vegetables An outstanding source of carotenoids (including beta-carotene), as well as vitamin C, calcium, and potassium, sweet potatoes (and other orange vegetables such as carrots, pumpkin, and butternut squash) can help reduce LDL cholesterol, lower high blood pressure, fight cataracts and age-related macular degeneration, and boost your resistance to colds and infections. The carotenoids in these vegetables also help those with diabetes by stabilizing their blood sugar levels and lowering insulin resistance, and they have been found to protect against inflammatory conditions such as asthma and arthritis. Bright orange fruits, such as apricots, mangoes, and oranges, are also a good source of beta-carotene.

Tomatoes Rich in the antioxidant vitamin C, tomatoes also contain a red pigment called lycopene, a powerful carotenoid that may help lower your risk of heart disease and cancer (especially prostate, breast, and skin cancer). Tomatoes also contain lutein and zeaxanthin—antioxidant-rich plant pigments that can play a role in reducing the risk of macular degeneration, a leading cause of partial blindness in people over the age of 50.

Walnuts, Almonds, and Other Nuts Walnuts, almonds, hazelnuts, pistachios, peanuts, and pecans are all excellent sources of protein, heart-healthy monounsaturated and polyunsaturated fats, vitamins, minerals, and fiber. When substituted for saturated fat in the diet, nuts can help lower total cholesterol as well as bad (LDL) cholesterol without affecting levels of good (HDL) cholesterol. Unlike other nuts, walnuts are high in alpha-linolenic acid (ALA), an omega-3 fat that has been shown to have antioxidant and anti-inflammatory properties and to help keep triglycerides, the bad fat associated with prediabetes, under control. Moreover, the polyphenols in walnuts may also help improve cognitive skills. Since all nuts are calorie dense, try to limit your total intake to 1 ounce (about ¼ cup) per day.

MEGARECIPES
FOR HEALTHY EATING

The recipes in this section were especially created to show you how easy it is to work more nutrient-rich foods into your daily meals so that eating healthy becomes second nature. Many of them contain four or more of the healthy MegaFoods listed previously (look for the boldface type in the ingredient lists). For example, we use antioxidant-rich blueberries to make a great salsa topping for steak, and we use cauliflower florets to add antioxidants and fiber to our mac and cheese. We add beta-carotene-rich sweet potatoes to the sauce for our meatballs and carrot juice to our chili.

Keep in mind that all of the recipes fit within our general South Beach Diet guidelines for healthy eating (for those of you currently on the South Beach Diet we have indicated the appropriate phase for each recipe). Because we know that all home cooks are time challenged, we've included a number of recipes that you can make in 30 minutes or less (just look for the clock icon). And when a dish does take a little longer, we have provided tips for making it ahead to refrigerate or freeze when possible. For example, it's well worth spending an hour on a weekend to make Tuscan Kale and Mushroom Soup or Better Beef Burgundy or Black Bean Chili with Tangerine-Avocado Salsa so you can enjoy one of these satisfying and extremely healthy dishes on a busy weeknight. And you'll also find variations for transforming one dish into another with some simple ingredient substitutions.

A final note: I love delicious, nutritious food and I find it encouraging that more and more parents are taking the time to teach their children some nutrition basics. If you have a family, I urge you to get your kids involved in simple shopping and cooking tasks. Let them pick out the broccoli or the mushrooms or the kale for these recipes. Discuss how these foods are grown and even create a backyard garden if you can. Teach them about organic produce, as Maria Rodale suggests in Chapter 3. Let them run the food processor. We know that children who learn about healthy foods early in life, and who help their parents in food preparation, will be healthier eaters—and healthier individuals—down the road.

BREAKFASTS

Sweet and Savory Breakfast Burritos with Sautéed Apples 262

Chickpea and Carrot Frittata 263

Pumpkin-Cranberry Breakfast Bread 264

Blueberry Buttermilk Muffins with Almonds 266

Toasted Pecan Muesli with Dried Fruit 268

APPETIZERS, SNACKS, AND SOUPS

Lemony Tomato Hummus with Carrot Chips 269

Salmon Mousse with Vegetable Dippers 270

Super Veggie Minestrone 272

Tuscan Kale and Mushroom Soup 274

MAIN DISHES

Chicken in Mexican Mole Sauce 275

MegaMeatballs and Sauce 276

Chicken Cutlets with Apricot Sauce and Pistachios 278

Sesame Flank Steak with Fresh Blueberry Salsa 279

Better Beef Burgundy 280

Spiced Pork Skewers with Napa Salad 282

Almond-Sunflower Cod with Tomato Tartar Sauce 284

Black Bean Chili with Tangerine-Avocado Salsa 286

Grilled Salmon with Cucumbers and Ginger Dressing 288

Stir-Fried Garlic Shrimp with Bok Choy 289

Mighty Mac and "Cheese" 290

Lentil-Bulgur Salad with Summer Squash and Walnuts 292

Layered Salad with Creamy Cilantro Dressing 294

SIDE DISHES

Apple-Baked Beans with Smoked Ham 296

Green and White Florets with Toasted Pumpkin Seeds 297

Broccolette with Brown Rice and Walnuts 298

Greens Gratin with Turkey Bacon 299

Golden Barley Pilaf with Herb-Roasted Carrots 300

Chunky Guacamole Salad 301

Quinoa and Tomato Salad with Goat Cheese 302

Sweet Potato Salad with Fresh Basil 303

DESSERTS

Multigrain Blueberry Cobbler 304

Chocolate Bark with Cranberries, Almonds, and Pecans 306

PHASE 2 # Sweet and Savory Breakfast Burritos with Sautéed Apples

HANDS-ON TIME: 35 minutes   **TOTAL TIME: 35 minutes**

This is a great make-ahead breakfast. The sautéed apples and the sweet potato mixture can both be prepared ahead so you can make one burrito at a time for breakfast. Or you can fill and roll all the burritos and refrigerate or freeze (wrapped individually in plastic wrap). Reheat in the microwave. Although the number of carbs in this filling dish may seem high, they are all "good carbs" and filled with dietary fiber: A single burrito has 14 grams of fiber, which is almost 50 percent of the suggested daily intake. Avoid using McIntosh apples; they turn into applesauce.

> 1 large or 2 small **sweet potatoes** (½ pound)
>
> 6 tablespoons nonfat (0%) plain Greek **yogurt**
>
> ½ teaspoon ground cumin
>
> 1 teaspoon **extra-virgin olive oil**
>
> 2 large sweet apples (such as Fuji or Pink Lady), peeled and cut into ½-inch dice
>
> 2 pinches ground cinnamon
>
> 6 (8-inch) **multigrain** wraps
>
> 6 tablespoons creamy natural **peanut butter**
>
> ¾ cup cooked or canned (rinsed) **black beans**

Pierce the sweet potatoes in several places and microwave until tender, 3 to 5 minutes (depending on the size of the potatoes). When cool enough to handle, peel and mash with the yogurt and cumin in a small bowl.

Meanwhile, in a large nonstick skillet, heat the oil over medium-high heat. Add the apples, sprinkle with the cinnamon, and cook until the apples brown, about 5 minutes. Add ¼ cup of water and reduce the heat to medium. Cover and cook until the apples are softened but not mushy, about 2 minutes. Remove from the heat, cover, and set aside.

To assemble, spread each wrap with 1 tablespoon peanut butter, then with 3 tablespoons of the sweet potato mixture. Spoon 2 tablespoons of the beans and a scant ¼ cup of the apples horizontally across the bottom half of the wrap (leaving a ½-inch border at the sides). Fold the bottom edge of the wrap up over the filling, fold in the two sides, then roll the burrito up.

MAKES 6 BURRITOS

Per burrito: 314 calories, 12 g fat, 1.5 g saturated fat, 13 g protein, 50 g carbohydrate, 14 g fiber, 320 mg sodium

Chickpea and Carrot Frittata

PHASE 2

HANDS-ON TIME: 20 minutes   TOTAL TIME: 40 minutes

A frittata is one of those dishes that can feel as much at home on the dinner table as it does on the brunch table, and leftovers make a great take-along lunch. This frittata is made with a combination of whole eggs and egg whites to provide more protein with less fat; chickpeas add fiber (and more high-quality protein).

4 teaspoons *extra-virgin olive oil*

1 large red onion, diced (about 1½ cups)

1 large *carrot,* shredded (about 1 cup)

1 can (15.5 ounces) *chickpeas,* rinsed and drained

½ teaspoon dried oregano

¼ teaspoon salt

5 large eggs

3 large egg whites

½ cup crumbled reduced-fat *feta cheese* (2 ounces)

Heat the oven to 350°F.

In a large nonstick, ovenproof skillet, heat 2 teaspoons of the oil over medium heat. Add the onion and carrot and cook, stirring frequently, until the vegetables are tender, about 10 minutes. Add the chickpeas and sprinkle with the oregano and salt. Stir to combine.

In a large bowl, whisk together the whole eggs and egg whites. Dribble the remaining 2 teaspoons oil around the side of the skillet and pour the egg mixture over the vegetables. Scatter the feta over the top and place the frittata in the oven.

Bake for 15 to 17 minutes, until the frittata is set. Cut the frittata into 6 wedges to serve warm or at room temperature.

MAKES 6 SERVINGS

Per serving: 212 calories, 9 g fat, 2.5 g saturated fat, 13 g protein, 20 g carbohydrate, 4 g fiber, 532 mg sodium

Pumpkin-Cranberry Breakfast Bread

HANDS-ON TIME: 15 minutes   TOTAL TIME: 1 hour plus cooling time

A moist, sweetly spiced pumpkin bread studded with cranberries and pumpkin seeds is a delicious, nutrient-rich way to start your day. If you can't find almond meal, no worries: simply process whole almonds (preferably unblanched, with the skin on) in a mini food processor or coffee/spice grinder until they are finely ground—do this in short bursts or pulses so you don't turn the almonds into a paste.

　1½ cups white **whole-wheat** flour, plus extra for the pan

　½ cup **almond** meal

　¼ cup *flaxmeal*

　2 teaspoons baking powder

　1 teaspoon baking soda

　½ teaspoon ground cinnamon

　½ teaspoon salt

　1 cup canned unsweetened **pumpkin** purée

　⅓ cup Truvía

　2 tablespoons agave nectar

　1 large egg

　1 large egg white

　1 tablespoon **extra-virgin olive oil**

　2 teaspoons grated orange zest

　⅓ cup dried cranberries

　¼ cup hulled **pumpkin seeds** (pepitas)

Heat the oven to 375°F. Coat a 9 x 5-inch loaf pan with cooking spray, dust with flour, then tap out the excess.

In a large bowl, whisk together the flour, almond meal, flaxmeal, baking powder, baking soda, cinnamon, and salt.

In a separate medium bowl, whisk together the pumpkin purée, Truvía, agave nectar, whole egg, egg white, oil, and orange zest. Fold the pumpkin mixture into the flour mixture until just moistened (do not overmix). Fold in the dried cranberries and pumpkin seeds.

Spoon the mixture into the loaf pan and smooth the top. Bake for 45 minutes, or until a toothpick inserted in the center comes out with just a few moist crumbs attached. Let cool in the pan for 10 minutes, then turn the loaf out onto a rack to cool completely before cutting into sixteen ½-inch slices.

MAKES 8 (2-SLICE) SERVINGS
Per serving: 223 calories, 9.5 g fat, 1 g saturated fat, 8 g protein, 39 g carbohydrate, 7 g fiber, 475 mg sodium

> TIP: The bread can be made a day ahead or be double-wrapped (in foil and then a resealable plastic bag) and frozen for up to 3 months.

PHASE 2 # Blueberry Buttermilk Muffins with Almonds

HANDS-ON TIME: 15 minutes   TOTAL TIME: 45 minutes plus cooling time

Buttermilk contributes tenderness to these muffins and canola oil adds richness (as well as good-for-you monounsaturated fats). And the combination of oats, whole-wheat flour, and wheat bran provides a good helping of whole grains; a small amount of all-purpose flour was added to lighten the texture, but you can make it with all whole-wheat if you prefer.

¾ cup quick-cooking **oats**

1 cup white **whole-wheat** flour

½ cup all-purpose flour

¼ cup **wheat bran**

2 tablespoons Truvía

1½ teaspoons ground cinnamon

1¼ teaspoons baking soda

¼ teaspoon grated nutmeg

¼ teaspoon salt

1¼ cups light (1.5%) **buttermilk**

2 large eggs, lightly beaten

¼ cup **canola oil**

1½ teaspoons pure vanilla extract

1¼ cups fresh or frozen (unthawed) **blueberries**

⅓ cup sliced **almonds**

Heat the oven to 375°F. Spread the oats in a baking pan and bake for 5 to 7 minutes, until lightly toasted. Leave the oven on but reduce the temperature to 350°F. Lightly coat a 12-cup muffin tin with cooking spray or line with paper liners.

In a large bowl, combine the toasted oats, whole-wheat flour, all-purpose flour, wheat bran, Truvía, cinnamon, baking soda, nutmeg, and salt.

In a medium bowl, whisk together the buttermilk, eggs, oil, and vanilla.

Make a well in the flour mixture. Add the buttermilk mixture and mix just to combine; do not overmix.

Gently fold the blueberries into the batter. Divide the batter evenly among the muffin cups. Top with almonds and gently press them into the batter. Bake for 25 minutes, or until a toothpick inserted in the centers comes out clean. Cool in the pan for 5 minutes and then transfer to a rack to cool completely.

MAKES 12 MUFFINS

Per muffin: 172 calories, 8 g fat, 1 g saturated fat, 5 g protein, 23 g carbohydrate, 3.5 g fiber, 190 mg sodium

Variation: Try these muffins with 1¼ cups fresh raspberries instead—they have some of the same healthful compounds as blueberries. If you do so, reduce the vanilla extract to 1 teaspoon and add ¼ teaspoon almond extract to the batter.

> **TIP:** Bake several batches of muffins and freeze them for easy grab-and-go breakfasts. For the best results, measure the ingredients and mix the batter for each batch separately. To freeze the muffins, arrange them on a baking sheet and pop in the freezer until frozen. Then transfer them to airtight freezer storage containers or bags

PHASE 2 — Toasted Pecan Muesli with Dried Fruit

HANDS-ON TIME: 10 minutes   TOTAL TIME: 25 minutes

Orange fruits—like mangoes, peaches, nectarines, and apricots—contain the antioxidant beta-carotene. They're a great addition to a simple, unsweetened breakfast cereal filled with fiber, minerals, and good fats. Muesli makes a great make-ahead snack since it stores well in a covered container in the refrigerator for up to 2 weeks.

1½ cups old-fashioned rolled *oats*

1 cup chopped *pecans*

½ cup *wheat germ*

¼ cup hulled unsalted *sunflower seeds*

½ cup finely chopped dried *mango,* dried *peaches,* or dried *apricots* (or a combination)

Fat-free *milk*

Heat the oven to 350°F. Spread the oats and pecans on a rimmed baking sheet and bake for 12 to 15 minutes, shaking the baking sheet occasionally, until the oats are lightly browned and the pecans are toasted and fragrant. Set aside to cool.

In a large bowl, stir together the toasted oats and pecans, wheat germ, sunflower seeds, and chopped fruit. Transfer the mixture to an airtight container and store in the refrigerator.

To serve: Scoop ½ cup of muesli into a cereal bowl and serve with ¼ cup milk.

MAKES 8 (½-CUP) SERVINGS

Per serving (with ¼ cup milk): 251 calories, 15 g fat, 1.5 g saturated fat, 8 g protein, 25 g carbohydrate, 5.5 g fiber, 34 mg sodium

Variation: Substitute cashews for the pecans and chopped hulled pumpkin seeds for the sunflower seeds.

Lemony Tomato Hummus with Carrot Chips

PHASE 2
PHASE 1
(see variation)

HANDS-ON TIME: 10 minutes   **TOTAL TIME:** 10 minutes

The trick to making nice chip-shaped scoopers for this smooth, rich-tasting hummus is to use extra-large carrots (usually sold loose, and without tops). Surprisingly, these so-called jumbo carrots can be sweeter and more flavorful than smaller, tops-on carrots.

2¼ cups canned **chickpeas,** rinsed and drained

4 oil-packed sun-dried **tomatoes,** plus 1 tablespoon of the oil

1 small garlic clove, peeled

¼ cup nonfat (0%) plain Greek **yogurt**

2 teaspoons grated lemon zest

2 tablespoons fresh lemon juice

½ teaspoon dark **sesame oil**

¼ teaspoon ground cumin

¼ teaspoon salt

2 jumbo **carrots** (about 6 ounces each)

In a food processor, combine the chickpeas, sun-dried tomatoes, tomato oil, and garlic and pulse to chop coarsely. Add the yogurt, lemon zest, lemon juice, sesame oil, cumin, and salt and process until smooth. If the mixture is too thick, add a couple of teaspoons of water to achieve a dipping consistency.

Shortly before serving, peel the carrots and cut them crosswise, at an extreme angle, into long oval "chips" ⅛ inch thick.

MAKES 2 CUPS

Per tablespoon (on 1 carrot chip): 29 calories, 1 g fat, 0.1 g saturated fat, 1 g protein, 5 g carbohydrate, 1 g fiber, 32 mg sodium

Variation: For Phase 1 of the South Beach Diet, serve the hummus with fennel and celery sticks instead of carrots.

PHASE I # Salmon Mousse with Vegetable Dippers

HANDS-ON TIME: 25 minutes   TOTAL TIME: 30 minutes plus chilling time

Creamy and delicious—and brimming with omega-3s and vitamin D—this salmon mousse gets a health and flavor kick from horseradish, which has the same nutritious compounds as other members of the cruciferous vegetable family.

1 cup nonfat or low-fat plain *yogurt*

1 envelope unflavored gelatin

1 can (16 ounces) pink *salmon,* drained

⅔ cup reduced-fat *sour cream*

1 jar (6 ounces) prepared *horseradish,* drained and squeezed dry (about ¼ cup)

3 tablespoons finely chopped red onion

1 tablespoon chopped fresh dill, or ½ teaspoon dried dill, crumbled

1 tablespoon Worcestershire sauce

½ teaspoon paprika

2 thick *broccoli* stalks (see Tips)

1 large red bell pepper, cut into ½-inch-wide strips

1 unpeeled cucumber, cut crosswise into slices

Line a strainer with cheesecloth or paper towels and set over a bowl. Spoon the yogurt into the strainer and drain for 10 minutes.

Meanwhile, place ½ cup cold water in a small saucepan, sprinkle the gelatin over it, and let soften for 1 minute. Heat the mixture over low heat, stirring, until the gelatin dissolves, about 3 minutes. Do not let it boil.

In a food processor, combine the drained yogurt, gelatin mixture, salmon, sour cream, horseradish, onion, dill, Worcestershire sauce, and paprika. Purée until smooth.

Lightly coat a 1-quart decorative mold, bowl, or loaf pan with cooking spray. Pour the mousse mixture evenly into the mold. Cover and refrigerate until set, at least 12 hours.

Just before serving, run a thin knife around the edges of the mold or bowl and invert the mousse onto a platter.

Peel the broccoli stalks and cut them crosswise, at an extreme angle, into long oval "chips" ⅛ inch thick. Arrange the broccoli chips, bell pepper strips, and cucumber slices around the mousse.

MAKES 15 (¼-CUP) SERVINGS

Per serving with vegetable dippers: 85 calories, 3 g fat, 1 g saturated fat, 9 g protein, 6 g carbohydrate, 1.5 g fiber, 196 mg sodium

> TIPS:
>
> • Save the florets from the heads of broccoli for the kids, since most prefer them to the stalks anyway. Or use them in our Super Veggie Minestrone (page 272).
>
> • You can serve the broccoli chips raw or boil them for about 45 seconds to soften them slightly. Take care not to cook them too long, because you still want a relatively crisp dipper.

Super Veggie Minestrone

HANDS-ON TIME: 40 minutes   TOTAL TIME: 50 minutes

In addition to all of the phytonutrients, vitamins, and minerals in this Italian-style vegetable and pasta soup, one serving supplies almost half of your recommended daily intake of fiber. Whole-wheat couscous replaces the traditional addition of white pasta. Make the soup on a weekend and freeze for weekday meals.

1 tablespoon ***extra-virgin olive oil***

1 small onion, finely chopped

2 ***carrots,*** halved lengthwise and thinly sliced crosswise

2 garlic cloves, thinly sliced

4 cups diced (1-inch) red ***cabbage*** (about ½ pound)

1 teaspoon ancho chile powder

½ teaspoon dried rosemary, crumbled

2 cups lower-sodium chicken broth

1 can (14.5 ounces) no-salt-added diced ***tomatoes***

1 can (15 ounces) no-salt-added ***red kidney beans,*** rinsed and drained

¼ teaspoon salt

3 cups small ***broccoli*** florets

½ cup thinly sliced, peeled ***broccoli*** stalks

½ cup whole-wheat couscous

2 tablespoons red wine vinegar

¼ cup grated Parmesan cheese

In a large saucepan or 5-quart Dutch oven, heat the oil over medium heat. Add the onion, carrots, and garlic and cook, stirring frequently, until the onion is tender, about 10 minutes. Add the cabbage, cover the pan, and cook until the cabbage has wilted, about 5 minutes.

Add the chile powder and rosemary and stir to coat. Add the chicken broth, tomatoes, beans, salt, and 2½ cups water and bring to a boil. Cook for 5 minutes.

Add the broccoli florets and stalks and cook until the broccoli is tender, 3 to 5 minutes. Stir in the couscous, cover, and remove from the heat. Let stand for 5 minutes for the couscous to soften. Uncover and stir in the vinegar. Serve with Parmesan.

MAKES 4 (2½-CUP) SERVINGS

Per serving: 276 calories, 5.5 g fat, 1.5 g saturated fat, 16 g protein, 45 g carbohydrate, 17 g fiber, 501 mg sodium

Variation: Make this with 3½ cups cut-up broccoli rabe instead of regular broccoli, and chickpeas instead of kidney beans. Swap in whole-wheat orzo for the couscous (but precook it in boiling water first).

Tuscan Kale and Mushroom Soup

HANDS-ON TIME: 15 minutes   TOTAL TIME: 50 minutes

Tuscan kale—also called Lacinato kale, dinosaur kale, and cavolo nero (black cabbage)—has dark-green, crinkly leaves that look like extra-long spinach leaves. Like other dark-green vegetables, kale has quite a lot of beta-carotene (hidden underneath the leaves' green pigments): Just one serving of this hearty, meaty-tasting soup provides over 700 percent of your daily requirement. And as a bonus, the dried shiitakes are contributing an impressive 59 percent of your daily need for vitamin D.

   2 ounces dried **shiitake mushrooms,** rinsed

   2 teaspoons **extra-virgin olive oil**

   3 garlic cloves, minced

   4 cups lower-sodium chicken or vegetable broth

   Pinch red pepper flakes

   1 bunch (¾ pound) Tuscan or regular **kale,** cut crosswise into ¼-inch-wide shreds

   ⅛ teaspoon salt

   1 can (15 ounces) no-salt-added **cannellini beans,** rinsed and drained

   8 teaspoons shredded reduced-fat sharp **Cheddar cheese**

In a small saucepan, combine the mushrooms and 2 cups water. Bring to a boil, cover, and remove from the heat. Let stand until the mushrooms are softened, about 15 minutes.

Meanwhile, in a large saucepan, heat the oil over medium-high heat. Add the garlic and cook until fragrant, about 45 seconds. Add 1 cup of the broth, the red pepper flakes, and kale. Sprinkle the kale with the salt, stir, cover, and let steam over medium-high heat for 5 minutes.

Stir in the beans and remaining 3 cups broth. Cover and simmer until the kale is tender, about 25 minutes.

Meanwhile, as soon as the mushrooms have softened, drain them and add the soaking liquid to the simmering soup.

Cut off and discard the mushroom stems and cut the caps crosswise into thin slice. Add them to the soup and let simmer until tender, about 5 minutes.

Top each serving with 2 teaspoons Cheddar.

MAKES 4 (2-CUP) SERVINGS

Per serving: 222 calories, 5 g fat, 1 g saturated fat, 13 g protein, 35 g carbohydrate, 8.5 g fiber, 572 mg sodium

Chicken in Mexican Mole Sauce

PHASE I

HANDS-ON TIME: 35 minutes   TOTAL TIME: 45 minutes

The delicious sauce for this chicken stew is chock-full of antioxidant nutrients, including flavonoids in the cocoa. You can double the recipe and freeze the extra.

2 teaspoons *extra-virgin olive oil*

1½ pounds boneless, skinless chicken breasts, cut into cubes

    Salt

1 medium red onion, chopped

2 green bell peppers, chopped

2 garlic cloves, minced

1 tablespoon mild chili powder

½ teaspoon ground cinnamon

1 can (14.5 ounces) diced *tomatoes* with green chiles

2 tablespoons creamy natural *peanut butter*

2 tablespoons unsweetened *cocoa powder*

2 scallions, chopped

In a Dutch oven, heat the oil and 2 tablespoons water. Add the chicken, season lightly with salt, and cook until opaque on the outside (but still pink on the inside), about 3 minutes. With a slotted spoon, transfer the chicken to a plate.

Add the onion, bell peppers, and garlic to the pan. Sprinkle with the chili powder and cinnamon, stir well, and cook for 1 minute. Add ¼ cup water, cover, and cook, stirring once or twice, until the onion softens, about 7 minutes.

Add the tomatoes, peanut butter, and cocoa powder and stir until the peanut butter is incorporated. With an immersion blender, pulse on and off a couple of times to thicken the sauce slightly, but leave it with some texture (or pulse about half the ingredients in a mini food processor or blender then return to the pan). Bring the sauce to a brisk simmer and return the chicken (and any juices on the plate) to the pan. Reduce to a low simmer, partially cover, and cook for 15 minutes, stirring often, to blend the flavors and cook the chicken through.

Serve sprinkled with the chopped scallions.

MAKES 4 (1½-CUP) SERVINGS

Per serving: 323 calories, 9.5 g fat, 1.5 g saturated fat, 44 g protein, 16 g carbohydrate, 4.5 g fiber, 364 mg sodium

PHASE 2 # MegaMeatballs and Sauce

HANDS-ON TIME: 30 minutes   TOTAL TIME: 1 hour

What's the surprise mega ingredient in the tomato sauce? A sweet potato. It adds thickness, natural sweetness, and an amazing amount of the antioxidant beta-carotene to a sauce that is already brimming with lycopene (another carotenoid phytonutrient) from the tomatoes. The meatballs gain their mega status with the addition of flaxmeal (high in healthful essential fatty acids) and meaty-tasting cremini mushrooms. Serve the meatballs and sauce over ½ cup whole-wheat couscous, whole-wheat pasta, or barley, if desired.

Sauce

1 small **sweet potato** (6 ounces)

2 teaspoons **extra-virgin olive oil**

1 small red onion, chopped

4 garlic cloves, chopped

1 can (28 ounces) no-salt-added diced or crushed **tomatoes**

1½ teaspoons dried basil

1½ teaspoons dried oregano

Meatballs

¼ cup **flaxmeal**

6 tablespoons shredded Parmesan cheese

1 teaspoon ground fennel seed

½ teaspoon salt

¼ teaspoon freshly ground black pepper

10 ounces **cremini mushrooms,** finely minced

3 scallions, minced

1 large garlic clove, grated or very finely minced

1¼ pounds extra-lean ground turkey breast

1 large egg

To make the sauce: Pierce the sweet potato in several places with a knife. Microwave on high power for 4 to 5 minutes, until tender. When cool enough to handle, peel and cut into chunks.

Meanwhile, in a large (at least 12-inch) nonstick skillet, heat the oil over medium-high heat. Add the onion and garlic and cook until the onion is softened and beginning to brown, 5 to 7 minutes. Stir in the tomatoes, basil, and oregano. Reduce the heat to low, cover, and simmer, stirring once or twice, while you make the meatballs.

To make the meatballs: In a large bowl, combine the flaxmeal, Parmesan, fennel seed, salt, and pepper. Stir in the mushrooms, scallions, and garlic. Add the turkey and egg and use your hands to mix well. With wet hands (the mixture will be very loose and sticky), form 24 meatballs, each about the size of a large golf ball.

In a mini food processor or a medium bowl, combine the sweet potato chunks, ½ cup water, and about 1 cup of the tomato sauce from the skillet. Process or mash to a smooth purée, then stir back into the skillet. Season with salt and pepper to taste.

Gently add the meatballs to the sauce, cover, and simmer for 10 minutes. Turn the meatballs over, cover, and simmer until cooked through, 10 to 15 minutes longer. Serve 4 meatballs per person with sauce spooned on top.

MAKES 6 SERVINGS

Per serving: 236 calories, 6.5 g fat, 1.5 g saturated fat, 31 g protein, 14 g carbohydrate, 4 g fiber, 389 mg sodium

TIPS:
- You can cook the dish ahead of time and store the meatballs in the sauce, refrigerated or frozen. Gently reheat in the microwave, on the stovetop, or in a covered casserole in the oven.

- Make a double batch of the sauce (in a large Dutch oven). Freeze half of it for use later.

PHASE 2

Chicken Cutlets with Apricot Sauce and Pistachios

HANDS-ON TIME: 30 minutes   TOTAL TIME: 30 minutes

The red wine–fruit sauce is rich with antioxidants, including resveratrol and flavonoids from the red wine. Even the small pinches of spices—known to be high in antioxidant activity—are making a contribution here. Since raisins are a high-sugar fruit that we recommend eating only occasionally, you can include them or not if you're on Phase 2 of the South Beach Diet.

4 chicken cutlets (about 5 ounces each)

Salt and freshly ground black pepper

3 teaspoons **extra-virgin olive oil**

1 garlic clove, minced

Pinch ground allspice

Pinch cayenne pepper

Pinch ground cinnamon

½ cup lower-sodium chicken broth

½ cup dry **red wine**

¼ cup sliced dried **apricots**

¼ cup chopped golden raisins (optional)

2 scallions, white and light green parts only, sliced

¼ cup chopped **pistachios**

Season the chicken lightly with salt and pepper. In a large nonstick skillet, heat 2 teaspoons of the oil over medium-high heat. Add the cutlets and cook until browned on one side, 2 minutes. Flip and cook for 1 to 2 minutes on the second side, until just cooked through but still juicy. Transfer to a plate and cover to keep warm.

Add the remaining 1 teaspoon oil to the pan. Add the garlic, sprinkle with the allspice, cayenne, and cinnamon and cook, stirring, for 30 seconds. Add the broth, wine, apricots, and raisins. Bring to a simmer, scraping the bottom of the pan to loosen any bits of chicken. Simmer, stirring occasionally, for 7 minutes to soften the fruit, cook off the alcohol, and concentrate the flavors. In the last minute of cooking, stir in the scallions and any juices from the chicken plate.

Serve each cutlet topped with 2 tablespoons of the sauce and 1 tablespoon of the pistachios.

MAKES 4 SERVINGS

Per serving: 311 calories, 9 g fat, 1.5 g saturated fat, 36 g protein, 17 g carbohydrate, 2 g fiber, 144 mg sodium

Sesame Flank Steak with Fresh Blueberry Salsa

HANDS-ON TIME: 25 minutes   TOTAL TIME: 30 minutes

The natural sweet-tart flavor of fresh blueberries goes perfectly with a simple roasted flank steak. The blueberries are matched with sweet red bell pepper, limes, and apricots, and mashing a few of the berries makes the salsa juicier. Be sure to roast, not broil, the steak.

2 tablespoons **sesame seeds**

1 teaspoon ground coriander

1 teaspoon ground cumin

½ teaspoon salt

1¼ pounds flank steak

4 teaspoons **extra-virgin olive oil**

3 tablespoons fresh lime juice

2 tablespoons apricot all-fruit spread

1 tablespoon Dijon mustard

2 cups fresh **blueberries**

½ cup finely diced red bell pepper

2 scallions, thinly sliced

Heat the oven to 450°F.

Place the sesame seeds in a spice grinder and pulse until finely ground (or grind with a mortar and pestle).

In a small bowl, combine the ground sesame seeds, coriander, cumin, and salt. Rub the mixture into one side of the flank steak and then rub 2 teaspoons of the oil over the spice mixture.

Place the meat on a rimmed baking sheet and roast for about 15 minutes for medium-rare, until the steak registers 135°F on an instant-read thermometer.

Meanwhile, in a large bowl, whisk together the lime juice, fruit spread, mustard, and remaining 2 teaspoons oil. Add 1 cup of the blueberries, the bell pepper, and scallions. Toss to combine. With a fork, coarsely mash the remaining 1 cup blueberries and stir into the bowl.

To serve, thinly slice the meat across the grain and on the diagonal. Serve topped with the blueberry salsa.

MAKES 4 SERVINGS

Per serving: 330 calories, 16 g fat, 4.5 g saturated fat, 32 g protein, 17 g carbohydrate, 2.5 g fiber, 446 mg sodium

PHASE 2   # Better Beef Burgundy

HANDS-ON TIME: 40 minutes   TOTAL TIME: 2 hours 10 minutes

This hearty beef, mushroom, and sweet potato stew is an absolute powerhouse of antioxidants. The beta-carotene levels alone are through the roof (over 1,000 percent of your daily needs!); and the wine, cocoa, and tomato paste contribute a megadose of lycopene and flavonoids. B vitamins (especially B$_{12}$ and niacin) are also in good supply.

- 1¾ cups **carrot** juice
- ¼ cup **tomato** paste
- ¼ cup white **whole-wheat** flour
- ½ teaspoon salt
- ¼ teaspoon freshly ground black pepper
- 1½ pounds top round steak, cubed
- 2 teaspoons unsweetened **cocoa powder**
- 7 teaspoons **extra-virgin olive oil**
- 1 large red onion, cut into ½-inch chunks
- 5 garlic cloves, minced
- 1¾ cups dry **red wine**
- 1 pound **cremini mushrooms,** trimmed and quartered
- 2 cups lower-sodium beef or chicken broth
- 2 bay leaves
- 1½ pounds **sweet potatoes,** peeled and cut into 1-inch cubes

In a measuring cup or small bowl, whisk together the carrot juice and tomato paste.

Combine the flour, salt, and pepper in a large resealable plastic bag. Add the cubes of beef, seal, and toss to coat well. Transfer the beef to a plate. Pour the excess flour mixture into a small bowl and stir in the cocoa.

In a Dutch oven or large saucepan, heat 3 teaspoons of the oil over medium-high heat. Add half the beef and cook, stirring, until browned all over but still pink inside, about 2 minutes. Transfer to a plate. Repeat with the remaining beef, using 2 more teaspoons of oil.

Add the remaining 2 teaspoons oil to the pan. Add the onion and garlic and cook, stirring, for 30 seconds. Add ½ cup of the wine and stir to loosen any browned bits from the bottom of the pan. Add the mushrooms, stir, and cook until the wine has mostly evaporated, about 2 minutes.

Sprinkle the reserved flour-cocoa mixture over the vegetables and stir to coat. Stir in the carrot juice mixture, remaining 1¼ cups wine, the broth, and bay leaves. Return the beef to the pan and bring to a boil. Reduce the heat to low, cover, and simmer for 1 hour 30 minutes. Add the sweet potatoes and return the stew to a simmer. Cover and cook until the sweet potatoes are tender, about 10 minutes. Discard the bay leaves before serving.

MAKES 8 (1½-CUP) SERVINGS

Per serving: 281 calories, 7 g fat, 1.5 g saturated fat, 23 g protein, 27 g carbohydrate, 3.5 g fiber, 344 mg sodium

> TIP: This is a great dish to make on a rainy Sunday afternoon. Freeze half of the stew and serve the other half for Sunday dinner or refrigerate and gently reheat the next day. If the entire stew is being made ahead, undercook the sweet potatoes by about 5 minutes so they won't overcook when you reheat.

Spiced Pork Skewers with Napa Salad

HANDS-ON TIME: 30 minutes   TOTAL TIME: 1 hour including standing time

This simple grilled pork dish is rich in B vitamins (most notably thiamin) and the mineral selenium, an antioxidant. A fresh salad of avocado, orange, and napa cabbage (the mildest of the cabbages) adds additional important health-promoting compounds such as beta-carotene, monounsaturated fats, and sulforaphane—a substance found in cruciferous vegetables that may have anticancer properties.

Pork

2 teaspoons paprika

1 teaspoon ground cumin

½ teaspoon garlic powder

¼ teaspoon cayenne pepper

1½ pounds center-cut pork loin, cut into 1-inch cubes

Salad

1 navel *orange*

1 head (1 pound) *napa cabbage,* thinly sliced

1 Hass *avocado,* finely diced

2 scallions, thinly sliced

1 tablespoon *extra-virgin olive oil*

¼ teaspoon salt

¼ teaspoon freshly ground black pepper

Pinch cayenne pepper

To make the pork: In a large bowl, combine the paprika, cumin, garlic powder, and cayenne. Add the pork and toss to coat. Cover the bowl and let sit at room temperature for 30 minutes. Thread the pork evenly onto four 12-inch skewers.

To make the salad: Grate the zest of the orange to get 2 teaspoons. Peel the orange, coarsely chop, and add to a large bowl along with any juice. Add the zest, cabbage, avocado, scallions, oil, salt, pepper, and cayenne. Toss well.

Lightly coat a grill rack or grill pan with cooking spray and heat to medium-high. Grill the pork skewers, turning frequently, until the pork is cooked through, 10 to 12 minutes.

Serve a pork skewer on top of or alongside the salad.

MAKES 4 SERVINGS

Per serving: 373 calories, 19 g fat, 5 g saturated fat, 38 g protein, 12 g carbohydrate, 5.5 g fiber, 239 mg sodium

Variation: For Phase 1 of the South Beach Diet, omit the orange from the salad.

> TIP: If you buy your meat from a butcher, be sure to get pork loin cut from the center, not from the shoulder end, which is higher in fat. The leaner meat will also be lighter in color; the fattier shoulder portion will be a darker red.

PHASE I Almond-Sunflower Cod
with Tomato Tartar Sauce

HANDS-ON TIME: 20   TOTAL TIME: 25 minutes

The cool, creamy texture of a fresh lemony tartar sauce made with Greek yogurt is the perfect counterpoint to crumb-coated baked fish. Using finely ground almonds instead of flour or bread crumbs is a good way to give fish a crispy coating that is also high in important nutrients. The almond–sunflower seed mixture provides one-third of your daily requirement for vitamin E, and the cod itself gives you nearly 100 percent of your daily need for selenium, an important antioxidant mineral.

Fish

3 ounces unblanched ***almonds,*** ground to a fine meal

2 tablespoons very finely minced ***sunflower seeds***

2 teaspoons grated lemon zest

1 large egg

2 large egg whites

4 skinless cod fillets (6 ounces each)

Salt and freshly ground black pepper

Tartar Sauce

½ cup nonfat (0%) plain Greek ***yogurt***

1 tablespoon mayonnaise

1 teaspoon grated lemon zest

1 teaspoon fresh lemon juice

⅛ teaspoon salt

A few grinds of black pepper

½ cup finely diced grape ***tomatoes***

Lemon wedges, for serving (optional)

To make the fish: Heat the oven to 350°F. Lightly coat a nonstick baking sheet with olive oil cooking spray.

In a shallow bowl, combine the almonds, sunflower seeds, and lemon zest. In another shallow bowl, lightly beat the whole egg and egg whites. Sprinkle the fish on both sides with salt and pepper. Dip the fish in the eggs, letting the excess drip off. Then dip the fish in the almond-sunflower mixture to lightly coat both sides and place skinned-side down on the baking sheet.

Bake the fillets for 13 to 15 minutes, until the topping is lightly browned and the fish just flakes when tested with a fork.

Meanwhile, make the tartar sauce: In a small serving bowl, combine the yogurt, mayonnaise, lemon zest, lemon juice, salt, and pepper. Stir in the tomatoes.

Dollop each serving of fish with 2 generous tablespoons of the tartar sauce and serve with lemon wedges, if desired.

MAKES 4 SERVINGS

Per serving: 291 calories, 14 g fat, 1.5 g saturated fat, 37 g protein, 6 g carbohydrate, 2.5 g fiber, 170 mg sodium

Black Bean Chili
with Tangerine-Avocado Salsa

HANDS-ON TIME: 35 minutes   TOTAL TIME: 1 hour 15 minutes

Creamy avocado and citrus-y tangerine tossed with scallions and cilantro make a great fresh topping for a bowl of black bean chili. Vegetables and fruits with the deepest colors have the most antioxidant activity, so it should be no surprise that black beans top the antioxidant charts for beans. This vegetarian chili is on the mild side, so if you are a fan of spicy food, add some chopped pickled jalapeños to the salsa.

Salsa

  1 *tangerine* or small *orange,* peeled, chopped, and seeded

  3 scallions, minced

  3 tablespoons chopped cilantro

  ¼ teaspoon ground cumin

  ¼ teaspoon freshly ground black pepper

  1 Hass *avocado,* diced

Chili

  2 teaspoons *extra-virgin olive oil*

  1¼ cups *carrot* juice

  1 large red onion, finely chopped

  2 large garlic cloves, minced

  2 green bell peppers, diced

  1 tablespoon mild chili powder

  2 cans (15.5 ounces each) no-salt-added *black beans,* rinsed and
    drained

  1 can (14.5 ounces) fire-roasted diced *tomatoes*

  1½ teaspoons dried oregano

  ¼ teaspoon salt

  6 tablespoons nonfat (0%) plain Greek *yogurt*

To make the salsa: In a large bowl, combine the tangerine or orange, scallions, cilantro, cumin, and black pepper and toss well. Add the avocado and gently toss. Cover and refrigerate while you make the chili.

To make the chili: In a large Dutch oven, heat the oil and ¼ cup of the carrot juice over medium-high heat. When the carrot juice starts to simmer, add the onion and garlic and stir to coat. Cook, stirring frequently, until the carrot juice has evaporated and the onion starts to sizzle, about 5 minutes.

Add the bell peppers and cook until slightly softened, about 2 minutes. Sprinkle with the chili powder and cook until fragrant, about 1 minute. Add the beans, tomatoes and their juices, oregano, salt, remaining 1 cup carrot juice, and 1 cup water. Bring to a boil, reduce to a simmer, and cook, partially covered, for 30 minutes to blend the flavors.

Serve the chili with 2 heaping tablespoons of salsa and a generous tablespoon of Greek yogurt.

MAKES 4 (2-CUP) SERVINGS

Per serving: 367 calories, 8 g fat, 1 g saturated fat, 18 g protein, 58 g carbohydrate, 17 g fiber, 451 mg sodium

> TIP: The chili can be made ahead and frozen, but the salsa should be made no more than 1 or 2 hours before serving.

Grilled Salmon
with Cucumbers and Ginger Dressing

HANDS-ON TIME: 20 minutes   TOTAL TIME: 1 hour 15 minutes including draining time

Grilled salmon, pungent arugula, and a crispy cucumber-onion salad are served with a Thai-style fresh ginger and tahini dressing—an incredibly tasty way to get your omega-3 fatty acids and vitamin D. This dish delivers almost 200 percent of your daily need for omega-3s, nearly 90 percent of vitamin D, and it also has impressive amounts of vitamin B_{12}, selenium, and niacin.

2 cucumbers, peeled, halved lengthwise, seeded, and thinly sliced crosswise

½ teaspoon salt

4 tablespoons rice vinegar

2 tablespoons fresh lime juice

2 tablespoons reduced-sodium soy sauce

2 tablespoons **tahini** or creamy natural **peanut butter**

1 teaspoon plus 1 tablespoon dark **sesame oil**

1 garlic clove, chopped

1 teaspoon minced fresh ginger

½ small red onion, very thinly sliced

4 **salmon** fillets, skin on (5 ounces each)

6 cups baby **arugula**

Place the cucumbers in a strainer set over a bowl; toss with the salt. Drain for at least 1 hour or up to 3 hours if you want to.

Meanwhile, in a blender, combine 2 tablespoons of the vinegar, 1 tablespoon of the lime juice, 1 tablespoon water, the soy sauce, tahini, 1 teaspoon of the sesame oil, the garlic, and ginger. Purée the dressing until well blended.

Toss the cucumbers with the onion and the remaining 2 tablespoons vinegar, 1 tablespoon lime juice, and 1 tablespoon sesame oil. Refrigerate until serving time.

Heat the grill to medium-high. Place the salmon skin-side down on the grill. Cook for 3 minutes, or until the skin shrinks and separates from the flesh. Flip and cook until the salmon is opaque throughout but still moist, about 4 minutes.

Divide the arugula among 4 plates. Top with the salmon. Drizzle the sesame-ginger dressing over the salmon and arugula, then top the salmon with the cucumber mixture.

MAKES 4 SERVINGS

Per serving: 356 calories, 19 g fat, 3 g saturated fat, 36 g protein, 11 g carbohydrate, 2 g fiber, 563 mg sodium

Stir-Fried Garlic Shrimp with Bok Choy   PHASE I

HANDS-ON TIME: 35 minutes   TOTAL TIME: 35 minutes

Spicy chili sauce gives a nice pungent boost to the sauce for this shrimp and bok choy stir-fry. Though the dish is simple, the nutrients are complex. A single serving is very high in beta-carotene, cancer-fighting phytonutrients, and antioxidants (such as the selenium from the shrimp)—not to mention providing more than 80 percent of your daily supply of vitamin B_{12}.

1¼ pounds large shrimp, peeled and deveined

4 scallions, thinly sliced, white and green parts kept separate

2 garlic cloves, minced

2 teaspoons *extra-virgin olive oil*

1½ pounds **bok choy,** sliced crosswise

4 teaspoons reduced-sodium soy sauce

2 teaspoons chili-garlic sauce such as sriracha

In a large bowl, combine the shrimp, scallion whites, and garlic.

In a wok or large nonstick skillet, heat the oil over medium-high heat. Add the shrimp mixture and cook, stirring occasionally, until the shrimp turn pink and are opaque throughout, 3 to 4 minutes. Transfer to a large clean bowl.

Return the pan to medium-high heat. Add the bok choy, cover, and cook, stirring occasionally, until crisp-tender, 3 to 4 minutes. Push the bok choy to one side of the pan and stir the soy sauce and chili-garlic sauce into the sauce in the bottom of the pan. Toss to coat the bok choy with the sauce.

Return the shrimp to the pan, toss to coat, and cook briefly to reheat. Stir in the scallion greens and serve hot.

MAKES 4 SERVINGS

Per serving: 183 calories, 5 g fat, 1 g saturated fat, 28 g protein, 6 g carbohydrate, 2 g fiber, 487 mg sodium

PHASE 2 # Mighty Mac and "Cheese"

HANDS-ON TIME: 15 minutes   TOTAL TIME: 40 minutes

*How do you make a mac and cheese that's not just better for you, but actually **good** for you? Well, first you use cauliflower to stand in for half the macaroni. Then you make a creamy orange sauce that just looks like it's all cheese but is actually mostly winter squash purée. Since we all eat with our eyes, the color of the sauce here goes a long way toward making you feel like you're eating something decadent. But don't worry, your taste buds will be happy, too. (And as a bonus, the kids will be getting more vegetables!)*

1 slice **100% whole-grain** bread, torn into pieces

2 tablespoons plus ¼ cup grated Parmesan cheese

1 ounce **pecans** (14 halves)

1½ cups **whole-wheat** elbow macaroni (half a 12-ounce box)

3 cups very small **cauliflower** florets (half a small head)

1 package (12 ounces) frozen **winter squash** purée, thawed

3 wedges (¾ ounce each) **light spreadable cheese**

1 teaspoon Dijon mustard

¼ teaspoon salt

Freshly ground black pepper

Heat the oven to 375°F. Coat a 9 x 9-inch baking dish with olive oil cooking spray.

In a mini food processor or blender, process the bread to make fine crumbs (or finely mince the bread with a knife). Transfer the crumbs to a bowl and stir in 2 tablespoons of the Parmesan. Add the pecans to the processor and finely grind (or finely mince with a knife). Stir into the crumb mixture.

Bring a large pot of salted water to a boil. Add the macaroni and cook for 4 minutes. Add the cauliflower and cook for 3 minutes. Reserving 2 tablespoons of the cooking water, drain the pasta and cauliflower and return to the pot.

Meanwhile, in a small saucepan, bring the squash purée to a simmer. Drop in the cheese wedges and stir until melted (don't worry if there are small lumps). Stir in the mustard, salt, and a couple of grinds of pepper.

Add the squash sauce and reserved cooking water to the drained pasta and cauliflower and toss well. Scrape the mixture into the baking dish. Top evenly with the crumb mixture.

Bake for 15 minutes, or until the topping is nicely browned. Let rest for 10 minutes before serving.

MAKES 4 SERVINGS

Per serving: 326 calories, 9.5 g fat, 2.5 g saturated fat, 15 g protein, 49 g carbohydrate, 7 g fiber, 486 mg sodium

Variation: Make this with 1½ cups unsweetened canned pumpkin purée instead of squash. Add ⅛ teaspoon grated nutmeg to the crumb topping.

PHASE 2
Lentil-Bulgur Salad
with Summer Squash and Walnuts

HANDS-ON TIME: 25 minutes   TOTAL TIME: 50 minutes

Meaty lentils, chewy bulgur, and fresh yellow summer squash are tossed in a light lemon-tarragon vinaigrette for a main-course salad. Though there's not a scrap of meat in the salad, the lentils, bulgur, and walnuts combine to deliver a good amount of protein. (And the walnuts are also contributing omega-3 fatty acids.)

¾ cup **lentils**

½ cup **bulgur**

A pinch plus ½ teaspoon salt

3 teaspoons **extra-virgin olive oil**

1 medium shallot, minced

2 small yellow squash, halved lengthwise and cut crosswise into ⅓-inch-thick half-moons

1 garlic clove, minced

1 teaspoon grated lemon zest

2 tablespoons chopped fresh tarragon leaves or 2 teaspoons dried

2 tablespoons fresh lemon juice

Freshly ground black pepper

⅓ cup chopped **walnuts**

In a small saucepan, combine the lentils and water to cover by 2 inches. Bring to a boil, reduce to a simmer, cover, and cook until just tender but not falling apart, 20 to 25 minutes. Drain well and cool slightly.

Meanwhile, in another small saucepan, cook the bulgur according to package directions, using a pinch of the salt. Drain off any remaining cooking liquid. Cool slightly.

In a large nonstick skillet, heat 2 teaspoons of the oil over medium-low heat. Add the shallot and cook, stirring, until softened, about 2 minutes. Add the squash, garlic, and lemon zest. Cook until the squash has softened, about 8 minutes.

In a salad bowl, combine the lentils, bulgur, sautéed squash, tarragon, lemon juice, remaining 1 teaspoon oil, remaining ½ teaspoon salt, and pepper to taste. Toss to combine. Serve warm or at room temperature, sprinkled with the walnuts.

MAKES 4 (2-CUP) SERVINGS

Per serving: 303 calories, 10 g fat, 1 g saturated fat, 16 g protein, 43 g carbohydrate, 9.5 g fiber, 304 mg sodium

Variation: Omit the lemon juice and lemon zest and use balsamic vinegar and grated orange zest instead.

> TIP: The bulgur and lentils can both be made several hours or even 1 day ahead. If making a day ahead, cover and refrigerate, but bring back to room temperature before dressing and serving.

PHASE I

Layered Salad
with Creamy Cilantro Dressing

HANDS-ON TIME: 35 minutes   TOTAL TIME: 35 minutes plus optional standing time

An American classic, this hearty salad gets completely assembled ahead of time, in layers (including the dressing), which keeps it fresh until serving time. Of course there's no reason why you can't eat the salad immediately; the fact that it can hold for hours is merely a convenience for the cook.

Cilantro Dressing

2 Hass *avocados,* scooped

½ cup packed cilantro leaves

⅓ cup spicy 100% vegetable juice (from a 5.5-ounce can)

3 tablespoons fresh lime juice

Salad

1½ cups small *cauliflower* florets, fresh or frozen

1 cup grape *tomatoes,* halved lengthwise

1 yellow bell pepper, diced

4 ounces smoked turkey in one piece, diced

2 cups shredded romaine lettuce

1 cup chopped *watercress*

1 can (15 ounces) no-salt-added *navy beans* or other small *white beans,* rinsed

¼ cup hulled unsalted *sunflower seeds*

To make the dressing: In a food processor, combine the avocado, cilantro, vegetable juice, and lime juice. Process to a smooth purée.

To make the salad: Steam the fresh cauliflower until crisp-tender, 5 to 7 minutes; or cook the frozen cauliflower according to package directions. Rinse under cold water to stop the cooking.

Meanwhile, spread the avocado dressing on the bottom of a 3-quart salad bowl. Arrange the tomatoes cut-side down on the dressing, completely covering it (see Tip).

Layer the following ingredients on top of the tomatoes in this order: bell pepper, cauliflower, turkey, romaine, watercress, and beans. Cover the salad well and refrigerate for up to 8 hours. Meanwhile, toast the sunflower seeds in a small dry skillet or in a toaster oven until lightly browned, 3 to 5 minutes. Store in an airtight container.

To serve, sprinkle the salad with the toasted sunflower seeds and toss everything together.

MAKES 4 (2-CUP) SERVINGS

Per serving: 325 calories, 17 g fat, 2.5 g saturated fat, 18 g protein, 30 g carbohydrate, 12 g fiber, 389 mg sodium

Variation: The lean protein in this dish can easily be varied. Try this with 6 ounces of cooked shrimp, lean Black Forest ham, extra-firm tofu (or baked tofu), or shredded chicken.

> TIP: Though it may seem an unimportant detail, be sure you place the tomatoes over the dressing with their cut sides down. The juices that leak out of the tomatoes will contribute to the dressing and also help keep the avocado purée from discoloring.

PHASE 2 # Apple-Baked Beans with Smoked Ham

HANDS-ON TIME: 10 minutes   TOTAL TIME: 1 hour 10 minutes

Traditional baked beans are made with tons of sugar and fatty pork. These much-better-for-you beans have a small amount of lean smoked ham and are mildly sweetened with apple-sauce, a good source of heart-healthy soluble fiber. The sauce for the beans also provides some important phytonutrients: lycopene in the tomato paste and flavonoids in the cocoa. The dish can be assembled in the morning, covered, and refrigerated until time to bake.

2 teaspoons **extra-virgin olive oil**

1 tablespoon unsweetened **cocoa powder**

1 cup unsweetened applesauce

2 tablespoons **tomato paste**

2 teaspoons Dijon **mustard**

⅛ teaspoon ground allspice

2 cans (15 ounces each) no-salt added **pinto beans,** rinsed and drained

¼ pound lean Black Forest ham in one piece, diced

Heat the oven to 325°F. Lightly coat an 8 x 8-inch baking dish with cooking spray.

In a medium bowl, stir together the oil and cocoa powder. Stir in the apple-sauce, tomato paste, mustard, and allspice.

Add the beans and ham and toss to coat. Scrape into the baking dish, cover, and bake for 1 hour, or until piping hot.

MAKES 6 (⅔-CUP) SERVINGS

Per serving: 169 calories, 2 g fat, 0 g saturated fat, 10 g protein, 27 g carbohydrate, 7 g fiber, 256 mg sodium

TIP: All of the ingredients that go into this dish are already cooked, so the time in the oven is really just to blend the flavors and get the dish hot. If you're in a hurry, you could put the beans in a hotter oven (350°F) for a shorter time (30 minutes).

Green and White Florets with Toasted Pumpkin Seeds

PHASE I

HANDS-ON TIME: 20 minutes   TOTAL TIME: 20 minutes

In the world of good-for-you vegetables, broccoli is a superstar. Not only is it one of the best sources of the health-protective sulfur compounds found in cruciferous vegetables, but it's also a good source of two antioxidant nutrients: vitamin C and beta-carotene.

1 large bunch **broccoli** (about 1½ pounds), cut into florets

½ head **cauliflower** (about ¾ pound), cut into florets

½ cup hulled **pumpkin seeds** (pepitas)

1 tablespoon **extra virgin olive oil**

1 tablespoon fresh lemon juice

    Salt and freshly ground black pepper

3 tablespoons chopped flat-leaf parsley

In a large pot of lightly salted boiling water, cook the broccoli and cauliflower until just crisp-tender, about 5 minutes. Drain well.

Meanwhile, in a dry skillet, stir the pumpkin seeds over medium heat until they brown and start to puff up a bit, 3 to 5 minutes. Transfer the seeds to a plate.

In a large skillet or wok, heat the oil over medium heat. Add the broccoli, cauliflower, and lemon juice and cook, stirring, for 1 minute. Season with salt and pepper. Add the parsley and pumpkin seeds and toss to combine. Serve hot.

MAKES 4 SERVINGS

Per serving: 126 calories, 7 g fat, 1 g saturated fat, 7 g protein, 12 g carbohydrate, 4.5 g fiber, 130 mg sodium

Variation: If you're a fan of cilantro, use it instead of parsley and add ground cumin to taste when you season the vegetables with salt and pepper.

Broccolette with Brown Rice and Walnuts

HANDS-ON TIME: 10 minutes   **TOTAL TIME:** 1 hour

Broccolette—also called broccolini or baby broccoli—is actually a cross between regular broc-coli and Chinese broccoli. It has a mild broccoli flavor and consists of thin stalks with small florets on the top. Similar looking, but much more pungent in flavor, is broccoli rabe. Because the two vegetables are the same shape, they can easily be substituted for one another in recipes.

½ cup **brown basmati rice**

1¼ cups lower-sodium chicken broth

Freshly ground black pepper

Pinch of smoked paprika (optional)

2 pounds **broccolette** or **broccoli rabe,** cut crosswise into 1-inch pieces

2 teaspoons **extra-virgin olive oil**

2 garlic cloves, very thinly sliced

¼ teaspoon salt

3 tablespoons chopped **walnuts**

In a small saucepan, combine the rice, chicken broth, ¼ teaspoon pepper, and the paprika (if using). Bring to a boil and stir once. Reduce to a simmer, cover, and cook until the rice is tender, about 45 minutes. Remove from the heat and let stand for 5 minutes.

Meanwhile, in a steamer set over 1 inch of boiling water, cook the brocco-lette until crisp-tender, 4 to 6 minutes; set aside.

In a large Dutch oven, heat the oil over medium-low heat. Add the garlic and cook, stirring, for 1 minute. Add the broccolette and salt and toss to coat. Stir in the cooked rice and toss well. Season to taste with pepper. Serve sprin-kled with the walnuts.

MAKES 4 SERVINGS

Per serving: 236 calories, 6.5 g fat, 1 g saturated fat, 12 g protein, 35 g carbohydrate, 4.5 g fiber, 335 mg sodium

TIP: This can turn into a super-fast side dish if you can buy freshly steamed plain brown rice from a local Chinese restaurant. Or you can make your own brown rice several hours ahead or earlier in the day.

Greens Gratin with Turkey Bacon

HANDS-ON TIME: 45 minutes   TOTAL TIME: 45 minutes

Any kind of cooking green is good for you, but those that taste a little peppery or bitter are actually the best nutrition-wise. The bitterness comes from compounds called isothiocyanates, which are powerful health-protective phytonutrients.

1¼ pounds cooking greens (such as **turnip greens, collards,** or **kale**), thick
    stems removed, leaves chopped

4 slices turkey bacon, cut into 1-inch pieces

2 teaspoons **extra-virgin olive oil**

1 small onion, chopped

2 garlic cloves, minced

½ cup fat-free evaporated **milk**

    Freshly ground black pepper

3 tablespoons grated Parmesan cheese

Heat the broiler.

In a deep flameproof skillet, bring a few inches of water to a boil. Add the greens and cook over medium-high heat until tender, 6 to 10 minutes. Drain and press to remove excess liquid.

Wipe the skillet dry and return to medium-high heat. Add the bacon and cook until crispy, 4 to 5 minutes. Transfer the bacon to a plate.

Add the oil, onion, and garlic to the pan and stir to coat the vegetables. Reduce the heat to medium, and cook, stirring, until the onion is softened, 4 to 6 minutes.

Return the bacon to the pan and add the evaporated milk. Bring to a simmer and cook until the liquid is slightly reduced, about 5 minutes. Season with pepper to taste. Add the greens and stir to combine. Sprinkle evenly with the cheese. Place the pan under the broiler for 2 to 3 minutes, or until the cheese is lightly browned.

MAKES 4 SERVINGS

Per serving: 140 calories, 7 g fat, 2 g saturated fat, 9 g protein, 13 g carbohydrate, 4 g fiber, 288 mg sodium

Golden Barley Pilaf with Herb-Roasted Carrots

HANDS-ON TIME: 10 minutes   **TOTAL TIME:** 50 minutes

The golden glow in this tasty grain pilaf comes from cooking the barley with a little bit of carrot juice. In addition to a beautiful color, the carrot juice adds a natural sweetness and a lot of beta-carotene.

1½ cups lower-sodium chicken or vegetable broth

½ cup *carrot* juice

¾ cup pearled *barley*

   Salt

8 ounces baby *carrots*

2 tablespoons *extra-virgin olive oil*

¼ teaspoon dried basil

¼ teaspoon dried thyme

   Freshly ground black pepper

2 tablespoons chopped fresh parsley

2 scallions, green parts only, sliced

1½ teaspoons red wine vinegar

Heat the oven to 400°F. Line a rimmed baking sheet with foil.

In a medium saucepan, bring the broth and carrot juice to a boil. Add the barley and a pinch of salt and stir. Reduce to a simmer, cover, and cook until the barley is tender, 40 to 45 minutes. Remove from the heat and let stand, covered, for 5 minutes.

Meanwhile, on the prepared baking sheet, toss the carrots with 1½ tablespoons of the oil, the basil, thyme, and pepper to taste. Spread in an even layer and roast, stirring every 10 minutes, for 25 to 30 minutes, or until tender.

Drain the barley of any excess liquid and transfer to a large serving bowl. Stir in the roasted carrots, parsley, scallion greens, vinegar, remaining 1½ teaspoons oil, and a generous pinch of salt. Serve warm or at room temperature.

MAKES 4 (¾-CUP) SERVINGS

Per serving: 240 calories, 7.5 g fat, 1 g saturated fat, 6 g protein, 39 g carbohydrate, 8 g fiber, 262 mg sodium

Variation: Omit the basil and thyme and use ½ teaspoon dried tarragon instead. Toss the barley with chopped fresh basil instead of parsley.

Chunky Guacamole Salad

HANDS-ON TIME: 20 minutes   TOTAL TIME: 30 minutes

In this Mexican-inspired salad, the peppery taste of the watercress is complemented by the creaminess of avocado and the fresh, tart flavors of lime juice and tomatoes. Watercress is a cruciferous vegetable and, like other members of that family, is rich in health-promoting phytonutrients.

2½ tablespoons fresh lime juice

1 tablespoon minced red onion

⅛ teaspoon plus ½ teaspoon salt

¼ cup chopped cilantro

3 tablespoons *extra-virgin olive oil*

2 scallions, chopped

1 garlic clove, minced

2 bunches (4 ounces each) *watercress,* thick stems discarded

Freshly ground black pepper

3 large *tomatoes,* diced, with juices reserved

2 Hass *avocados,* diced

In a large salad bowl, whisk together the lime juice, onion, and ⅛ teaspoon of the salt. Set aside at room temperature for 10 minutes. Whisk in the cilantro, oil, scallions, and garlic.

Add the watercress to the salad bowl and toss gently to coat with the dressing. Sprinkle with pepper to taste and the remaining ½ teaspoon salt. Add the tomatoes (and their juices) and avocados, tossing gently.

MAKES 8 (1-CUP) SERVINGS

Per serving: 120 calories, 10 g fat, 1.5 g saturated fat, 2 g protein, 7 g carbohydrate, 3.5 g fiber, 199 mg sodium

PHASE 2

Quinoa and Tomato Salad with Goat Cheese

HANDS-ON TIME: 20 minutes   TOTAL TIME: 25 minutes

This fresh-tasting salad is similar to a tabbouleh (Middle Eastern bulgur salad) in the sense that the vegetables and herbs outweigh the grain. Because quinoa has a good balance of all eight essential amino acids (usually found only in meat, poultry, and seafood), it is an exceptionally good plant source of protein.

¾ cup **quinoa**

4 plum **tomatoes,** coarsely chopped

1 medium cucumber, peeled, seeded, and diced

4 scallions, thinly sliced

6 tablespoons chopped flat-leaf parsley

4 tablespoons chopped fresh mint leaves

2 tablespoons fresh lemon juice

1 tablespoon **extra-virgin olive oil**

¼ teaspoon salt

¼ teaspoon freshly ground black pepper

3 ounces reduced-fat **goat cheese** or **feta cheese,** crumbled (see Tip)

In a small saucepan, cook the quinoa according to package directions. Drain any excess liquid.

Meanwhile, in a large bowl, combine the tomatoes, cucumber, scallions, parsley, and mint.

When the quinoa is done, add to the bowl and toss everything together. Let sit for 10 minutes.

Meanwhile, in a small bowl, whisk together the lemon juice, oil, salt, and pepper. Pour the dressing over the salad and toss well. Serve at room temperature or chilled, topped with the cheese.

MAKES 4 (1½-CUP) SERVINGS
Per serving: 214 calories, 8 g fat, 2 g saturated fat, 9 g protein, 29 g carbohydrate, 4 g fiber, 234 mg sodium

Variation: Give the dish a Mexican twist: Use cilantro instead of mint and lime juice instead of lemon juice. If you like spicy food, add 1 minced serrano chile to the dressing.

TIP: If you can't find reduced-fat goat cheese, make this with regular, but reduce the amount to 2 ounces.

Sweet Potato Salad with Fresh Basil

PHASE 2

HANDS-ON TIME: 10 minutes   TOTAL TIME: 25 minutes

When you're in the mood for a great potato salad, this is the one to have. Sweet potatoes alone are a spectacular source of beta-carotene, but if you throw in some fresh basil, scallion greens, and red bell pepper, then you have almost 1,200 percent of the recommended daily intake for this antioxidant in a single serving.

2 medium *sweet potatoes* (1½ pounds), peeled and cut into 1-inch cubes

⅓ cup low-fat plain *yogurt*

1 small red bell pepper, diced

2 scallions, thinly sliced

3 tablespoons chopped fresh basil

1 teaspoon red wine vinegar

¼ teaspoon salt

⅛ teaspoon freshly ground black pepper

In a medium saucepan, combine the sweet potatoes and cold water to cover. Bring to a boil and cook until tender, 8 to 10 minutes. Drain, run under cold water to cool, and drain again.

In a large bowl, combine the sweet potatoes, yogurt, bell pepper, scallions, basil, vinegar, salt, and black pepper. Serve at room temperature or chilled.

MAKES 4 (GENEROUS ¾-CUP) SERVINGS
Per serving: 123 calories, 0.5 g fat, 0.3 g saturated fat, 3 g protein, 27 g carbohydrate, 4 g fiber, 198 mg sodium

PHASE 2 # Multigrain Blueberry Cobbler

HANDS-ON TIME: 20 minutes   TOTAL TIME: 1 hour

In this delicious cobbler, blueberries (which are high in powerful antioxidants called antho-cyanins) are baked under a multigrain biscuit dough and served with a dollop of nonfat Greek yogurt.

- 4 cups (about 1½ pounds) fresh **blueberries** (see Variation)
- 3 tablespoons agave syrup
- 1 teaspoon fresh lemon juice
- ¾ cup plus 2 tablespoons white **whole-wheat** flour
- 2 tablespoons **flaxmeal**
- 1 tablespoon chopped hulled **pumpkin seeds, sunflower seeds,** or **sesame seeds**
- 1 tablespoon Truvía
- 1½ teaspoons baking powder
- 1 teaspoon grated lemon zest
- ½ teaspoon ground cinnamon
- ⅛ teaspoon salt
- 5 tablespoons (2½ ounces) cold trans-fat-free margarine (vegetable oil spread), cut into bits
- ¼ cup plus 2 tablespoons 1% **milk**
- ½ cup nonfat (0%) plain Greek **yogurt**

Heat the oven to 350°F.

Place the blueberries in an 8 x 8-inch baking dish. Drizzle with the agave syrup and lemon juice and stir to coat.

In a medium bowl, combine the flour, flaxmeal, seeds, Truvía, baking powder, lemon zest, cinnamon, and salt. With a pastry blender or 2 knives, cut the margarine into the flour mixture until it resembles coarse meal. Stir in the milk to make a slightly sticky, soft dough.

Drop the dough by large spoonfuls over the fruit, covering as much of the fruit as you can. Bake for 35 to 40 minutes, until the top is golden and the berries are hot and bubbling. Serve immediately or at room temperature.

For each serving, spoon a portion of the cobbler topping, blueberries, and juices into a dessert bowl and top with 1 tablespoon Greek yogurt.

MAKES 8 SERVINGS

Per serving: 208 calories, 9 g fat, 1 g saturated fat, 5 g protein, 32 g carbohydrate, 5 g fiber, 218 mg sodium

Variation: When fresh blueberries are not in season, make this with 2 bags (12 ounces each) frozen blueberries (not thawed).

> TIP: The cobbler can also be doubled and made in a 9 x 13-inch pan to make 16 servings. The baking time will be the same.

PHASE 2

Chocolate Bark
with Cranberries, Almonds, and Pecans

HANDS-ON TIME: 15 minutes   **TOTAL TIME:** 25 minutes

Just a small bite of this delicious chocolate treat provides important health benefits: antioxidants in the cranberries and chocolate, and good unsaturated fats in the pecans and almonds. Make the effort to find bittersweet chocolate chips, since the darker the chocolate, the higher the levels of antioxidants. The bark will keep for 2 weeks stored in the refrigerator.

6 tablespoons coarsely chopped **almonds**

6 tablespoons coarsely chopped **pecans**

6 tablespoons coarsely chopped dried **cranberries**

9 ounces **bittersweet chocolate chips**

In a small bowl, combine the almonds, pecans, and cranberries.

Line a baking sheet with foil. In a medium bowl set over hot, not boiling, water, melt the chocolate chips. Remove from the heat and stir in the cranberry-nut mixture.

Spread the mixture evenly over the baking sheet. Refrigerate for 10 minutes, or until firm but not brittle. Cut or break into about 30 jagged pieces and serve, or store in an airtight container for later.

MAKES 15 (2-PIECE) SERVINGS
Per serving: 65 calories, 5.5 g fat, 2 g saturated fat, 1 g protein, 6 g carbohydrate, 1 g fiber, 0 mg sodium

Variation: This is an extremely easy recipe to play with. Try chopped dried apricots instead of cranberries, or cashews instead of almonds, for example, using the same amounts indicated above.

MASTER SHOPPING LIST
FOR A HEALTHY DIET

The following list shows the wide variety of wholesome foods that you and your family can enjoy as you strive to create healthier meals. You can either photocopy this list or download it from southbeachdiet.com/wakeupcall. Remember: Look for bargains, shop for produce in season, and freeze foods for future use. If you are following the South Beach Diet and are on Phase 1 or 2 of the weight-loss program, shop accordingly for the phase you're on.

VEGETABLES

Fresh, frozen, or canned without added sugar

Artichoke hearts
Artichokes
Arugula
Asparagus
Beets
Bok choy
Broccoli
Broccolini
Broccoli rabe
Brussels sprouts
Cabbage (green, red, napa, savoy)
Calabaza
Cassava
Capers
Carrots
Cauliflower
Celeriac (celery root)
Celery
Chayote
Collard greens
Corn

Cucumbers
Daikon radish
Eggplant
Endive
Escarole
Fennel
Fiddlehead ferns
Garlic
Grape leaves
Green beans
Hearts of palm
Jícama
Kale
Kohlrabi
Leeks
Lettuce (all varieties)
Mushrooms (all varieties)
Mustard greens
Okra
Onions
Parsley
Peas, green
Pepperoncini
Peppers (all varieties)

VEGETABLES—*continued*

Pickles (dill or artificially sweetened)

Pimientos

Pumpkin

Radicchio

Radishes

Rhubarb

Sauerkraut

Scallions

Sea vegetables (seaweed, nori)

Shallots

Snap peas

Snow peas

Spinach

Sprouts (alfalfa, bean, broccoli, lentil, radish, sunflower)

Squash, spaghetti

Squash, summer

  yellow

  zucchini

Squash, winter

Sweet potatoes

Swiss chard

Taro

Tomatoes (all varieties)

Tomato juice

Turnips (greens and roots)

Vegetable juice and vegetable juice blends

Water chestnuts

Watercress

Wax beans

Yams

BEANS AND OTHER LEGUMES

Fresh, frozen, or canned without added sugar

Adzuki beans

Black beans

Black-eyed peas

Broad beans

Butter beans

Cannellini beans

Chickpeas (garbanzo beans)

Cranberry beans

Edamame

Fava beans

Great Northern beans

Italian beans

Kidney beans

Lentils (any variety)

Lima beans

Mung beans

Navy beans

Pigeon beans

Pinto beans

Refried beans (fat-free, canned)

Soybeans

Split peas

White beans

FRUITS

Fresh, frozen, or canned without added sugar

Apples

Apricots

Avocados

Bananas

Blackberries

Blueberries

Boysenberries

Cactus pear fruits (prickly pears)

Cantaloupe

Cherries

Clementines

Cranberries

Elderberries

Gooseberries

Grapefruit

Grapes

Honeydew melons

Kiwifruit

Loganberries

Mandarin oranges

Mangoes

Mulberries

Nectarines

Oranges

Papayas

Peaches

Pears

Plums

Pomegranate seeds

Pomelos

Prunes

Raspberries

Strawberries

Tangelos

Tangerines

LEAN PROTEIN

Lean meat has 10 g or less of total fat and 4.5 g or less of saturated fat per 100 g portion.

Beef (remove all visible fat)

Bottom round

Eye of round

Flank steak

Ground beef

    Extra lean

    Lean sirloin

Hot dogs (look for 97% fat-free or 3–6 g of fat per serving)

London broil

Pastrami, lean

Sirloin steak

T-bone steak

Tenderloin (filet mignon)

Top loin

Top round

Poultry

Choose cuts without the skin or remove it when cooking or before eating.

Chicken breast, all cuts

Cornish hen

Duck breast

Ground breast of chicken

Ground breast of turkey

Hot dogs (look for 97% fat-free or 3–6 g of fat per serving)

Turkey bacon

Turkey breast, all cuts

Turkey pastrami

Turkey sausage, low-fat (3–6 g of fat per 60 g serving)

Seafood

Limit your intake of fish high in mercury, such as marlin, swordfish, shark, tilefish, orange roughy, king mackerel, bigeye and ahi tuna, and canned albacore tuna (use light tuna instead).

Fish (all types)

Salmon roe

Shellfish (all types)

Pork

Canadian bacon

Ham, boiled

Hot dogs (look for 97% fat-free or 3–6 g of fat per serving)

Loin, chop or roast

Tenderloin

LEAN PROTEIN—*continued*

Veal

Chop

Leg cutlet

Leg roast

Top round

Lamb (remove all visible fat and eat occasionally)

Center cut

Chop

Loin (chop or roast)

Game Meats

Buffalo

Elk

Ostrich

Venison

Deli Meats

Reduced-fat or natural, preferably reduced sodium

Chicken breast

Ham, boiled or smoked

Roast beef

Turkey breast, regular or smoked

SOY-BASED MEAT SUBSTITUTES AND MEAT ALTERNATIVES

Unless otherwise stated, look for products that have 6 g or less of fat per 2–3 oz serving.

Seiten

Soy bacon

Soy burgers

Soy chicken, unbreaded

Soy crumbles

Soy hot dogs

Soy sausage, patties or links

Tempeh

Tofu (all varieties)

Yuba (bean curd in sticks or sheets)

WHOLE GRAINS

Bagels, small whole grain

Barley

Bread, 100% whole-grain, including homemade breads made with whole grains (buckwheat, whole wheat, spelt, whole oats, bran, rye)

Bran

Multigrain

Oat

Rye

Sprouted grain

Whole wheat

Buckwheat

Cereal, cold (choose low-sugar with 5 g or more of fiber per serving; serving sizes vary so be sure to check the label to determine the recommended amount)

Cereal, hot (choose whole-grain and slow-cooking varieties—not instant—with at least 3 g of fiber and no more than 2 g of sugar; serving sizes vary so be sure to check the label to determine the recommended amount)

Couscous, whole wheat or Israeli

Crackers, whole grain (3 g or more of fiber per ounce and no trans fats)

English muffin, whole grain (most contain 2.5 g of fiber per half muffin; varieties with 3 g of fiber are the best choice)

Farro

Flaxmeal (ground flaxseed)

Flour

    Garbanzo flour

    Soy flour

    Spelt flour

    White whole-wheat flour

    Whole-wheat flour

    Whole-wheat pastry flour

Matzo, whole wheat

Pasta

    Whole wheat (3 g or more of fiber per ½ cup)

    Soy (3 g or more of fiber per ½ cup)

Phyllo dough and shells, whole wheat

Pita (most contain 2.5 g of fiber per half pita; varieties with 3 g of fiber are the best choice)

Popcorn

    Air-popped

    Microwave, plain, no trans fats

    Stove-top, cooked with canola oil

Quinoa

Rice

    Basmati

    Brown

    Converted

    Parboiled

    Wild

Rice noodles

Shirataki noodles

Soba noodles

Tortilla, 100% whole grain (3 g or more of fiber per ounce, no trans fats)

Wheat germ

DAIRY, CHEESE, AND EGGS

Dairy (fat-free or reduced-fat) and milk alternatives

Almond milk

Buttermilk, nonfat or light (1.5%)

Greek yogurt, nonfat (0%)

Kefir, nonfat and low-fat plain

Milk, 1% or fat-free

Sour cream, light or reduced fat

Soy milk, low-fat plain, vanilla, or artificially sweetened (4 g or less of fat per 8 oz. serving; avoid varieties that contain high-fructose corn syrup)

Whipped cream, light

Yogurt (artificially sweetened, low-fat, or nonfat; avoid varieties that contain high-fructose corn syrup)

Cheese (fat-free or reduced-fat)

For hard cheese, look for varieties that have 6 g or less of fat per oz.

American

Blue cheese (such as gorgonzola)

Cheddar

Cottage cheese, 1%, 2%, or fat-free

Cream cheese, fat-free or light

Farmer cheese (and light farmer cheese)

Feta

Goat cheese (chèvre)

Mozzarella

Parmesan

Provolone

Queso fresco

Ricotta, part-skim

Sheep's milk cheese

String cheese, part-skim

Swiss

Eggs

The use of whole eggs is not limited unless otherwise directed by your doctor. Egg whites and egg substitutes are OK.

HEALTHY OILS AND OTHER FATS

Monounsaturated Oils

Canola oil

Olive oil (particularly extra-virgin)

Polyunsaturated Oils or a Blend of Monounsaturated and Polyunsaturated

Corn

Flaxseed

Grapeseed

Peanut

Safflower

Sesame

Soybean

Sunflower

Other Good Fat Choices

Mayonnaise, regular or low-fat (avoid varieties made with high-fructose corn syrup or other added sugars)

Olives (green or black)

Salad dressing (buy those that contain 3 g of sugar or less per 2 Tbsp; the best choices contain canola or olive oil—dressings labeled "low-carb" should only be purchased if they meet these guidelines)

Trans fats–free spreads

Vegetable oil spread (margarine)—choose brands that do not contain trans fats

NUTS AND SEEDS

Limit to ¼ cup per day. Dry roasted recommended.

Almonds

Brazil nuts

Cashews

Chestnuts

Edamame, dry roasted

Filberts

Flaxseed

Hazelnuts

Macadamias

Peanut butter, natural, and other nut butters

Peanuts (dry roasted or boiled)

Pecans

Pine nuts (pignoli)

Pistachios

Pumpkin seeds

Sesame seeds

Soy nuts

Sunflower seeds

Walnuts

SEASONINGS AND CONDIMENTS

Check labels for added sugar or monosodium glutamate (MSG). "Low-carb" condiments should be used only if they are trans fats–free and contain no added sugar.

Broth (preferably reduced-sodium and fat-free)

Cocktail sauce, sugar-free

Cooking sprays, nonstick (such as olive oil, canola oil)

Espresso powder

Extracts (almond, vanilla, or others)

Horseradish

Hot sauce

Ketchup, sugar-free

Lemon juice

Lime juice

Liquid smoke

Miso

Mustard, sugar free

Pepper (black, cayenne, red, white)

Salsa (check the label for added sugar)

Shoyu

Soy sauce

Spices and spice blends (use only those that contain no added sugar)

Steak sauce

Taco sauce

Tamari

Tomato paste

Worcestershire sauce

BEVERAGES

Almond milk, unsweetened

Buttermilk, nonfat or light (1.5%)

Club soda

Beer, light

Coffee, caffeinated or decaffeinated

Milk, 1% or fat-free

Powdered drink mixes, sugar-free

Seltzer

Soda, sugar free (caffeinated or caffeine free)

Soymilk, low-fat plain, vanilla, or artificially sweetened (4 g or less of fat per 8 oz serving; avoid varieties that contain high-fructose corn syrup)

Tea, caffeinated (black, green, white, oolong) or herbal (such as peppermint, chamomile, orange blossom)

Tomato juice

Vegetable juice blends

Wine, red or white

SUGAR-FREE TREATS

Some sugar-free products may be made with sugar alcohols (isomalt, lactitol, mannitol, sorbitol, or xylitol) and may have associated side effects of gastrointestinal distress if consumed in excessive amounts. Limit to 75–100 calories per day.

Candies, hard, sugar-free

Chocolate powder, no sugar added

Chocolate syrup, sugar-free

Cocoa powder, unsweetened baking type, labeled 100% cacao

Fudgsicles, no sugar added

Gelatin, sugar-free

Gum, sugar-free

Jams and jellies, sugar-free

Popsicles, sugar-free

Syrups, sugar-free

SUGAR SUBSTITUTES

Some sugar substitutes may be made with sugar alcohols (isomalt, lactitol, mannitol, sorbitol, or xylitol) and may have associated side effects of gastrointestinal distress if consumed in large amounts.

Agave nectar (limit to 2 Tbsp daily)

Aspartame (NutraSweet, Equal)

Saccharin (Sweet'N Low)

Stevia

Stevia and erythritol (Truvía)

Sucralose (Splenda)

SPECIAL TREAT

Chocolate, dark (choose brands that contain at least 70% cacao and the least amount of sugar)

ONLINE RESOURCES

Knowledge is essential to achieving a healthy lifestyle. Readers who want to delve deeper into some of the topics discussed in this book can explore the following Web sites.

DISEASE-SPECIFIC INFORMATION

Alz.org
The Alzheimer's Association offers insight and information on this debilitating neurological disorder, as well as important tips for caregivers.

Americanheart.org
Are you or a loved one at risk for heart disease? For information on the prevention and treatment of heart disease, high blood pressure, and stroke, check out the American Heart Association online.

Arthritis.org
Sponsored by the Arthritis Foundation, this site provides information on treating osteoarthritis, rheumatoid arthritis, and other related conditions—including safe ways to exercise and find pain relief—and features the latest research.

Cancer.org
A healthy lifestyle can help reduce your risk for developing many different types of cancer. Visit the American Cancer Society Web site for information on all types of cancer, as well as information on how to prevent it.

Diabetes.org
Type 2 diabetes has become an epidemic in the developing world. The American Diabetes Association Web site provides the latest information on how to prevent and treat this disease.

Lungusa.org
One of the best ways to prevent cancer and heart disease is to *quit smoking*. Visit the American Lung Association Web site for facts about lung diseases and tips for smokers who want to quit.

Womenshealth.gov/publications/our-publications/fact-sheet/autoimmune-diseases.cfm
This US government site answers commonly asked questions about different autoimmune conditions, including lupus, irritable bowel syndrome, and thyroid disease.

OBESITY PREVENTION

CDC.gov/obesity
This Centers for Disease Control and Prevention site provides comprehensive information on the obesity epidemic, including the latest statistics, research findings, and national trends.

Childrenshospital.org/owl
The Optimal Weight for Life (OWL) Program at Children's Hospital Boston is a multidisciplinary clinic dedicated to treating children who are overweight or obese and those with or at risk for type 2 diabetes.

Healthiergeneration.org
The William J. Clinton Foundation and the American Heart Association teamed up to create the Alliance for a Healthier Generation, whose Web site offers an action plan for combating childhood obesity.

Hopenyu.org/early-childhood/strategies-for-families
New York University's Child Study Center features the Harris Obesity Prevention Effort (HOPE), whose research focuses on helping parents and educators of young children promote healthy lifestyle habits and prevent obesity and related health problems.

Obesity.org/resources-for/consumer.htm
The Obesity Society is an organization of scientists and medical professional dedicated to researching and treating obesity. Visit its Web site for treatment options, statistics, and health facts for the lay public.

Southbeachdiet.com
The site for all you need to know about the South Beach Diet. It features weight-loss tools, including a mobile app, meal plans, recipes, and exercise information, and support from registered dietitians and an active community of South Beach Diet followers.

GLUTEN AWARENESS

Celiac.com
This site provides comprehensive information about celiac disease and gluten intolerance. It also cautions consumers against products that claim to be gluten free but are not.

Celiacdiseasecenter.columbia.edu
Directed by Peter H.R. Green, MD, the Celiac Disease Center at Columbia University is one of the first medical-school-supported centers devoted to the treatment and study of celiac disease. Its Web site provides the latest medical information on this condition for both physicians and patients.

Celiac.nih.gov
The National Institute of Diabetes and Digestive and Kidney Diseases sponsors the Celiac Disease Awareness Campaign site to educate people about the symptoms of celiac disease. You'll find information on eating gluten free as well as the latest research on this condition.

Glutenfreeceliacweb.com
Founded by a patient with celiac disease, this Web site provides information about places to find gluten-free products and restaurants catering to gluten-intolerant customers.

Thesavvyceliac.com
This site has news and tips for the gluten-intolerant community.

HEALTHIER SCHOOL MEALS

Betterschoolfood.org
Founded by a group of parents, educators, and health professionals, Better School Food offers information on the principles of healthy eating and teaches parents how to advocate for more nutritious school meals.

ChefAnn.com
Chef Ann Cooper, better known as the "Renegade Lunch Lady," is an outspoken advocate for improving the quality of school lunches—"one school lunch at a time." This site gives parents and professionals the latest information on ways to bring healthier, better-tasting food into school cafeterias.

JamieOliver.com/foundation
As part of his ongoing "Food Revolution," chef and author Jamie Oliver provides parents with information on improving food in schools and making healthier lunches. He also offers updates on pending legislation pertaining to childhood obesity.

School-lunch.org
This Web site is devoted to monitoring school lunch programs nationwide and also provides specific information on how to improve nutrition in schools.

Schoollunchlady.com
Founded by Susan S. Brooks, RD, MA, this site has information for nutritionists and parents who are interested in making significant changes to school lunch programs.

Smarterlunchrooms.org
Cornell University's Food and Brand Lab encourages healthier eating in school lunchrooms
    through research, education, and outreach.

Yum-o.org
Author and TV personality Rachael Ray supports this nonprofit site, which is designed to
    encourage kids and their families to develop a healthy relationship with food and cooking
    and to improve the quality of meals in schools and at home.

IMPROVING THE FAMILY DINING TABLE

Eatright.org
This American Dietetic Association Web site provides basic information on nutrition and meal
    planning, including food safety at home, food allergies, and ideas for quick family meals.

Mindlesseating.org
Dr. Brian Wansink (author of *Mindless Eating*) sponsors this site to help people better
    understand their eating behaviors and ultimately make healthier food choices.

Thefamilydinnerproject.org
The grassroots Family Dinner Project organization describes itself as a "movement of food,
    fun, and conversation about things that matter." Its goal is to encourage families to share
    a family meal, as well as to share their experiences and their insights on the benefits of
    family dinners.

ORGANIC AND LOCALLY GROWN PRODUCE

Apps.ams.usda.gov/farmersmarkets
Use the locator on this US Department of Agriculture site to find a farmers' market near you.

Communitygarden.org
Want to garden but don't have your own outdoor space? The American Community Garden
    Association shows you how to organize and maintain a garden in your neighborhood.

Coopdirectory.org
Food co-ops are organizations that are operated and controlled by members to provide high-
    quality (often organic) food at the best prices. Check out this site for more information.

Localharvest.org
Use this site to locate farmers' markets, family farms, and other sources of sustainably grown
    food in your area, and to find restaurants that cook with locally produced food.

Organicgardening.com
Sponsored by *Organic Gardening* magazine, this site provides tips on how to make your garden
    and yard thrive using only organic products and sustainable growing methods. It features
    articles on natural pest control, landscaping, cooking the food you grow, and other topics.

Rodaleinstitute.org
The Rodale Institute's mission: "Through Organic Leadership we improve the health and well-
    being of people and the planet." On this site, you can learn about sustainable farming,
    the benefits of organic food, the impact of government policy on farming and the food
    supply, and more.

PROMOTING AN ACTIVE LIFESTYLE

Americawalks.org
The mission of America Walks is to "make America a great place for walking" and to promote
    "safe, convenient, accessible walking conditions for all." Visit this site and become an
    advocate for a healthier lifestyle.

CDC.gov/nccdphp/dnpa/kidswalk
Sponsored by the Centers for Disease Control and Prevention, this Web site has resources on
    KidsWalk-to-School, a community-based program that encourages parents to walk their
    kids to and from school to promote more physical activity during the day.

Fitness.gov

The President's Council on Fitness, Sports and Nutrition is on a mission to engage, educate, and empower Americans of all ages and abilities to adopt a healthy, active lifestyle.

Kidnetic.com

Designed for kids, this self-proclaimed "cool" site encourages them to engage in physical activity and is filled with good information on food and fitness.

Letsmove.gov

Let's Move! is a program developed by First Lady Michelle Obama with the goal of solving the epidemic of childhood obesity within a generation. Its Web site provides information on how to incorporate nutrition and fitness into your family's life.

Walkable.org

Leave the car at home, drive less, and walk more. How? Check out this site, which promotes the concept of walkable communities.

IMPROVING SLEEP

NHLBI.nih.gov/health/public/sleep

This government-sponsored Web site provides the latest research on sleep disorders, including sleep apnea, narcolepsy, and insomnia.

Sleepapnea.org

The nonprofit American Sleep Apnea Association is dedicated to "reducing injury, disability, and death from sleep apnea and to enhancing the well-being of those affected by this common disorder." The group's Web site has tips on diagnosing sleep apnea as well as treatment options.

Sleepfoundation.org

Sleep disorder professionals provide basic information on getting a better night's sleep on this National Sleep Foundation site. It includes the latest studies and news on sleep and helps you find a sleep disorder specialist in your area.

Yoursleep.aasmnet.org

This site, from the American Academy of Sleep Education, offers in-depth information on sleep disorders and the health risks of sleep deprivation, as well as a review of over-the-counter and prescription treatments. Parents can also find excellent advice on childhood sleep disorders and how to ensure that children get a good night's sleep.

SELECT BIBLIOGRAPHY

CHAPTER I: THE TICKING TIME BOMB

Adams MK, Simpson JA, et al. Abdominal obesity and age-related macular degeneration. *Am J Epidemiol* 2011;173(11):1246–1255.

Capewell S, Lloyd-Jones DM. Optimal cardiovascular prevention strategies for the 21st century. *JAMA* 2010;304(18):2057–2058.

Centers for Disease Control and Prevention. "U.S. Obesity Trends by State, 1985–2009." http://www.cdc.gov/obesity/data/trends.html#State.

Ford ES, Ajani UA, Croft JB, et al. Explaining the decrease in U.S. deaths from coronary disease, 1980–2000. *N Engl J Med* 2007;356:2388–2398.

Fraser A, Tilling K, et al. Association of maternal weight gain in pregnancy with offspring obesity and metabolic and vascular traits in childhood. *Circulation* 2010;121(23):2557–2564.

Hasselbalch AL. Genetics of dietary habits and obesity: A twin study. *Dan Med Bull* 2010;57(9):B4182.

Huang TT, Glass TA. Transforming research strategies for understanding and preventing obesity. *JAMA* 2008;300(15):1811–1813.

Jia H, Lubetkin EI. Obesity-related quality-adjusted life years lost in the U.S. from 1993 to 2008. *Am J Prev Med* 2010;39(3):220–227.

Juonala M, Magnussen CG, et al. Influence of age on associations between childhood risk factors and carotid intima-media thickness in adulthood: The Cardiovascular Risk in Young Finns Study, the Childhood Determinants of Adult Health Study, the Bogalusa Heart Study, and the Muscatine Study for the International Childhood Cardiovascular Cohort (i3C) Consortium. *Circulation* 2010;22(24):2514–2520.

Kipping RR, Jago R, et al. Obesity in children. Part 1: Epidemiology, measurement, risk factors, and screening. *BMJ* 2008;337:a1824.

———. Obesity in children. Part 2: Prevention and management. *BMJ* 2008;337:a1848.

Ludwig DS, Pollack HA. Obesity and the economy: From crisis to opportunity. *JAMA* 2009;301(5):533–535.

Nemetz PN, Roger VL, et al. Recent trends in the prevalence of coronary disease: A population-based autopsy study of nonnatural deaths. *Arch Intern Med* 2008;168(3):264–270.

Ng SF, Lin RC, et al. Chronic high-fat diet in fathers programs β-cell dysfunction in female rat offspring. *Nature* 2010;467(7318):963–966.

Ogden CL, Carroll MD, et al. High body mass index for age among US children and adolescents, 2003–2006. *JAMA* 2008;299(20):2401–2405.

Pratt CA, Stevens J, et al. Childhood obesity prevention and treatment: Recommendations for future research. *Am J Prev Med* 2008;35(3):249–252.

Roger VL, Go AS, et al. Heart disease and stroke statistics—2011 update: A report from the American Heart Association. *Circulation* 2011;123(6):e240.

Steinberger J, Daniels SR, et al. Progress and challenges in metabolic syndrome in children and adolescents: A scientific statement from the American Heart Association Atherosclerosis, Hypertension, and Obesity in the Young; Committee of the Council on Cardiovascular Disease in the Young; Council on Cardiovascular Nursing; and Council on Nutrition, Physical Activity, and Metabolism. *Circulation* 2009;119(4):628–647.

The NS, Suchindran C, et al. Association of adolescent obesity with risk of severe obesity in adulthood. *JAMA* 2010;304(18):2042–2047.

Tzotzas T, Evangelou P, et al. Obesity, weight loss and conditional cardiovascular risk factors. *Obes Rev* 2011;12(5):e282–289.

White House Task Force on Childhood Obesity. *Solving the Problem of Childhood Obesity within a Generation.* May 2010. http://www.letsmove.gov/white-house-task-force-childhood-obesity-report-president.

CHAPTER 2: GETTING OLD BEFORE OUR TIME

Agatston AS, Janowitz WR, et al. Quantification of coronary artery calcium using ultrafast CT. *J Am Coll Cardiol* 1990;15:827–832.

Agatston AS, Janowitz WR, et al. Ultrafast computed tomography-detected coronary calcium reflects the angiographic extent of coronary arterial atherosclerosis. *Am J Cardiol* 1994;74:1272–1274.

Agarwal S, Morgan T, et al. Coronary calcium score and prediction of all-cause mortality in diabetes. *Diabetes Care* 2011;34(5):1219–1224.

Akram K, O'Donnell RE, Agatston AS, et al. Influence of symptomatic status on the prevalence of obstructive coronary artery disease in patients with zero calcium score. *Atherosclerosis* 2009;3:533–537.

Aude W, Agatston AS, et al. A randomized trial comparing the National Cholesterol Education Program Step 2 Diet to a study diet lower in carbohydrates and higher in protein and monounsaturated fat. *Arch Int Med* 2004;164:2141–2146.

Berenson GS. Cardiovascular risk begins in childhood: A time for action. *Am J Prev Med* 2009;37(1 Suppl):S1–2.

Berenson GS, Srinivasan SR, et al. Association between multiple cardiovascular risk factors and atherosclerosis in children and young adults: The Bogalusa Heart Study. *New Eng J Med* 1998;338(23):1650–1656.

Blaha MJ, DeFilippis AP, Agatston, AS, et al. The relationship between insulin resistance and incidence and progression of coronary artery calcification: The Multi-Ethnic Study of Atherosclerosis (MESA). *Diabetes Care* 2011;34(3):749–751.

Broyles S, Katzmarzyk PT, et al. The pediatric obesity epidemic continues unabated in Bogalusa, Louisiana. *Pediatrics* 2010;125(5):900–905.

Budoff MJ, Georgiou D, Agatston AS, et al. Ultrafast computed tomography as a diagnostic modality in the detection of coronary artery disease: A multi center study. *Circulation* 1996;93:898–904.

Cesar L, Suarez SV, Agatston AS, Webster KA, et al. An essential role for diet in exercise-mediated protection against dyslipidemia, inflammation and atherosclerosis in ApoE / mice. *PLoS One* 2011;6(2):e17263.

Dowd JB, Zajacova A, et al. Predictors of inflammation in U.S. children aged 3–16 years. *Am J Prev Med* 2010;39(4):314–320.

Emerging Risk Factors Collaboration, Seshasai SR, et al. Diabetes mellitus, fasting glucose, and risk of cause-specific death. *N Engl J Med* 2011;364(9):829–841.

Farhat T, Iannotti RJ, et al. Overweight, obesity, youth, and health-risk behaviors. *Am J Prev Med* 2010;38(3):258–267.

Hassenstab JJ, Sweat V, et al. Metabolic syndrome is associated with learning and recall impairment in middle age. *Dement Geriatr Cogn Disord* 2010;29(4):356–362.

Janowitz WR, Agatston AS, et al. Comparison of serial quantitative evaluation of calcified coronary artery plaque by ultrafast CT in persons with and without obstructive CAD. *Am J Cardiol* 1991;68(1):1–6.

Le J, Zhang D, et al. Vascular age is advanced in children with atherosclerosis-promoting risk factors. *Circ Cardiovasc Imaging* 2010;3(1):8–14.

Moffat T. The "childhood obesity epidemic": Health crisis or social construction? *Med Anthropol Q* 2010;24(1):1–21.

Obarzanek E, Wu CO, et al. Prevalence and incidence of hypertension in adolescent girls. *J Pediatr* 2010;157(3):461–467.

Pletcher MJ, Bibbins-Domingo K, et al. Nonoptimal lipids commonly present in young adults and coronary calcium later in life: The CARDIA (Coronary Artery Risk Development in Young Adults) Study. *Ann Intern Med* 2010;153(3):137–146.

Powell LM, Szczypka G, et al. Trends in exposure to television food advertisements among children and adolescents in the United States. *Arch Pediatr Adolesc Med* 2010;164(9):794–802.

Preis SR, Massaro JM, et al. Abdominal subcutaneous and visceral adipose tissue and insulin resistance in the Framingham heart study. *Obesity (Silver Spring)* 2010;18(11):2191–2198.

Rubin J, Chang HJ, Agatston AS, et al. Association between high-sensitivity C-reactive protein and coronary plaque subtypes assessed by 64-slice coronary computed tomography angiography in an asymptomatic population. *Circ Cardiovasc Imaging* 2011;4(3):201–209.

Rubin J, Nasir K, Agatston AS, et al. Coronary calcium score and outcomes. *Curr Cardiovasc Imaging Rep* 2010;3:342–349.

Tonstad S, Butler T, et al. Type of vegetarian diet, body weight, and prevalence of type 2 diabetes. *Diabetes Care* 2009;32(5):791–796.

Xu WL, Atti AR, et al. Midlife overweight and obesity increase late-life dementia risk: A population-based twin study. *Neurology* 2011;76(18):1568–1574.

CHAPTER 3: THE PERILS OF PROGRESS

Cordain, L. *The Paleo Diet: Lose Weight and Get Healthy by Eating the Foods You Were Designed to Eat.* Hoboken, NJ: Wiley, 2010.

Diamond, J. *Guns, Germs, and Steel: The Fates of Human Societies.* New York: W.W. Norton, 1997.

Eaton, SB. *The Paleolithic Prescription: A Program of Diet and Exercise and a Design for Living.* New York: HarperCollins, 1989.

Rodale, M. *Organic Manifesto: How Organic Food Can Heal Our Planet, Feed the World, and Keep Us Safe.* Emmaus, PA: Rodale Books, 2010.

CHAPTER 4: WHAT'S WRONG (AND RIGHT) WITH "DIETS"

Arnold JM, Yusuf S, et al. Prevention of heart failure in patients in the Heart Outcomes Prevention Evaluation (HOPE) Study. *Circulation* 2003;107(9):1284–1290.

See also references for Part 3.

CHAPTER 5: EAT TO LIVE . . . WELL

Benetou V, Trichopoulou A, et al. Conformity to traditional Mediterranean diet and cancer incidence: The Greek EPIC cohort. *Br J Cancer* 2008;99(1):191–195.

Beunza JJ, Toledo E, et al. Adherence to the Mediterranean diet, long-term weight change, and incident overweight or obesity: The Seguimiento Universidad de Navarra (SUN) cohort. *Am J Clin Nutr* 2010;92(6):1484–1493.

De Lorgeril M, Renaud S, et al. Mediterranean alpha-linolenic acid-rich diet in secondary prevention of coronary heart disease. *Lancet* 1994;343(8911):1454–1459.

Giugliano F, Maiorino MI, et al. Adherence to Mediterranean diet and erectile dysfunction in men with type 2 diabetes. *J Sex Med* 2010;7(5):1911–1917.

Hu FB, Stampfer MJ, et al. Dietary fat intake and the risk of coronary heart disease in women. *N Engl J Med* 1997;337(21):1491–1499.

Jakobsen MU, Dethlefsen C, et al. Intake of carbohydrates compared with intake of saturated fatty acids and risk of myocardial infarction: importance of the glycemic index. *Am J Clin Nutr* 2010;91(6):1764–1768.

Leidy HJ, Tang M, et al. The effects of consuming frequent, higher protein meals on appetite and satiety during weight loss in overweight/obese men. *Obesity (Silver Spring)* 2011;19(4):818–824.

Mahoney CR, Taylor HA. Effect of breakfast composition on cognitive processes in elementary school children. *Physiol Behav* 2005;85(5):635–645.

McKeown NM, Troy LM, et al. Whole- and refined-grain intakes are differentially associated with abdominal visceral and subcutaneous adiposity in healthy adults: The Framingham Heart Study. *Am J Clin Nutr* 2010;92(5):1165–1171.

Mozaffarian D, Katan MB, et al. Trans fatty acids and cardiovascular disease. *N Engl J Med* 2006;354(15):1601–1613.

Oh K, Hu FB, et al. Dietary fat intake and risk of coronary heart disease in women: 20 years of follow-up of the Nurses' Health Study. *Am J Epidemiol* 2005;161(7):672–679.

O'Neil CE, Nicklas TA, et al. Whole-grain consumption is associated with diet quality and nutrient intake in adults: The National Health and Nutrition Examination Survey, 1999–2004. *J Am Diet Assoc* 2010;110(10):1461–1468.

Park Y, Subar AF, et al. Dietary fiber intake and mortality in the NIH-AARP Diet and Health Study. *Arch Intern Med* 2011. Epub ahead of print.

Salas-Salvadó J, Bulló M, et al. Reduction in the incidence of type 2 diabetes with the Mediterranean diet: Results of the PREDIMED-Reus nutrition intervention randomized trial. *Diabetes Care* 2011;34(1).14–19.

Trichopoulou A, Bamia C, et al. Conformity to traditional Mediterranean diet and breast cancer risk in the Greek EPIC (European Prospective Investigation into Cancer and Nutrition) cohort. *Am J Clin Nutr* 2010;92(3):620–625.

See also references for Part 3.

CHAPTER 6: NEW CONCERNS ABOUT GLUTEN

Brar P, Kwon GY, et al. Change in lipid profile in celiac disease: Beneficial effect of gluten-free diet. *Am J Med* 2006;119(9):786–790.

Briani C, Samaroo D, et al. Celiac disease: From gluten to autoimmunity. *Autoimmun Rev* 2008;7(8):644–650.

Geary N, Garcia O. *The Food Cure for Kids: A Nutritional Approach to Your Child's Wellness.* Guilford, CT: Lyons Press, 2010.

Green, Peter HR. *Celiac Disease: A Hidden Epidemic.* New York: William Morrow, 2010.

Makovický P, Rimárová K. The importance of and options available for screening of celiac disease. *Vnitr Lek* 2011;57(2):183–187.

CHAPTER 7: THE POWER OF THE DINING TABLE

Aatola H, Koivistoinen T, et al. Lifetime fruit and vegetable consumption and arterial pulse wave velocity in adulthood: The Cardiovascular Risk in Young Finns Study. *Circulation* 2010;122(24):2521–2528.

Aberg MA, Pedersen NL, et al. Cardiovascular fitness is associated with cognition in young adulthood. *Proc Natl Acad Sci USA* 2009;106(49):20906–20911.

Anderson SE, Whitaker RC. Household routines and obesity in US preschool-aged children. *Pediatrics* 2010;125(3):420–428.

Bernstein AM, Bloom DE, et al. Relation of food cost to healthfulness of diet among US women. *Am J Clin Nutr* 2010;92(5):1197–1203

Collins CE, Okely AD, et al. Parent diet modification, child activity, or both in obese children: An RCT. *Pediatrics* 2011;127(4):619–627.

Esposito K, Maiorino MI, et al. Prevention and control of type 2 diabetes by Mediterranean diet: A systematic review. *Diabetes Res Clin Pract* 2010;89(2):97–102.

Fitzpatrick E, Edmunds LS, et al. Positive effects of family dinner are undone by television viewing. *J Am Diet Assoc* 2007;107(4):666–671.

Fulkerson JA, Kubik MY, et al. Are there nutritional and other benefits associated with family meals among at-risk youth? *J Adolesc Health* 2009;45(4):389–395.

Gillman MW, Rifas-Shiman SL, et al. Family dinner and diet quality among older children and adolescents. *Arch Fam Med* 2000;9(3):235–240.

Gorman N, Lackney JA, et al. Designer schools: The role of school space and architecture in obesity prevention. *Obesity* (Silver Spring) 2007;15(11):2521–2530.

Hammons AJ, Fiese BH. Is frequency of shared family meals related to the nutritional health of children and adolescents? *Pediatrics* 2011;127(6):e1565–1574.

Harris Interactive. "Three in Ten Americans Love to Cook, While One in Five Do Not Enjoy It or Don't Cook." Harris Poll 93, July 27, 2010.

Henderson, CC. The State of Nutrition and Physical Activity in Our Schools. Environment and Human Health, 2004. http://www.ehhi.org/reports/obesity/obesity_report04.pdf.

Hollar D, Messiah SE, Agatston AS, et al. Healthier options for public schoolchildren program improves weight and blood pressure in 6- to 13-year-olds. *J Am Diet Assoc* 2010:110(2):261–267.

Mhurchu CN. Food costs and healthful diets: The need for solution-oriented research and policies. *Am J Clin Nutr* 2010;92(5):1007–1008.

National Center on Addiction and Substance Abuse at Columbia University. "The Importance of Family Dinners VI," September 2010. http://www.casacolumbia.org/upload/2010/2010 0922familydinners6.pdf.

Park S, Sappenfield WM, et al. The impact of the availability of school vending machines on eating behavior during lunch: The Youth Physical Activity and Nutrition Survey. Am Diet Assoc 2010;110(10):1532–1536.

Pereira MA, Erickson E, et al. Breakfast frequency and quality may affect glycemia and appetite in adults and children. *J Nutr* 2011;141(1):163–168.

Raynor HA, Kilanowski CK, et al. A cost-analysis of adopting a healthful diet in a family-based obesity treatment program. *J Am Diet Assoc* 2002;102(5):645–656.

Singh GK, Siahpush M, et al. Neighborhood socioeconomic conditions, built environments, and childhood obesity. *Health Aff (Millwood)* 2010;29(3):503–512.

Smith KJ, Gall SL, et al. Skipping breakfast: Longitudinal associations with cardiometabolic risk factors in the Childhood Determinants of Adult Health Study. *Am J Clin Nutr* 2010;92(6):1316–1325.

Sweitzer SJ, Briley ME, et al. Lunch is in the bag: Increasing fruits, vegetables, and whole grains in sack lunches of preschool-aged children. *J Am Diet Assoc* 2010;110(7):1058–1064.

Thomas M, Desai KK, et al. How credit card payments increase unhealthy food purchases: Visceral regulation of vices. *Journal of Consumer Research* 2011:38(1).

US Council of Economic Advisors. Teens and their parents in the 21st century: An examination of trends in teen behavior and the role of parental involvement. Washington, DC, 2000. http://clinton3.nara.gov/WH/EOP/CEA/html/Teens_Paper_Final.pdf.

CHAPTER 8: THE HIGH COST OF INACTIVITY

Agatston A. *The South Beach Diet Supercharged.* Emmaus, PA: Rodale Books, 2008.

Association for Pet Obesity. "Fat Pets Getting Fatter According to Latest Survey." http://www.petobesityprevention.com/fat-pets-getting-fatter-according-to-latest-survey.

Auchincloss AH, Diez Roux AV, et al. Neighborhood resources for physical activity and healthy foods and incidence of type 2 diabetes mellitus: The Multi-Ethnic study of Atherosclerosis. *Arch Intern Med* 2009;169(18):1698–1704.

Babraj JA, Vollaard NB, et al. Extremely short duration high intensity interval training substantially improves insulin action in young healthy males. *BMC Endocr Disord* 2009;9:3.

Barros RM, Silver EJ, et al. School recess and group classroom behavior. *Pediatrics* 2009;123(2):431–436.

Bassett DR Jr, Wyatt HR, et al. Pedometer-measured physical activity and health behaviors in US adults. *Med Sci Sports Exerc* 2010;42(10):1819–1825.

Bassuk SS, Manson JE. Physical activity and cardiovascular disease prevention in women: A review of the epidemiologic evidence. *Nutr Metab Cardiovasc Dis* 2010;20(6):467–473.

Church TS, Blair SN, et al. Effects of aerobic and resistance training on hemoglobin A1c levels in patients with type 2 diabetes: A randomized controlled trial. *JAMA* 2010;304(20):2253–2262.

Eliassen AH, Hankinson SE, et al. Physical activity and risk of breast cancer among postmenopausal women. *Arch Intern Med* 2010;170(19):1758–1764.

Erickson KI, Voss MW, et al. Exercise training increases size of hippocampus and improves memory. *Proc Natl Acad Sci USA* 2011;108(7):3017–3022.

Farrell SW, Fitzgerald SJ, et al. Cardiorespiratory fitness, adiposity, and all-cause mortality in women. *Med Sci Sports Exerc* 2010;42(11):2006–2012.

Gibala MJ, McGee SL. Metabolic adaptations to short-term high-intensity interval training: A little pain for a lot of gain? *Exerc Sport Sci Rev* 2008;36(2):58–63.

Guthold R, Cowan MJ, et al. Physical activity and sedentary behavior among schoolchildren: A 34-country comparison *J Pediatr* 2010;157(1):43–49.

Hamilton MT, Hamilton DG, et al. Role of low energy expenditure and sitting in obesity, metabolic syndrome, type 2 diabetes, and cardiovascular disease. *Diabetes* 2007;56(11):2655–2667.

Healy GN, Matthews CE, et al. Sedentary time and cardio-metabolic biomarkers in US adults: NHANES 2003–06. *Eur Heart J* 2011;32(5):590–597.

Ingul CB, Tjonna AE, et al. Impaired cardiac function among obese adolescents: Effect of aerobic interval training. *Arch Pediatr Adolesc Med* 2010;164(9):852–859.

Katzmarzyk PT. Physical activity, sedentary behavior, and health: Paradigm paralysis or paradigm shift? *Diabetes* 2010;59(11):2717–2725.

Lee DC, Sui X, et al. Comparisons of leisure-time physical activity and cardiorespiratory fitness as predictors of all-cause mortality in men and women. *Br J Sports Med* 2011;45(6):504–510.

Levine JA. Health-chair reform: Your chair —comfortable but deadly. *Diabetes* 2010;59(11):2715–2716.

Marshall S, Gyi D. Evidence of health risks from occupational sitting: Where do we stand? *Am J Prev Med* 2010;39(4):389–391.

Martinez-Gomez D, Tucker J, et al. Associations between sedentary behavior and blood pressure in young children. *Arch Pediatr Adolesc Med* 2009;163(8):724–730.

Morris JN, Heady JA, et al. Coronary heart disease and physical activity of work. *Lancet* 1953; Nov 21;265(6795):1053–1057; contd.

———. Coronary heart disease and physical activity of work. *Lancet* 1953; Nov 28;265(6796):1111–1120; concl.

Nieman DC, Henson DA, et al. Upper respiratory tract infection is reduced in physically fit and active adults. *Br J Sports Med* 2010.

O'Keefe JH, Vogel R, et al. Achieving hunter-gatherer fitness in the 21st century: Back to the future. *Am J Med* 2010;123(12):1082–1086.

———. Exercise like a hunter-gatherer: A prescription for organic physical fitness. *Prog Cardiovasc Dis* 2011;53(6):471–479.

Owen CG, Nightingale CM, et al. Family dog ownership and levels of physical activity in childhood: Findings from the Child Heart and Health Study in England. *Am J Public Health* 2010;100(9):1669–1671.

Patel AV, Bernstein L, et al. Leisure time spent sitting in relation to total mortality in a prospective cohort of US adults. *Am J Epidemiol* 2010;172(4):419–429.

Powell LM, Szczypka G, et al. Trends in exposure to television food advertisements among children and adolescents in the United States. *Arch Pediatr Adolesc Med* 2010;164(9):794–802.

Reeves MJ, Rafferty AP, et al. The impact of dog walking on leisure-time physical activity: Results from a population-based survey of Michigan adults. *J Phys Act Health* 2011;8(3):436–444.

Sirard JR, Patnode CD, et al. Dog ownership and adolescent physical activity. *Am J Prev Med* 2011;40(3):334–337.

Thomas IM, Sayers SP, et al. Bike, walk, and wheel: A way of life in Columbia, Missouri. *Am J Prev Med* 2009;37(6 Suppl 2):S322–328.

Trigona B, Aggoun Y, et al. Preclinical noninvasive markers of atherosclerosis in children and adolescents with type 1 diabetes are influenced by physical activity. *J Pediatr* 2010;157(4):533–539.

Tudor-Locke C, Johnson WD, et al. Frequently reported activities by intensity for US adults: The American Time-Use Survey. *Am J Prev Med* 2010;39(4):e13–20.

Vandelanotte C, Sugiyama T, et al. Associations of leisure-time Internet and computer use with overweight and obesity, physical activity and sedentary behaviors: Cross-sectional study. *J Med Internet Res* 2009;11(3):e28.

Wolin KY, Yan Y, et al. Physical activity and colon cancer prevention: A meta-analysis. *Br J Cancer* 2009;100(4):611–616.

CHAPTER 9: WAKE UP AND GET SOME SLEEP!

Beebe DW, Byars KC. Adolescents with obstructive sleep apnea adhere poorly to positive airway pressure (PAP), but PAP users show improved attention and school performance. *PLoS One* 2011;6(3):e16924.

Beebe DW, Ris MD, et al. The association between sleep disordered breathing, academic grades, and cognitive and behavioral functioning among overweight subjects during middle to late childhood. *Sleep* 2010;33(11):1447–1456.

Bixler EO, Vgontzas AN, et al. Sleep disordered breathing in children in a general population sample: Prevalence and risk factors. *Sleep* 2009;32(6):731–736.

Brunetti L, Tesse R, et al. Sleep-disordered breathing in obese children: The southern Italy experience. *Chest* 2010;137(5):1085–1090.

Ferrie JE, Shipley MJ, et al. A prospective study of change in sleep duration: Associations with mortality in the Whitehall II cohort. *Sleep* 2007;30(12):1659–1666.

Gimble JM, Sutton GM, et al. Prospective influences of circadian clocks in adipose tissue and metabolism. *Nat Rev Endocrinol* 2011;7(2):98–107.

Gooley JJ, Chamberlain K, et al. Exposure to room light before bedtime suppresses melatonin onset and shortens melatonin duration in humans. *J Clin Endocrinol Metab* 2011;96(3):E463–472.

Javaheri S, Storfer-Isser A, et al. Association of short and long sleep durations with insulin sensitivity in adolescents. *J Pediatr* 2011;158(4):617–623.

Johansson K, Neovius M, et al. Effect of a very low energy diet on moderate and severe obstructive sleep apnoea in obese men: A randomised controlled trial. *BMJ* 2009;339:b4609.

King CR, Knutson KL, et al. Short sleep duration and incident coronary artery calcification. *JAMA* 2008;300(24):2859–2866.

Landhuis CE, Poulton R, et al. Childhood sleep time and long-term risk for obesity: A 32-year prospective birth cohort study. *Pediatrics* 2008;122(5):955–960.

Lytle LA, Pasch KE, et al. The relationship between sleep and weight in a sample of adolescents. *Obesity (Silver Spring)* 2011;19(2):324–331.

Nedeltcheva AV, Kilkus JM, et al. Insufficient sleep undermines dietary efforts to reduce adiposity. *Ann Intern Med* 2010;153(7):435–441.

Patel SR, Malhotra A, et al. Association between reduced sleep and weight gain in women. *Am J Epidemiol* 2006;164(10):947–954.

Prinz P. Sleep, appetite, and obesity: What is the link? *PLoS Med* 2004;1(3):e61.

Seegers V, Petit D, et al. Short sleep duration and body mass index: A prospective longitudinal study in preadolescence. *Am J Epidemiol* 2011;173(6):621–629.

Spruyt K, Molfese DL, et al. Sleep duration, sleep regularity, body weight, and metabolic homeostasis in school-aged children. *Pediatrics.* 2011;127(2):e345–352.

Taheri S, Lin L, et al. Short sleep duration is associated with reduced leptin, elevated ghrelin, and increased body mass index. *PLoS Med* 2004;1(3):e62.

Wolk R, Shamsuzzaman AS, et al. Obesity, sleep apnea, and hypertension. *Hypertension* 2003;42(6):1067–1074.

Wolk R, Somers VK. Obesity-related cardiovascular disease: Implications of obstructive sleep apnea. *Diabetes Obes Metab* 2006;8(3):250–260.

———. Sleep and the metabolic syndrome. *Exp Physiol* 2007;92(1):67–78.

PART 2: THE SOUTH BEACH DIET WAKE-UP PROGRAM

See references for Part 1 and Part 3.

PART 3: MEGAFOODS AND MEGARECIPES FOR HEALTHY EATING

Banel DK, Hu FB. Effects of walnut consumption on blood lipids and other cardiovascular risk factors: A meta-analysis and systematic review. *Am J Clin Nutr* 2009;90(1):56–63.

Basu A, Rhone M, et al. Berries: Emerging impact on cardiovascular health. *Nutr Rev* 2010;68(3):168–77.

Bazzano LA, Thompson AM, et al. Non-soy legume consumption lowers cholesterol levels: A meta-analysis of randomized controlled trials. *Nutr Metab Cardiovasc Dis* 2011;21(2):94–103.

Borriello A, Cucciolla V, et al. Dietary polyphenols: Focus on resveratrol, a promising agent in the prevention of cardiovascular diseases and control of glucose homeostasis. *Nutr Metab Cardiovasc Dis* 2010;20(8):618–625.

Buil-Cosiales P, Irimia P, et al. Dietary fibre intake is inversely associated with carotid intima-media thickness: A cross-sectional assessment in the PREDIMED study. *Eur J Clin Nutr* 2009;63(10):1213–1219.

Carpentier S, Knaus M, et al. Associations between lutein, zeaxanthin, and age-related macular degeneration: An overview. *Crit Rev Food Sci Nutr* 2009;49(4):313–326.

Castañer O, Fitó M, et al. The effect of olive oil polyphenols on antibodies against oxidized LDL: A randomized clinical trial. *Clin Nutr* 2011. Epub ahead of print.

Darvesh AS, Carroll RT, et al. Oxidative stress and Alzheimer's disease: Dietary polyphenols as potential therapeutic agents. *Expert Rev Neurother* 2010;10(5):729–745.

Djoussé L, Hopkins PN, et al. Chocolate consumption is inversely associated with prevalent coronary heart disease: The National Heart, Lung, and Blood Institute Family Heart Study. *Clin Nutr* 2011;30(1):38–43.

Djoussé L, Pankow JS, et al. Influence of saturated fat and linolenic acid on the association between intake of dairy products and blood pressure. *Hypertension* 2006;48(2):335–341.

Elwood PC, Strain JJ, et al. Milk consumption, stroke, and heart attack risk: Evidence from the Caerphilly cohort of older men. *J Epidemiol Community Health* 2005;59(6):502–505.

Erdman JW Jr, Ford NA, et al. Are the health attributes of lycopene related to its antioxidant function? *Arch Biochem Biophys* 2009;483(2):229–235.

Erlund I, Koli R, et al. Favorable effects of berry consumption on platelet function, blood pressure, and HDL cholesterol. *Am J Clin Nutr* 2008;87(2):323–331.

Etminan M, Takkouche B, et al. The role of tomato products and lycopene in the prevention of prostate cancer: A meta-analysis of observational studies. *Cancer Epidemiol Biomarkers Prev* 2004;13(3):340–345.

Faghih S, Abadi AR, et al. Comparison of the effects of cows' milk, fortified soy milk, and calcium supplement on weight and fat loss in premenopausal overweight and obese women. *Nutr Metab Cardiovasc Dis* 2010.

Fang N, Li Q, et al. Inhibition of growth and induction of apoptosis in human cancer cell lines by an ethyl acetate fraction from shiitake mushrooms. *J Altern Complement Med* 2006;12(2):125–132.

Faridi Z, Njike VY, et al. Acute dark chocolate and cocoa ingestion and endothelial function: A randomized controlled crossover trial. *Am J Clin Nutr* 2008;88(1):58–63.

Greenberg JA, Chow G, et al. Caffeinated coffee consumption, cardiovascular disease, and heart valve disease in the elderly (from the Framingham Study). *Am J Cardiol* 2008;102(11):1502–1508.

He K, Liu K, et al. Associations of dietary long-chain n-3 polyunsaturated fatty acids and fish with biomarkers of inflammation and endothelial activation (from the Multi-Ethnic Study of Atherosclerosis [MESA]). *Am J Cardio* 2009;103(9):1238–1243.

He M, van Dam RM, et al. Whole-grain, cereal fiber, bran, and germ intake and the risks of all-cause and cardiovascular disease-specific mortality among women with type 2 diabetes mellitus. *Circulation* 2010;121(20):2162–2168.

Hearst R, Nelson D, et al. An examination of antibacterial and antifungal properties of constituents of shiitake (*Lentinula edodes*) and oyster (*Pleurotus ostreatus*) mushrooms. *Complement Ther Clin Pract* 2009;15(1):5–7.

Heiss C, Kelm M. Chocolate consumption, blood pressure, and cardiovascular risk. *Eur Heart J* 2010;31(13):1554–1556.

Hudthagosol C, Haddad EH, et al. Pecans acutely increase plasma postprandial antioxidant capacity and catechins and decrease LDL oxidation in humans. *J Nutr* 2011;141(1):56–62.

Huxley R, Lee CM, et al. Coffee, decaffeinated coffee, and tea consumption in relation to incident type 2 diabetes mellitus: A systematic review with meta-analysis. *Arch Intern Med* 2009;169(22):2053–2063.

Jenkins DJ, Chiavaroli L, et al. Adding monounsaturated fatty acids to a dietary portfolio of cholesterol-lowering foods in hypercholesterolemia. *CMAJ* 2010;182(18):1961–1967.

Joseph JA, Shukitt-Hale B, et al. Grape juice, berries, and walnuts affect brain aging and behavior. *J Nutr* 2009;139(9):1813S–1817S.

Kaminski BM, Steinhilber D, et al. Phytochemicals resveratrol and sulforaphane as potential agents for enhancing the anti-tumor activities of conventional cancer therapies. *Curr Pharm Biotechnol* 2011.

Kendall CW, Josse AR, et al. Nuts, metabolic syndrome and diabetes. *Br J Nutr* 2010; 104(4):465–473.

Kim J, Lee HJ, et al. Naturally occurring phytochemicals for the prevention of Alzheimer's disease. *J Neurochem* 2010;112(6):1415–1430.

Krikorian R, Shidler MD, et al. Blueberry supplementation improves memory in older adults. *J Agric Food Chem* 2010;58(7):3996–4000.

López S, Bermúdez B, et al. Distinctive postprandial modulation of β cell function and insulin sensitivity by dietary fats: Monounsaturated compared with saturated fatty acids *Am J Clin Nutr* 2008;88(3):638–644.

López-Miranda J, Pérez-Jiménez F, et al. Olive oil and health: Summary of the II international conference on olive oil and health consensus report, Jaén and Córdoba (Spain) 2008. *Nutr Metab Cardiovasc Dis* 2010;20(4):284–294.

Maki KC, Reeves MS, et al. Green tea catechin consumption enhances exercise-induced abdominal fat loss in overweight and obese adults. *J Nutr* 2009;139(2):264–270.

Mandel SA, Amit T, et al. Understanding the broad-spectrum neuroprotective action profile of green tea polyphenols in aging and neurodegenerative diseases. *J Alzheimers Dis* 2011.

Mercken EM, de Cabo R. A toast to your health, one drink at a time. *Am J Clin Nutr* 2010;92(1):1–2.

Mitchell DC, Lawrence FR, et al. Consumption of dry beans, peas, and lentils could improve diet quality in the US population. *J Am Diet Assoc* 2009;109(5):909–913.

Monagas M, Khan N, et al. Effect of cocoa powder on the modulation of inflammatory biomarkers in patients at high risk of cardiovascular disease. *Am J Clin Nutr* 2009;90(5):1144–1150.

Nagao A. Absorption and function of dietary carotenoids. *Forum Nutr* 2009;61:55–63.

Pan A, Yu D, et al. Meta-analysis of the effects of flaxseed interventions on blood lipids. *Am J Clin Nutr* 2009;90(2):288–297.

Razquin C, Martinez JA, et al. A 3 years follow-up of a Mediterranean diet rich in virgin olive oil is associated with high plasma antioxidant capacity and reduced body weight gain. *Eur J Clin Nutr* 2009;63(12):1387–1393.

Riediger ND, Othman RA, et al. A systemic review of the roles of n-3 fatty acids in health and disease. *J Am Diet Assoc* 2009;109(4):668–679.

Riso P, Martini D, et al. Effect of broccoli intake on markers related to oxidative stress and cancer risk in healthy smokers and nonsmokers. *Nutr Cancer* 2009;61(2):232–237.

Sabaté J, Oda K, et al. Nut consumption and blood lipid levels: A pooled analysis of 25 intervention trials. *Arch Intern Med* 2010;170(9):821–827.

Seeram NP. Berry fruits for cancer prevention: Current status and future prospects. *J Agric Food Chem* 2008;56(3):630–635.

Singh KK, Mridula D, et al. Flaxseed: A potential source of food, feed and fiber. *Crit Rev Food Sci Nutr* 2011;51(3):210–222.

Stevenson DG, Eller FJ, et al. Oil and tocopherol content and composition of pumpkin seed oil in 12 cultivars. *J Agric Food Chem* 2007;55(10):4005–4013.

Wennberg M, Bergdahl IA, et al. Fish consumption and myocardial infarction: A second prospective biomarker study from northern Sweden. *Am J Clin Nutr* 2011;93(1):27–36.

Wu JN, Ho SC, et al. Coffee consumption and risk of coronary heart diseases: A meta-analysis of 21 prospective cohort studies. *Int J Cardiol* 2009;137(3):216–225.

Ylönen K, Alfthan G, et al. Dietary intakes and plasma concentrations of carotenoids and tocopherols in relation to glucose metabolism in subjects at high risk of type 2 diabetes: The Botnia Dietary Study. *Am J Clin Nutr* 2003;77(6):1434–1441.

Yung LM, Leung FP, et al. Tea polyphenols benefit vascular function. *Inflammopharmacology* 2008;16(5):230–234.

Zhang Z, Lanza E, et al. A high legume low glycemic index diet improves serum lipid profiles in men. *Lipids* 2010;45(9):765–775.

INDEX

Underscored page references indicate boxed text. **Boldface** references indicate photographs.

Advertising, to children, 38, 39, 40
Agatston Score, 17. *See also* Calcium Score
Agatston Urban Nutrition Initiative (AUNI), 109, 121–22
Aging
  inflammation and, 10, 22
  junk foods promoting, 63
  premature, 15–16, 19–20, 32–36, 124
  sleep habits and, 159
Agricultural revolution, 42–43, 103, 129
Agriculture, government policies on, 54
Alcohol
  health effects of, 80–81
    sleeplessness, 145, 245
    snoring, 247
  with restaurant meals, 219, 222
Almon, Marie, 119
Almonds
  Almond-Sunflower Cod with Tomato Tartar Sauce, 284–85
  Blueberry Buttermilk Muffins with Almonds, 179, 266–67
  Chocolate Bark with Cranberries, Almonds, and Pecans, 181, 306
Alzheimer's disease, 5, 21, 27, 88, 123, 255
Amino acids, 89, 90, 98
Angina, 154
Anti-inflammatory drugs, 84
Antioxidant drinks, 63
Antioxidants, 27, 28, 29
  exercise and, 28, 29, 125
  food sources of, 28, 29, 63, 77, 254–55, 257, 258
Appetite suppressant pills, 62
Apples
  Apple-Baked Beans with Smoked Ham, 296
  Sweet and Savory Breakfast Burritos with Sautéed Apples, 179, 262
Apricots
  Chicken Cutlets with Apricot Sauce and Pistachios, 212, 278
Arthritis, 7, 21, 29, 36, 76, 84, 98, 99, 125, 133, 148, 158, 226, 242, 257
Asthma, 3, 33, 36, 76, 82, 248, 257
Atherosclerosis, 5, 8, 9, 10, 17, 19, 24, 30–31, 32, 33–36, 136, 154, 257
AUNI. *See* Agatston Urban Nutrition Initiative

Avocados
  Black Bean Chili with Tangerine-Avocado Salsa, 193, 286–87
  Chunky Guacamole Salad, 212, 301
  health benefits of, 254
  Layered Salad with Creamy Cilantro Dressing, 294–95

Baby food, homemade, 100–101
Back extension with rotation, 236, **236**
Baked goods, types to eliminate, 172
Bannister, Roger, 140
Barley
  Golden Barley Pilaf with Herb-Roasted Carrots, 300
  health benefits of, 257
Basil
  Sweet Potato Salad with Fresh Basil, 303
Beans
  Apple-Baked Beans with Smoked Ham, 296
  Black Bean Chili with Tangerine-Avocado Salsa, 193, 286–87
  canned, 213
  cooking, 210
  health benefits of, 254
  on shopping list, 308
Bedroom. *See also* Sleep
  de-cluttering, 170, 174–75
  enhancing sleep in, 242–43
Bedtime snacks, 244
Bedtime wind-down routine, 245–47, 250–51
Beef. *See also* Meats
  Better Beef Burgundy, 280–81
  Sesame Flank Steak with Fresh Blueberry Salsa, 279
Belly fat, 10, 16, 17, 22, 23–24, 25, 25–26, 70, 75, 81, 102, 126
Beriberi, 46, 75
Berries. *See also specific berries*
  antioxidants in, 63, 76
  health benefits of, 254–55
Beverages
  on shopping list, 313
  sugar in, 201
  types to eliminate, 172
Bike, stationary, 232, 233
Biological clocks, 159

Blood chemistries, as indicator of health, 68–70
Blood pressure. *See also* High blood pressure
  lowering, 85, 137, 151, 256, 257
  in vegetarians, 93
Blood sugar
  dips in
    in reactive hypoglycemia, 23
    from sugar, 200
    from undereating, 177
  fruit juice and, 77
  in metabolic syndrome, 26
  stabilizing
    on Phase 1 of South Beach Diet, 68, 183
    with snacks, 180
  swings in
    fiber controlling, 78, 79
    foods causing, 24, 76
    hunger and cravings from, 67, 75, 154,
      155, 183, 184, 185
    in metabolic syndrome, 102
    protein preventing, 89, 199
Blueberries
  Blueberry Buttermilk Muffins with
    Almonds, 179, 266–67
  health benefits of, 254–55
  Multigrain Blueberry Cobbler, 181, 304–5
  Sesame Flank Steak with Fresh Blueberry
    Salsa, 279
Body mass index (BMI), 70
Bok choy
  Stir-Fried Garlic Shrimp with Bok Choy,
    193, 289
Bone health, protein for, 89
Brain
  exercise improving, 123–24
  hippocampus of, 123, 124
Bread
  Pumpkin-Cranberry Breakfast Bread, 179,
    264–65
  with restaurant meals, 217–18
  white, 46, 61
  whole grain, 196
Breakfast
  experiment on carbs in, 74
  guidelines for, 178–80
  on-the-go, 192
  recipes for, 262–68
  research on carbs in, 74
Breast cancer, 27, 80, 82, 125, 126, 256, 257
Broccolette
  Broccolette with Brown Rice and Walnuts,
    298
Broccoli
  Green and White Florets with Toasted
    Pumpkin Seeds, 297
Bulgur
  Lentil-Bulgur Salad with Summer Squash
    and Walnuts, 193, 292–93

Burkitt, Denis, 78
Burritos
  Sweet and Savory Breakfast Burritos with
    Sautéed Apples, 179, 262
Buying clubs, 204

Cabbage
  Spiced Pork Skewers with Napa Salad, 282–83
Cabbage Soup Diet, 58
Caffeine
  sleeplessness from, 145, 244–45, 248–49
  for staying awake, 160–61
Calcified plaque, 17
Calcium Score, 17, 18, 27, 154
Calorie counting, avoiding, 95, 177, 217
Calorie expenditure
  of hunter-gatherers, 128–29
  technology reducing, 129–30
Calorie-restricted diets, 57, 58, 59, 60
Calories
  burned by nonexercise activity, 131
  empty, 24, 46, 61, 72, 75, 77, 80, 95, 172,
    201, 203
  extra, in restaurant meals, 216
  overconsumption of, malnutrition and, 62
  overemphasis on, in American diet, 60,
    61, 62
Cancer, 5. *See also* Breast cancer
  alcohol and, 80, 257
  diabetes and, 27
  dietary fats and, 84, 88
  predictors of death from, 10
  preventing, 36, 76, 125–26, 255, 256, 257,
    258
  risk factors for, 6, 7, 21, 29
Candy, types to eliminate, 172
Carbohydrates
  bad, 183, 185
  evaluating quality of, 95
  good, 184
    vs. bad, 73–74, 77
    fruits and vegetables, 76–77, 177
    introducing children to, 77–78
    on Phase 2 of South Beach Diet, 69
    in snacks, 180–81
    whole grains, 75, 177, 196–97
  processed, 97, 103, 107
  in traditional heart-healthy diets, 72
  in vegetarian diet, 92–93
Cardiovascular conditioning, 224, 227. *See
    also* Exercise
Carotid arteries, 16–17, 18, 35
Carrots
  Chickpea and Carrot Frittata, 210, 263
  Golden Barley Pilaf with Herb-Roasted
    Carrots, 300
  Lemony Tomato Hummus with Carrot
    Chips, 193, 269

Cataracts, foods preventing, 255, 257
Cauliflower
    Green and White Florets with Toasted
        Pumpkin Seeds, 297
    Mighty Mac and "Cheese," 193, 290–91
Celiac disease, 97–99, 102–3, 104, 104, 105,
    106, 107
Chediak, Alejandro, 153, 157–61, 164
Cheese
    Greens Gratin with Turkey Bacon, 299
    Mighty Mac and "Cheese," 193, 290–91
    Quinoa and Tomato Salad with Goat
        Cheese, 302
    on shopping list, 311
    types to eliminate, 172
Cheeseburgers, 213, 214
Chek, Paul, 138, 139
Chernow, Ron, 117
Chicken
    Chicken Cutlets with Apricot Sauce and
        Pistachios, 212, 278
    Chicken in Mexican Mole Sauce, 275
    organic, 91
Chicken nuggets, 213, 214
Chickpeas, 210
    Chickpea and Carrot Frittata, 210, 263
    Lemony Tomato Hummus with Carrot
        Chips, 193, 269
Childhood, diseases starting in, 4–5
Children
    advertising directed toward, 38, 39, 40
    atherosclerosis in, 33–36, 136
    benefits of family meals for, 113–17
    breakfast skipping by, 178
    diabetes in, 6, 22–23, 33, 36, 136, 178
    dining out guidelines for, 220–21
    effect of maternal obesity on, 6–7
    exercise for, 167, 226, 227, 238–39
    future health risks for, 14
    improving nutrition for, 13
    inactivity among, 136–37
    introducing healthy foods to, 12, 77–78,
        86–87, 209
    involving, in
        de-cluttering, 176
        food preparation, 215, 259–60
        meal planning and shopping, 208–9
    malnutrition in, 62
    mealtime ground rules for, 188–89
    modeling healthy lifestyle for, 166–67
    overweight and obesity in, 6, 33, 34, 35,
        36, 37–40, 113, 136, 144, 152, 153,
        167, 176, 201
    playground equipment for, 175, 176
    schools promoting health of, 11
    sleep apnea in, 37, 149, 152–53
    sleep deprivation in, 144–45, 156, 160
    sleep-wake cycles of, 159

solving sleep problems of, 248–49
    treats for, 39, 172, 173, 209
    trying new foods, 114–15
Chili
    Black Bean Chili with Tangerine-Avocado
        Salsa, 193, 286–87
Chocolate, dark
    Chocolate Bark with Cranberries,
        Almonds, and Pecans, 181, 306
    health benefits of, 59, 85, 181, 255–56
    on shopping list, 313
Cholesterol
    effect of chocolate on, 85
    foods lowering, 76, 78, 254, 255, 256,
        257, 258
    HDL
        alcohol and, 81
        exercise boosting, 225
        metabolic syndrome and, 26
        trans fats lowering, 87
    high
        from breakfast skipping, 178
        in children, 36
        from fast food, 48
        from restaurant meals, 110, 220
    interacting with other risk factors, 18–19
    LDL
        inactivity increasing, 126
        reduced, in vegetarians, 93
        saturated and trans fats increasing, 84,
            87
Churchill, Winston, 152–53
Cilantro
    Layered Salad with Creamy Cilantro
        Dressing, 294–95
Clothing, for exercise, 232, 234
Clutter
    removing, 169–76
    as symptom of inner turmoil, 169
Cobbler
    Multigrain Blueberry Cobbler, 181, 304–5
Cocoa powder, health benefits of, 256
Coconut oil, 47, 84–85
Cod
    Almond-Sunflower Cod with Tomato
        Tartar Sauce, 284–85
Coffee
    caffeine in, 244
    health benefits of, 255
Cognitive behavioral therapy, for sleep
        problems, 161
Cognitive function, effect of good carbs on,
        74
Cola, caffeine in, 244
Colds, exercise preventing, 127
Colorectal cancer, exercise preventing,
        125–26
Comfort, eating for, 183, 186

Communal meals, 117. *See also* Family meals
Community Supported Agriculture (CSA)
    group, 206
Condiments
    on shopping list, 312–13
    types to eliminate, 172
Cooking at home. *See* Home cooking
Cooking programs, in school, 109–10
Core strengthening. *See also* Exercise
    everyday movements for, 240
    exercises for, 138, 224, 225, 227, 230–31,
        233–34, 234–37, **234–37**
Coronary artery disease. *See also*
        Atherosclerosis; Heart disease
    beginning in childhood, 5
    cranberries preventing, 255
    decline in deaths from, 8
    inflammation and, 21
    patient story about, 111–12
    in young adults, 8, 9
Cortisol, 154, 155, 183, 186
CPAP machine, for sleep apnea, 150
Cranberries
    Chocolate Bark with Cranberries,
        Almonds, and Pecans, 181, 306
    health benefits of, 255
    Pumpkin-Cranberry Breakfast Bread, 179,
        264–65
Cravings
    causes of, 23, 75, 184, 185, 200
    controlling, 66, 67, 68, 69, 177, 183
C-reactive protein (CRP), 10, 201, 256
Crete, fast food in, 48
Crisscross, 235, **235**
Cross-training, 138
Cruciferous vegetables, health benefits of,
    76, 255
CT heart scan, 9, 16, 17
Cucumbers
    Grilled Salmon with Cucumbers and
        Ginger Dressing, 288

Dairy products
    absence of, in hunter-gatherer diet, 42,
        96, 104
    low-fat, 192, 256
    origin of, 43
    protein in, 89
    on shopping list, 311
    types to eliminate, 172
    USDA guidelines for eating, 177
Dark Chocolate Ice Cream Diet, 58–59, 60
Death, premature, 26, 27, 149
Death rates, fiber lowering, 79
De-cluttering, 169–76, 186
Dementia, 27, 29, 36, 123, 124
Depression, 40, 84, 98, 99, 144, 147, 148,
    151, 158

Desserts
    guidelines for, 39, 181–82, 222
    recipes for, 304–6
    in South Beach Diet, 68, 69
Diabetes, type 1, 23, 33, 98
Diabetes, type 2
    alcohol and, 81
    in children, 6, 22–23, 33, 36, 136, 178
    C-reactive protein and, 256
    deaths from, 10, 26–27
    diagnosis of, 26
    in dogs, 133
    foods preventing or controlling, 79, 84,
        191, 254, 255, 256, 257
    health-care costs for, 38
    holistic community approach to, 10–11
    increase in, 3, 8, 42, 100
    low testosterone and, 25
    mouse studies on, 30–31
    patient story about, 111, 112
    preventing, 36, 125, 191
    risk factors for, 22, 33, 37, 51, 88, 126,
        144, 201, 220, 241, 246
    in vegetarians, 92, 93
Diet(s)
    for aesthetics vs. healthy lifestyle, 70
    calories and nutrients in, 60–61
    fad, 56–60
    healthy guidelines for, 177–78
    mouse studies on, 30–32, 35
    observational studies on, 34–35
    poor
        effect on health, 3, 4
        premature aging from, 32–36, 125
Dining out. *See* Restaurant meals
Dining rituals, benefits of, 108–9
Dining table. *See also* Family meals
    de-cluttering, 170
Diseases, chronic
    effect of good fats on, 88
    effect of lifestyle on, 4–5, 9, 10, 41
    epidemic of, 42
    good nutrition preventing, 79
    individuals at low risk for, 70
    inflammation and, 21–22, 27, 84, 157
    overwhelming health-care system, 5
    vegetarianism reducing, 93
Djokovic, Novak, 106–7
Dog walking, 132–33

Eating disorders, 113, 114
Eating out. *See* Restaurant meals
Eating slowly, importance of, 187, 190
Eating triggers, 182–83, 186
Eggs
    for breakfast, 178–79
    Chickpea and Carrot Frittata, 210, 263
    on shopping list, 311

Electronic devices
  interfering with mealtime, 187
  interfering with sleep, 170, 174–75, <u>249</u>,
    250
Elliptical machine, 224, 232, 233
Emotional eating, 183, 186
Empty calories, 24, 46, 61, 72, 75, 77, <u>80</u>, 95,
    <u>172</u>, <u>201</u>, 203
Endocrine disruptors, 51
Endurance athletes
  starch as fuel for, 61–62
Erectile dysfunction, <u>25</u>
Ethnic-themed meals, 193
Everyday activities, for increasing movement,
    224, 237–40
Exercise
  addictive nature of, 124
  benefits of, 9, 10, 29, 121, 123–27, <u>127</u>,
    186, 225–26, 245–46
  best forms of, 138–39
  cautions about, 135
  for children, <u>167</u>, 226, 227, <u>238–39</u>
  community promotion of, 141
  excuses for avoiding, 225
  home, equipment for, 142
  inadequate recommendations for, 133–34
  interval training, 139–40
  lack of (see Inactivity)
  from nonexercise activity thermogenesis
    (NEAT), 131
  in physical education programs, 120–21
  space for, 170, 175
  tips for starting, 226–27
  types of, 224–25
  in Wake Up and Move 2-Week Quick-Start
    Plan, 224, 228–29, <u>230–31</u>, 232–37
  walking, 131–32, <u>132–33</u>, 134, 135,
    139–40, 141
  in workplace, 141–42

Fad diets, 56–60
Family meals
  benefits of, 108, 113–17, 122, 186
  demise of, 47, 108
  parental ground rules for, <u>188–89</u>
  tips for enjoying, 186–87, 190
Farmers' markets, 13, 53, 205–6
Fast food
  advertising of, 38
  avoiding, 202–3, 211, <u>220</u>
  better choices of, <u>218–19</u>
  at birthday parties, <u>115</u>
  for family meals, 109
  government policies enabling, 54
  harmful health effects of, 25, 48, 125, 165
  homemade, 213–14
  money spent on, 110
  oxidant stress from, 125

proliferation of, 47–48
sodium in, 91, 93–94
during travel, 222
types to avoid, <u>219</u>
Fast-food, sedentary lifestyle. See also
    Sedentary lifestyle; Sitting
  effects on health, 4, 5, 8, 10, 12, 32, 48
Fat, belly. See Belly fat
"Fat and fit" individuals, 69–70
Fat burning, during exercise, 140
Fats, dietary
  bad, 79, 84–88, 177
    types to eliminate, <u>173</u>
  evaluating quality of, 95
  good, 82–83, 88, 192, 254
    on Phase 1 of South Beach Diet, 66, <u>68</u>
    on shopping list, 312
  restricted in traditional diets, 71, 72
  studies on, 79, 82, 88
Fertilizers, 50, 53
Fiber
  for breakfast, 178
  for cholesterol reduction, 254, 255
  deficient in American diet, 78, 199
  for diabetes prevention, 257
  in fruits and vegetables, 76, 77
  in good carbohydrates, 73, <u>184</u>
  health benefits of, 78–79
  insoluble, 78–79
  in snacks, 180–81
  soluble, 78
  in whole grains, 75
Fish. See also Cod; Salmon; Shellfish
  buying, 210
  mercury in, 210
  omega-3-rich, 82, 257
Fish oil supplements, 83
Flaxseeds, 82, 83, 256
Flour
  types to eliminate, <u>173</u>
  white, 45, 74–75
Food co-ops, 53, <u>101</u>, 204–5, 210
Food industry, promoting unhealthy eating,
    39, 40
Food labels, reading, <u>196</u>, <u>197</u>, 199, 202,
    203, <u>208–9</u>
Food production, evolution of, 42–48
Food shopping
  on budget, 202–7, 210
  with children, <u>208–9</u>
  guidelines for, 198–99, 202
  list for, <u>184</u>, 196–98, 307–13
  technology affecting, 46–47
  during travel, 223
Food sources, importance of knowing,
    90–92, 95
Food variety, importance of, 253
Fox, Melanie, 118–19

Free radicals, 27, 28, 29, <u>81</u>, 253
French paradox, <u>81</u>
Frittata
    Chickpea and Carrot Frittata, 210, 263
Fruit juices, 77
Fruits. *See also specific fruits*
    canned, 207
    consumed by children, 114, 115–16
    cultivation of, 43–44
    cutting costs on, 204–7
    eating variety of, 66, 95
    eliminated on Phase 1 of South Beach Diet,
        66, <u>68</u>
    frozen, 206–7
    in hunter-gatherer diet, 96
    importance of, 76, 77, 191
    natural sugar in, <u>201</u>
    phytonutrients in, 63, 66
    on shopping list, 308–9
    Toasted Pecan Muesli with Dried Fruit,
        268
    types to eliminate, <u>173</u>
    USDA guidelines for eating, 177
Functional exercise, 9, 138–39. *See also* Core
    strengthening

Garden, edible, 175
Garlic
    Stir-Fried Garlic Shrimp with Bok Choy,
        193, 289
Geary, Natalie, 33
"Generation S," 8. *See also* Sickest generation
Ghrelin, 155
Ginger
    Grilled Salmon with Cucumbers and
        Ginger Dressing, 288
Gluten
    absent from Phase 1 of South Beach Diet,
        99, 102–3
    celiac disease and (*see* Celiac disease)
    increased consumption of, <u>105</u>
    in restaurant meals, 218
    sources of, 97
Gluten-free baby foods, <u>100–101</u>
Gluten-free products, 106
Gluten intolerance, 99, 103, 105, <u>105</u>, 106,
    107
Gluten Solution, South Beach Diet, 103–7
Grain cultivation, history of, 43
Grains. *See also* Whole grains
    absent from hunter-gatherer diet, 96, 103
    refined, introduction of, 45
    USDA guidelines for eating, 177
Greens
    Greens Gratin with Turkey Bacon, 299
Grocery shopping. *See* Food Shopping
Guacamole
    Chunky Guacamole Salad, 212, 301

Ham
    Apple-Baked Beans with Smoked Ham,
        296
Harkavy, Ira, 121
Haub, Mark, 59
Health-care costs, obesity-related, 38
Health-care system, effect of chronic diseases
    on, 5
Healthier Options for Public Schoolchildren
    (HOPS) program, 13, 37, 118–20,
    121, <u>136–37</u>
Health indicators, best, 68–70
Healthy eating, essential principles of, 72,
    94–95, 191–92
Healthy foods, public demand for, 49
Heart attack(s)
    alcohol and, <u>81</u>
    causes of, 5, 9, 17, 24
    predictors of, 16, 17
    preventing, 70, <u>81</u>, 125, 256
    risk factors for, 18–19, 20, 24, <u>25</u>, 26, 37,
        38, 94, 149, 154
    sleep and, 151
    studies on, 82, 134–35
    in young adults, 8
Heart disease. *See also* Coronary artery
    disease
    alcohol and, <u>80</u>, 257
    atherosclerotic plaque and, 8
    in children, <u>6–7</u>, 36, <u>220</u>
    C-reactive protein and, 256
    decreased deaths from, 8
    diabetes and, <u>201</u>
    in dogs, <u>133</u>
    erectile dysfunction and, <u>25</u>
    French paradox and, <u>81</u>
    health-care costs for, 38
    imaging techniques for assessing, 16–18,
        35, 36
    inactivity increasing, 126
    increase in, 3
    patient story about, 15–16, 18
    postpregnancy, <u>6</u>
    predictors of death from, 10
    preventing, 36, 79, 82, 138, 254, 258
    studies on, 82
    reduced, in vegetarians, <u>93</u>
    saturated fat and, 84, 85
    sleep apnea and, 9–10, 148, 149
    sleep deprivation and, 144, 154, 241
    trans fats increasing, 88
Heart-healthy diets, misconceptions about,
    71–72
Heart scan, noninvasive computed
    tomography (CT), 9, 16, 17
Heart valve disease, 255
Hibbeln, Joseph, 84

High blood pressure
  in children, 36, _220_
  in dogs, _133_
  from fast food, 48
  with metabolic syndrome, 26
  preventing or lowering, 76, 82, 125, 255,
    256, 257
  from restaurant meals, 110, 111
  sleep apnea and, 148, 149
  from sodium, 94
  sugar and, _200–201_
Hippocampus, 123, 124
Hollar, Danielle, 119
Home cooking. _See also_ Family meals;
    Sample Meal Plan for Healthy Week
  benefits of, 53–54, 112–13
  guidelines for, 211–14
  importance of, 191, 253
  involving children in, _215_
  recipes for, 259 (_see also specific recipes_)
Home environment
  as healthful for children, 38–39
  toxins in, 52
HOPS program. _See_ Healthier Options for
    Public Schoolchildren (HOPS) program
Hummus
  Lemony Tomato Hummus with Carrot
    Chips, 193, 269
Hunger, 24, 75, 154, 155, 179–80, 182, _184_,
    _185_, _189_, 199
Hunter-gatherers, 42, 43, 44, 48, 83, 96–97,
    103, _104_, 128–29, 135, 138, 139, 144,
    _146_, 186
Hypertension. _See_ Blood pressure; High
    blood pressure
Hypoglycemia, reactive, 23, 24

Immune system, 26, _127_, 144, 256, 257
Inactivity
  among children, _136–37_
  health risks from, 126–28
  insomnia from, 245
  technology promoting, 129–30
Industrial revolution, 129
Infectious diseases, 43
Inflammation
  in aging process, 10, 26, 124
  from belly fat, 26
  chronic diseases and, 21–22, 27, 84, 157
  effect on stem cells, 30
  markers of, 10
  omega-6 fatty acids and, 83
  omega-9 fatty acids and, 82–83
  oxidant stress and, 27–29
  as survival mechanism, 20–21, 26
Insomnia. _See also_ Sleep problems
  causes of, 158, _248_
  incidence of, 148
  remedies for, 160–61, 245–46

Insulin resistance, 22–23, 24, 25, _25_, 26,
    36, 257
Interval training, 139–40
Interval walking, 224–25, 228–29, _230–31_,
    232–33

Janowitz, Warren, 17
Juices, fruit, 77
Junk food, 11, 53, 59, 169, 203
  advertising for, 38, 39
  eaten by children, 33, 39, 108, _136_, _208_,
    _221_
  eliminating, 39, _166_, _176_
  ill effects of, 63

Kale
  Tuscan Kale and Mushroom Soup, 274
Katzmarzyk, Peter T., 133–34
Kidney disease, 37, 38, 91, 94, _133_
Kidneys, effect of protein on, 89, 90
Kitchen
  de-cluttering, 170, 174
  foods to remove from, 39, _172–73_
  foods to stock, 196–98, 307–13

Labels, food. _See_ Food labels
Lactose intolerance, _100_, _104–5_
Leftovers, 192, 193
Leg circle, _235_, **235**
Leg kick, _236_, **236**
Legumes. _See also_ Beans; Lentils
  buying, 210
  health benefits of, 78, 254
  in healthy diet, 192
  on shopping list, 308
Lentils, 210, 254
  Lentil-Bulgur Salad with Summer Squash
    and Walnuts, 193, 292–93
Leptin, 155
Levine, James A., 130–32
Lifestyle
  changing
    case history about, 11–12
    efforts to promote, 12–13
  healthy
    committing to, 165–68
    for disease prevention, 36
    Phases 2 and 3 of South Beach Diet for,
      67
  South Beach Diet as, 67
  toxic
    assessing, 165
    beginning in womb, _6–7_
    effects on health, 3, 4–5, 8, 9, 10, 14,
      29–30, 143, 163
    as societal problem, 11
    understanding origins of, 41–42
Light exposure, affecting sleep, 246–47, 250
Lombardo, Michelle, 119

Low-fat products, drawbacks of, 72
Ludwig, David, 37–40, <u>201</u>
Lyon Diet Heart Study, 82

Macaroni
  Mighty Mac and "Cheese," 193, 290–91
Macular degeneration, 5, 21, 29, 88, 255,
    257, 258
Malnutrition
  in children, 62
  in history, 46, 60–61, 75
Mattress, when to replace, 243
Mayo, Charles, 152
Meals. *See also* Dining out; Family meals;
    specific meals
  recommended number of, 177–78, 191
Meatballs
  MegaMeatballs and Sauce, 193, 276–77
Meatless meals, 193
Meats
  from grass- vs. grain-fed animals, 90
  in hunter-gatherer diet, 96–97
  lean, 97
  saturated fat in, 84
  types to eliminate, <u>173</u>
Mediterranean diet, 48, 67, 82
MegaFoods, 66, 214, 253, 254–58, 259
MegaRecipes, 66, 214, 253, 259–61. *See also*
    specific recipes
Melatonin, sleep and, 160, 174, 246, 247, 250
Memory, exercise improving, 124
Memory loss, foods preventing, 76, 88, 255, 257
Menu planning, 192–95, <u>208</u>
Menus, restaurant, 217
Metabolic syndrome, 9, 22, <u>25</u>, 26, 33, 102,
    103, 157
Microwave oven, 47
Milk, 42, 43, 96, <u>201</u>
Milk allergy, <u>104</u>
Miracle diets, 56–60
Monounsaturated fats, 82, 199, 254, 258,
    266, 282, 312
Morris, Jerry, 134–35
Motion-tracking research, 131
Motivation, for healthy lifestyle, 165–68
Mouse studies, on diet, 30–32, <u>35</u>
Movement, from everyday activities, 224,
    237–40
Muesli
  Toasted Pecan Muesli with Dried Fruit,
    268
Muffins
  Blueberry Buttermilk Muffins with
    Almonds, 179, 266–67
Muscle building, protein for, 88–89
Muscle loss, from sleep deprivation, 156
Mushrooms
  health benefits of, 256–57
  Tuscan Kale and Mushroom Soup, 274

Napa cabbage
  Spiced Pork Skewers with Napa Salad,
    282–83
Napping, 151, 152–53, 160
NEAT (nonexercise activity thermogenesis),
    131
Netter Center for Community Partnerships,
    109, 121, 122
Nonalcoholic fatty liver disease, in children,
    <u>6</u>
Nonexercise activity thermogenesis (NEAT),
    131
"Normal weight obesity" individuals, 70
Nurses' Health Study, <u>35</u>, 82, 125
Nutrition
  anti-inflammatory and anti-aging effects
    of, 10
  confusion about, 56
  food production depleting, 44
  good, basics of, 72–73
  importance to overall health, 9, 10
  improving, for children, 13
  observational studies on, <u>34–35</u>
Nutrition education, in schools, 118–20,
    121–22
Nuts. *See also* Almonds; Pecans; Pistachios;
    Walnuts
  in dinners, 213
  health benefits of, 258
  omega-9 fatty acids in, 82
  on shopping list, 312

Oatmeal, 179, 180
Oats, 257
Obama, Michelle, 13
Obesity
  in children, <u>6–7</u>, 33, 34, 36, 37–40, 144,
    <u>152</u>, <u>153</u>, <u>201</u>
  contributors to, 51, 72, 88, 111, 131, 144,
    156, 190, <u>200</u>
  dementia risk from, 27
  in dogs, <u>133</u>
  from fast food, 48
  health-care costs from, 38
  holistic community approach to, 10–11
  parental, effect on children's health, <u>6–7</u>
  as pregnancy risk, <u>6</u>
  prevalence of, 4, 26, <u>100</u>
  preventing, 84, 140, 191
  sleep apnea from, 148, 149
  in vegetarians, <u>92</u>
Obesity epidemic, 5, 13, 33, 37–40, 41, 42,
    46, 54, 129, <u>136</u>, 156
Obstructive sleep apnea, 148–49. *See also*
    Sleep apnea
Oils
  on shopping list, 312
  types to eliminate, <u>173</u>
Okinawa, diet in, 48, 77

Olive oil, health benefits of, 254
Oliver, Jamie, 211
Omega-3 fatty acids
  anti-inflammatory effects of, 84
  sources of, 82, 83, 90, 91, 97, 256
  types of, 83
Omega-3 fish oils, 63
Omega-6 fatty acids
  imbalance of, 83–84
  in meats, 90, 93, 96–97
Omega-9 fatty acids, 82–83
Orange vegetables, health benefits of, 257
Organic food, 50–51, 52–55, 100, 101
Organic Manifesto, 50
Outdoor space, de-cluttering, 171, 175
Overweight. *See also* Obesity
  in children, 33, 34, 35, 36, 113, 136, 152,
    153, 167, 176
  in dogs, 133
  health risks from, 6, 27
  prevalence of, 3, 26
Oxidant stress, 10, 20, 26, 27–29, 30, 125
Oxidation, "rusting" from, 63, 124

Palm oil, 47, 84–85
Parents
  involving children in food preparation,
    259–60
  as promoters of healthy eating, 38, 39, 40
  tips for, 164, 166–67, 176, 188–89, 208–9,
    215, 220–21, 238–39, 248–49
Pasta
  types to eliminate, 173
  whole-wheat, 213, 218
Pecans
  Chocolate Bark with Cranberries,
    Almonds, and Pecans, 181, 306
  Toasted Pecan Muesli with Dried Fruit, 268
Pellagra, 46
Pesticides, 50, 51, 100
Pets
  dog walking, 132–33
  interfering with sleep, 249
Phase 1 of South Beach Diet, 57, 58, 64,
    68–69, 183
  as gluten free, 99, 102–3
  overview and purpose of, 66–67
  recipes
    Almond-Sunflower Cod with Tomato
      Tartar Sauce, 284–85
    Chicken Cutlets with Apricot Sauce and
      Pistachios, 212, 278
    Chunky Guacamole Salad, 212, 301
    Green and White Florets with Toasted
      Pumpkin Seeds, 297
    Greens Gratin with Turkey Bacon, 299
    Grilled Salmon with Cucumbers and
      Ginger Dressing, 288

Layered Salad with Creamy Cilantro
      Dressing, 294–95
    Lemony Tomato Hummus with Carrot
      Chips, 193, 269
    Salmon Mousse with Vegetable Dippers,
      270–71
    Spiced Pork Skewers with Napa Salad,
      282–83
    Stir-Fried Garlic Shrimp with Bok Choy,
      193, 289
    Tuscan Kale and Mushroom Soup, 274
Phase 2 of South Beach Diet, 192
  overview of, 69
  recipes
    Apple-Baked Beans with Smoked Ham,
      296
    Better Beef Burgundy, 280–81
    Black Bean Chili with Tangerine-
      Avocado Salsa, 193, 286–87
    Blueberry Buttermilk Muffins with
      Almonds, 179, 266–67
    Broccolette with Brown Rice and
      Walnuts, 298
    Chicken Cutlets with Apricot Sauce and
      Pistachios, 212, 278
    Chicken in Mexican Mole Sauce, 275
    Chickpea and Carrot Frittata, 210, 263
    Chocolate Bark with Cranberries,
      Almonds, and Pecans, 181, 306
    Golden Barley Pilaf with Herb-Roasted
      Carrots, 300
    Lemony Tomato Hummus with Carrot
      Chips, 193, 269
    Lentil-Bulgur Salad with Summer
      Squash and Walnuts, 193, 292–93
    MegaMeatballs and Sauce, 193,
      276–77
    Mighty Mac and "Cheese," 193, 290–91
    Multigrain Blueberry Cobbler, 181,
      304–5
    Pumpkin-Cranberry Breakfast Bread,
      179, 264–65
    Quinoa and Tomato Salad with Goat
      Cheese, 302
    Sesame Flank Steak with Fresh
      Blueberry Salsa, 279
    Spiced Pork Skewers with Napa Salad,
      282–83
    Super Veggie Minestrone, 210, 272–73
    Sweet and Savory Breakfast Burritos
      with Sautéed Apples, 179, 262
    Sweet Potato Salad with Fresh Basil,
      303
    Toasted Pecan Muesli with Dried Fruit,
      268
  when to start, 67, 68–69
Phase 3 of South Beach Diet, 67, 69
Physical education, in schools, 39, 120–21

Phytonutrients, 63, 66, 76, 253, 254
Pilates, 138
Pistachios
    Chicken Cutlets with Apricot Sauce and
        Pistachios, 212, 278
Plant foods, knowing source of, 91
Plant proteins, 90
    complete vs. incomplete, 89
Plaques, atherosclerotic. *See* Atherosclerosis
Pollan, Michael, 88, 95
Polyphenols, 63
Polysomnogram, for diagnosing sleep apnea,
        149, 150
Pomegranates, antioxidants in, 63
Pork. *See also* Ham
    Spiced Pork Skewers with Napa Salad,
        282–83
Posture
    correct, 240
    for interval walking, 229
Potatoes, types to eliminate, 173
Poultry. *See also* Chicken; Turkey; Turkey
        bacon
    types to eliminate, 173
Prediabetes, 6, 7, 9, 22, 126, 128, 191, 216,
        258
Pregnancy risks, from overweight and
        obesity, 6
Prepared foods, 49, 112, 213
Processed foods
    limiting, 177
    sodium in, 91, 93, 94
    sugar in, 200, 201
    in supermarkets, 199
    as unhealthy, 24, 29, 72, 73, 79, 83, 109
Protein
    animal
        in hunter-gatherer diet, 96–97
        nutrient value of, 90–91
    evaluating quality of, 95
    lean
        best sources of, 90, 93, 97
        for breakfast, 178–79
        cutting costs on, 207, 210
        in healthy diet, 192, 199
        overview of, 88–90
        on Phase 1 of South Beach Diet, 66, 68
        in restaurant meals, 217
        on shopping list, 309–10
        USDA guidelines for eating, 177
    in snacks, 180–81
Pumpkin
    Pumpkin-Cranberry Breakfast Bread, 179,
        264–65
Pumpkin seeds
    Green and White Florets with Toasted
        Pumpkin Seeds, 297
    health benefits of, 256

Quinoa, 75, 97, 213
    Quinoa and Tomato Salad with Goat
        Cheese, 302

Reactive hypoglycemia, 23, 24
Recess, benefits of, 136–37
Recipes. *See* MegaRecipes; *specific recipes*
Red wine
    Better Beef Burgundy, 280–81
    health benefits of, 81, 257
Restaurant meals
    extra calories in, 216
    guidelines for, 216–22
    hazards of, 110–12
Restless leg syndrome, 148, 242
Resveratrol, in red wine, 81, 257, 278
Rice
    Broccolette with Brown Rice and Walnuts,
        298
    types to eliminate, 173
    white vs. brown, 75, 218
Robotic surgery, 130
Rodale, Maria, 49, 50–55, 260
Roosevelt, Franklin, 152–53
Running, ill effects of, 135, 138
"Rusting" process
    causes of, 26, 27–29, 63, 124
    effect on vessels and organs, 9, 10
    exercise controlling, 125
    premature aging from, 19–20, 124
    premature death from, 27

Salad dressings, types to eliminate, 172
Salads
    Chunky Guacamole Salad, 212, 301
    Layered Salad with Creamy Cilantro
        Dressing, 294–95
    Lentil-Bulgur Salad with Summer Squash
        and Walnuts, 193, 292–93
    Quinoa and Tomato Salad with Goat
        Cheese, 302
    Spiced Pork Skewers with Napa Salad,
        282–83
    Sweet Potato Salad with Fresh Basil, 303
Salmon
    Grilled Salmon with Cucumbers and
        Ginger Dressing, 288
    health benefits of, 257
    Salmon Mousse with Vegetable Dippers,
        270–71
    wild vs. farmed, 90–91
Salsa
    Black Bean Chili with Tangerine-Avocado
        Salsa, 193, 286–87
    Sesame Flank Steak with Fresh Blueberry
        Salsa, 279
Salt sensitivity, 94

Sample Meal Plan for a Healthy Week, 192, 194–95
Satiety, from slow eating, 190
Saturated fats, 84–85, 87, 177
School cooking programs, 109–10
School lunches, 13, 39, 49, 61, 62, 108, 117–20
Schools
    changing starting times of, 156, 159
    nutrition education in, 118–20, 121–22
    physical education in, 39, 120–21
    role of, in promoting health, 10–11
Screen time. *See also* Television
    limiting, for children, 137, 238–39
Scurvy, 61
Seasonings, on shopping list, 312–13
Sedentary lifestyle. *See also* Fast-food, sedentary lifestyle; Sitting
    among children, 136, 137
    health risks from, 126–27, 224
Seeds. *See also* Flaxseeds; Pumpkin seeds; Sesame seeds; Sunflower seeds
    health benefits of, 256
    on shopping list, 312
Sesame seeds
    health benefits of, 256
    Sesame Flank Steak with Fresh Blueberry Salsa, 279
Setbacks, dealing with, 251
Sex, sleeplessness after, 246
Shellfish
    Stir-Fried Garlic Shrimp with Bok Choy, 193, 289
Shopping list, for healthy diet, 184, 196–98, 307–13
Shrimp
    Stir-Fried Garlic Shrimp with Bok Choy, 193, 289
"Sickest generation," 5, 8–9
Sickness. *See also* Diseases, chronic
    causes and effects of, 3
Side bend, 237, **237**
Signorile, Joseph, 139
Sitting. *See also* Fast-food, sedentary lifestyle; Sedentary lifestyle
    hazards of, 126–27, 130–31, 133, 134, 135
Sleep
    anti-inflammatory and anti-aging effects of, 10, 29
    importance of, 9–10, 143–44, 146, 147, 157
    increasing, for children, 11, 167
    lost, making up for, 161
    napping, 151, 152–53, 160
    non-REM vs. REM, 146–47
    theories on need for, 146
Sleep apnea, 9–10, 36, 37, 143, 148–51, 152–53, 153, 157, 158, 242, 247, 248

Sleep deprivation
    in children, 144–45, 156, 160
    health effects of, 144, 153–56, 183
    symptoms of, 157–58
    in United States, 143, 144–45
Sleep medications, 160, 161, 242
Sleep problems. *See also* Insomnia
    causes of, 145, 148, 241–42, 247
        assessing, 242, 249
    in children, 248–49
    effects of, 241, 246
    remedies for, 164, 242–47, 250–51
Sleep-wake cycles, 159
Slow cooker, 179, 212
Slow eating, importance of, 187, 190
Smoking
    ill effects of, 20, 29, 245
    studies on, 34
Smoking-cessation programs, 110
Smoothies, breakfast, 179
Snacks
    bedtime, 244
    for children, 220
    guidelines for, 180–81
    importance of, 177, 178, 191
    poor choices of, 178, 183
    recipes for, 269–71
    for travel, 222–23
    types to eliminate, 173
Snoring, 148, 149, 150, 152, 153, 242, 247, 248. *See also* Sleep apnea
Sodium, 91–94, 173, 177, 207
Soil devastation, from fertilizers, 53
Soups
    Super Veggie Minestrone, 210, 272–73
    Tuscan Kale and Mushroom Soup, 274
    type to eliminate, 173
South Beach Diet, 56, 57, 58, 112, 141, 151, 181, 182, 192, 217
    candidates for, 68–70
    as lifestyle, 67, 70
    mouse studies on, 31, 32
    origins of, 9
    perceived as low-carb, 73
    phases of, 68-69 (*see also specific phases*)
    recipes suitable for, 259
    shopping list for, 307–13
    success stories about, 11–12, 64–65, 86–87
    for vegetarians, 92
South Beach Diet Gluten Solution, 103–7
South Beach Diet Wake-Up Program
    committing to, 165–68
    expected health benefits from, 164, 251
    goals of, 163
    lifestyle assessment before, 165
    strategies in, 14, 163–64

Soy-based meat substitutes, on shopping list, 310
Soy milk, type to eliminate, <u>173</u>
Sports equipment, 171
Spurlock, Morgan, 60
Squash
    Lentil-Bulgur Salad with Summer Squash and Walnuts, 193, 292–93
Stationary bike, 232, 233
Stearic acid, 85
Steel roller mill, invention of, 45
Stem cells, 29–32
Stress
    eating from, 183, 186
    from sleeplessness, 154–55
Stroke(s), 5, 17, 24, 26, 37, 94, 125, 144, 149, 151, 154, 256
Substance abuse, 116
Sugar
    added to foods, 199, <u>200–201</u>, 202
    controlling cravings for, 66, 67, <u>68</u>
    cravings from, 75, 183
    ignorance about dangers of, 71
    limiting, 177
Sugar experiment, <u>200–201</u>
Sugar-free treats, on shopping list, 313
Sugar substitutes, on shopping list, 313
Sunflower seeds
    Almond-Sunflower Cod with Tomato Tartar Sauce, 284–85
    health benefits of, 82, 256
Sun protection, during outdoor exercise, 232
Super Dads, 12, 156
Supermarkets, birth of, 46
Super Moms, 12–13, 36, 78, 113, 156, 167–68, 203, 204, 211
    stories of, <u>86–87</u>, <u>100–101</u>, <u>114–15</u>
Super Size Me, 60
Sweeteners, types to eliminate, <u>173</u>
Sweet potatoes
    for french fries, 214
    health benefits of, 77, 257
    substituted for white potatoes, 77, 217
    Sweet Potato Salad with Fresh Basil, 303

Tangerines
    Black Bean Chili with Tangerine-Avocado Salsa, 193, 286–87
Target heart rate, 140
Tea
    caffeine in, 244
    health benefits of, 255
Technology
    advantages of, 41, 48–49
    health consequences of, 42–49
    reducing calorie expenditure, 129–30
    unhealthy lifestyle and, 10

Television
    limiting, for children, 12, 38, 40, <u>87</u>, <u>238</u>
    overeating and, 187
    preventing sleep, 145, 161, 170, 174, 175, 250
    time spent on, 134, <u>137</u>
Testosterone, belly fat reducing, <u>25</u>
Toe dip, <u>234</u>, **234**
Toffler, Alvin, 41
Tomatoes
    Almond-Sunflower Cod with Tomato Tartar Sauce, 284–85
    health benefits of, 258
    Lemony Tomato Hummus with Carrot Chips, 193, 269
    nutrient depletion in, 44
    Quinoa and Tomato Salad with Goat Cheese, 302
Toxins, in home environment, 52
Trans fats, 47, 84, 85–88, <u>173</u>
Travel
    eating challenges during, 16
    healthy eating during, 222–23
Treadmill desks, 131–32, 141
Treadmill walking, 139–40, 224, 232, 233
Treats, for children, 39, <u>172</u>, <u>173</u>, <u>209</u>
Triglycerides
    factors increasing, <u>81</u>, <u>92</u>, 126, <u>201</u>
    factors lowering, 83, 256, 258
    in metabolic syndrome, 26
Turkey
    MegaMeatballs and Sauce, 193, 276–77
Turkey bacon
    Greens Gratin with Turkey Bacon, 299
Twinkie Diet, 59–60

University-community partnerships, for good nutrition, 121–22
USDA dietary guidelines, 177

Vazzana, Andrea, 164
Vegans, 90, <u>92</u>, <u>100</u>
Vegetables. *See also specific vegetables*
    canned, 207
    for children, 12, 114, 115–16
    cruciferous, 76, 255
    cultivation of, 43–44
    cutting costs on, 204–7
    eating variety of, 66, 95
    frozen, 206–7
    in hunter-gatherer diet, 96
    importance of, 76, 77, 191
    natural sugar in, <u>201</u>
    orange, health benefits of, 257
    in Phase 1 of South Beach Diet, 66, <u>68</u>
    phytonutrients in, 63, 66
    on shopping list, 307–8
    starchy, 76–77
    USDA guidelines for eating, 177

Vegetarians, 90, 92–93, 100
Visceral fat, 22, 23, 24, 26, 70. *See also* Belly fat
Vitamin C deficiency, scurvy from, 61
Vitamin supplements, overemphasis on, 62–63

Waist circumference, 26, 68, 70, 178
Wake Up and Move 2-Week Quick-Start Plan, 140, 224, 228–29, 230–31, 232–37
Walking, 131–32, 134, 135, 139–40, 141. *See also* Interval walking; Treadmill walking
  with dog, 132–33
Walking shoes, 229
Walnuts
    Broccolette with Brown Rice and Walnuts, 298
    health benefits of, 258
    Lentil-Bulgur Salad with Summer Squash and Walnuts, 193, 292–93
    omega-3 fatty acids in, 82, 83
Warehouse clubs, 204
Washington, George, 117
Watercress
    Chunky Guacamole Salad, 212, 301
Water drinking, during exercise, 232
Waters, Alice, 118
Webster, Keith, 30
Weight, effect of sleep on, 154–56
Weight gain
    causes of
        carbohydrates, 72, 92, 103
        fast food, 60
        pregnancy, 6
        restaurant meals, 110, 111, 220
        sleep apnea, 153, 153
        sleeplessness, 154, 155, 157, 241, 246, 247
        stress hormones, 155
    exercise preventing, 121, 189
Weight loss
    dairy foods for, 256
    emphasis on, vs. good nutrition, 72–73

fad diets for, 56–60
from healthy lifestyle, 165
lean protein for, 89
on Phase 2 of South Beach Diet, 69
quick
    infatuation with, 62
    on Phase 1 of South Beach Diet, 66, 68
for sleep apnea, 150–51
Wheat
    avoidance of, in South Beach Gluten Solution, 105, 107
    gluten in, 97
    grinding of, 45
    health benefits of, 257
    insoluble fiber in, 78
White bread, 46, 61
White flour, 45, 74–75
Whole grains
    eliminated on Phase 1 of South Beach Diet, 66
    health benefits of, 257
    importance of, 74–75, 191, 196–97
    insoluble fiber in, 78
    natural sugar in, 201
    parts of, 45
    reading labels on, 196, 197, 199
    on shopping list, 310–11
    USDA guidelines for eating, 177
Wii exercise activities, for children, 238–39
Willett, Walter, 35
Wine
    on Phase 2 of South Beach Diet, 69
    red
        Better Beef Burgundy, 280–81
        health benefits of, 81, 257
Women, as guardians of family health, 13. *See also* Super Moms
Work, night shift, sleep problems from, 145, 148
Workplaces
    automation of, 130
    exercise in, 141–42
Worry, sleeplessness from, 145, 250–51

VISIT SOUTHBEACHDIET.COM

For more weight-loss tools, great recipes, customized meals plans, and support from registered dietitians and a vibrant community of South Beach Diet followers, visit www.SouthBeachDiet.com.